IDIOT'S GUIDES®

AS EASY AS IT GETS!

Krav Maga

by Kevin Lewis and David Michael Gilbertson

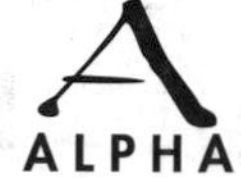

A member of Penguin Random House LLC

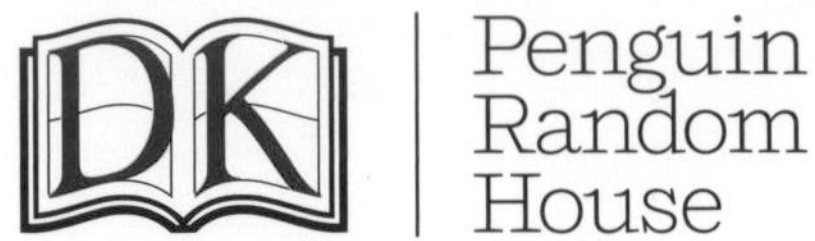

Publisher: Mike Sanders
Associate Publisher: Billy Fields
Acquisitions Editor: Jan Lynn
Development Editors: Kayla Dugger and Alexandra Elliott
Cover and Book Designers: William Thomas and Christine Keilty
Photographer: Zach Coco
Prepress Technician: Brian Massey
Proofreader: Monica Stone
Indexer: Celia McCoy

First American Edition, 2016
Published in the United States by DK Publishing
6081 E. 82nd Street, Indianapolis, Indiana 46250

A Penguin Random House Company

16 17 18 19 10 9 8 7 6 5 4 3 2 1

001-291438-AUGUST2016

Published in the United States by Dorling Kindersley Limited.

ISBN: 978-1-46545-116-3

Library of Congress Catalog Card Number: 2015959228

Printed and bound in China

idiotsguides.com

CONTENTS

PART 3

KRAV MAGA TECHNIQUES 51

INTRODUCTION

Krav Maga is a self-defense system that provides realistic defenses against a variety of attacks. No matter your age or fitness level, you can achieve proficiency in a short period of time in Krav Maga.

Whether the threat involves an armed or unarmed assailant or even multiple assailants, the ultimate goal and the greatest profit of Krav Maga is it allows you to protect yourself and get home safe. To defend against and neutralize physical attacks, the system combines decisive and aggressive responses with the body's instinctive reactions to stress so you're prepared no matter the situation.

To ensure effectiveness, Krav Maga provides techniques that emphasize simple problem-solving principles, as well as training drills to practice. Through these, you're given the tools necessary to fight when your attention is divided, when your vision is impaired, and when you just want to give up. Plus, Krav Maga's "open" system keeps it relevant—as attacks change, the system adapts with new techniques. So no matter the challenge, you can learn to turn on your warrior instincts and fight your way out of an attack. This is what makes Krav Maga the best street-fighting self-defense system in the world.

Acknowledgments

We would like to honor and give our respect to the late Imi Lichtenfeld for developing the Krav Maga system of problem-solving—which is realistic, practical, and easily transferable to the masses—and for being an example of how a man of integrity can be a positive force of change in the world. We also wish to thank our Chief Instructor Darren Levine for his years of mentorship and friendship. We acknowledge the amazing team at Penguin Random House—Jan, Kayla, Bill, and Christine—for making this project possible and pushing us to new limits. We would like to thank the very talented Zach Coco for taking great photographs, as well as thank our models Tammy, Jarrett, Noi, and Chad for playing along and getting behind the cameras at a moment's notice. We would also like to give special thanks to our friends and families for putting up with us during this process. From our first Krav Maga classes to the last word written in this book, you stuck by our sides, had our backs, and pushed us forward when we needed it, so we could carry on Imi's dream of showing the world that every person can walk in peace. Thank you!

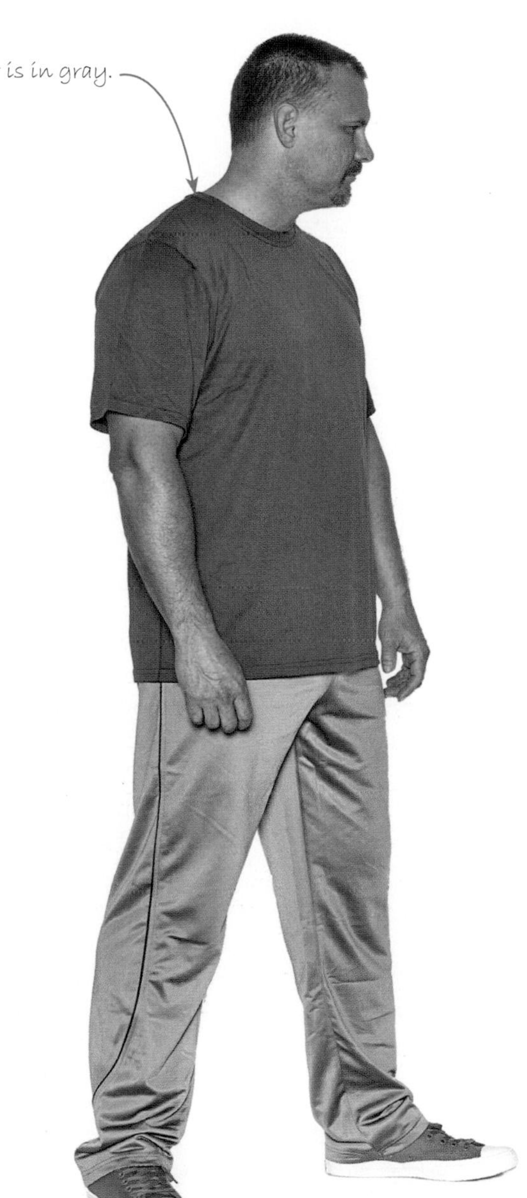

The attacker is in gray.

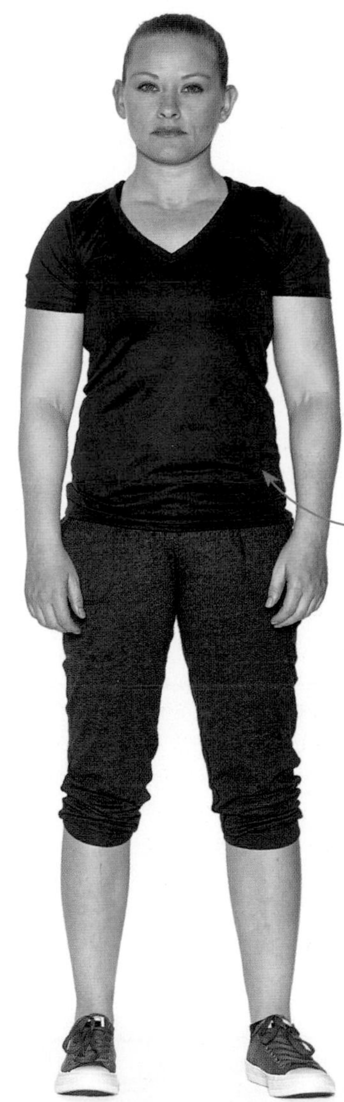

The defender has a colored shirt.

TECHNIQUE NOTE

Certain techniques in this book involve two people, with one acting as the attacker and the other as the defender. For clarity, the attacker is always dressed in a gray shirt.

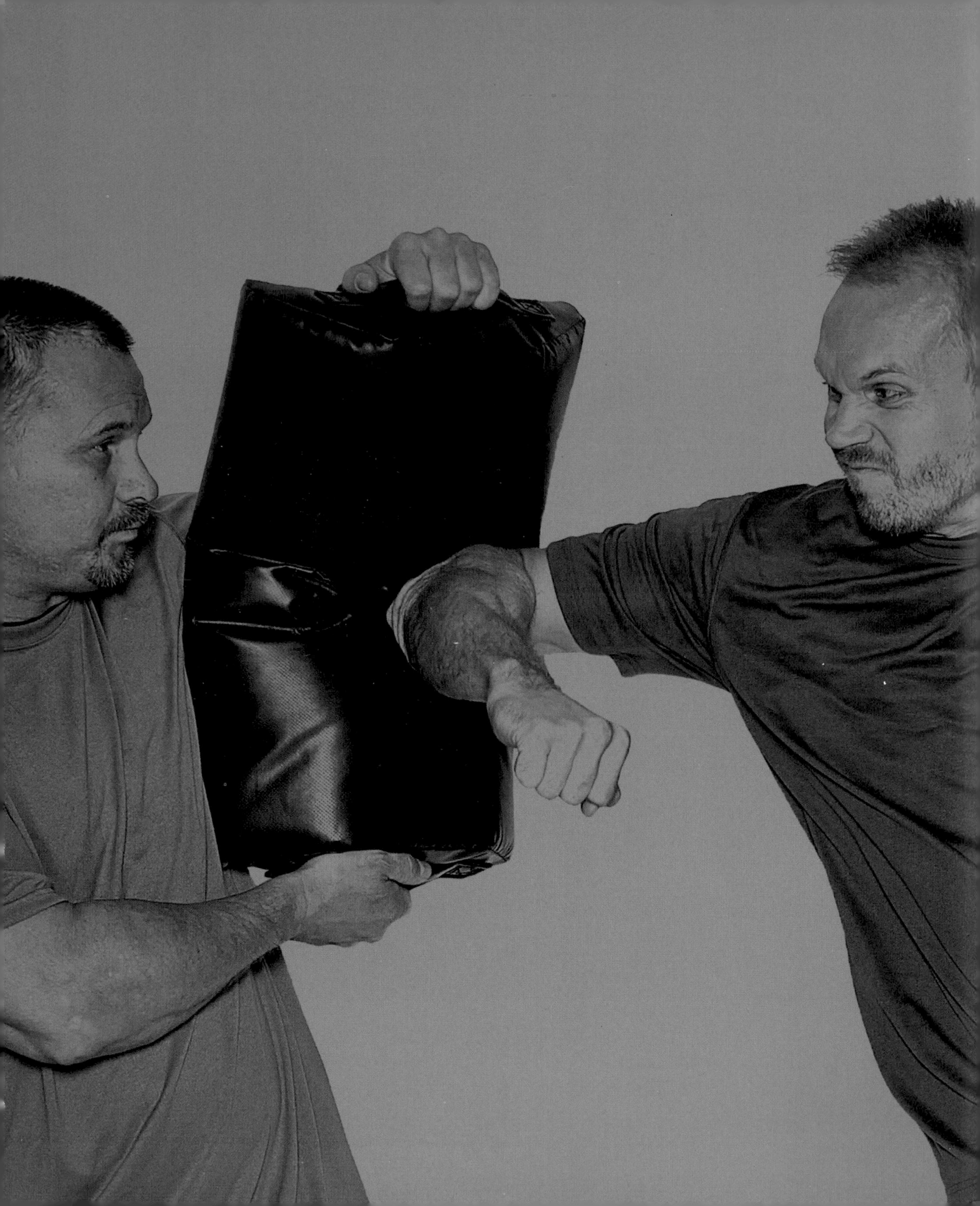

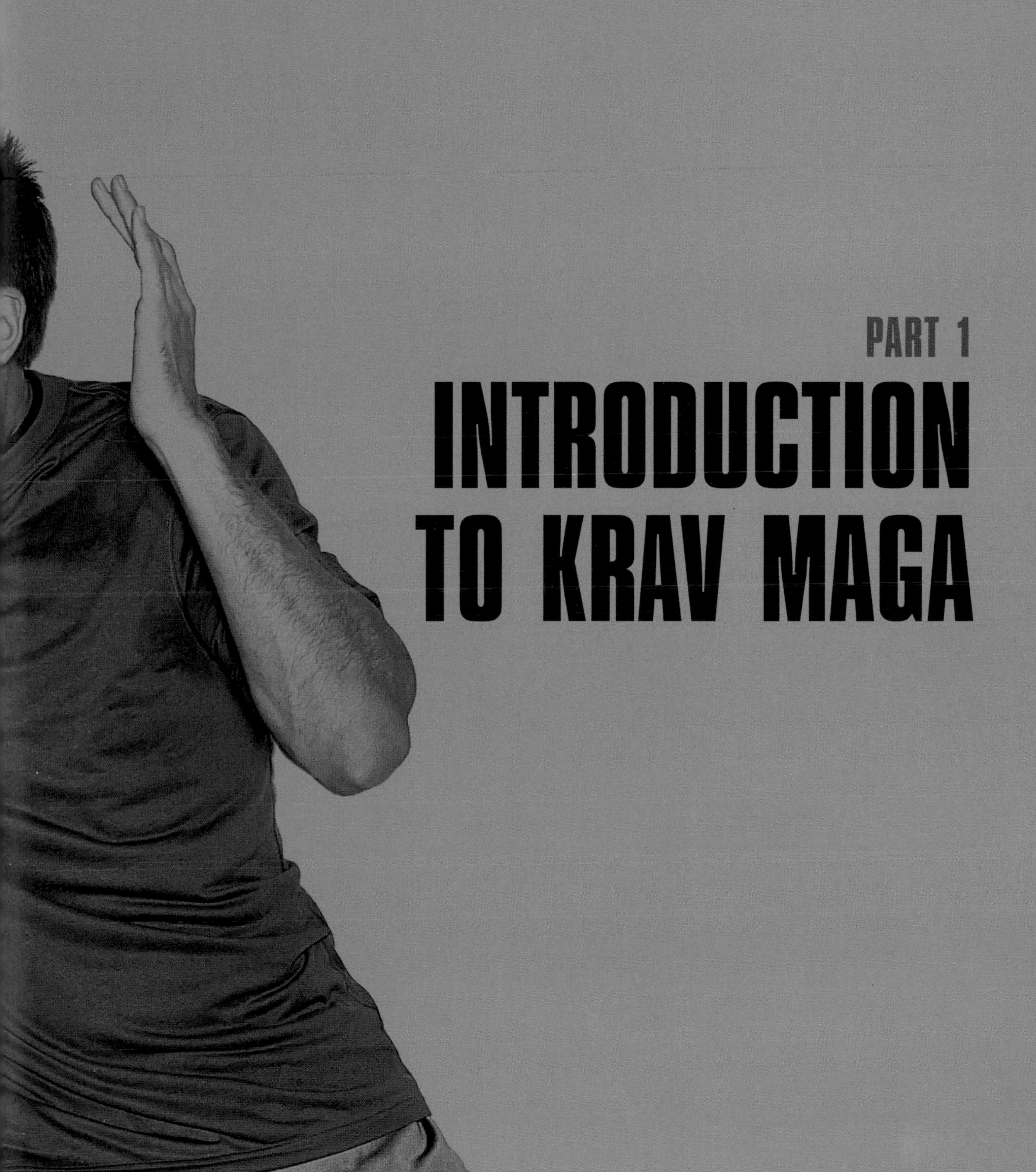

PART 1

INTRODUCTION TO KRAV MAGA

WHAT IS KRAV MAGA?

Krav Maga is an aggressive, reality-based self-defense system that virtually anyone can practice, regardless of size, age, or athletic level.

Defining Krav Maga

Meaning "contact combat" in Hebrew, Krav Maga is a street-fighting system best known for its efficiency in defending against real-world attacks with brutal counterattacks. It emphasizes targeting the most vulnerable parts of the attacker's body while employing basic principles to keep defenders safe. Krav Maga incorporates movements and techniques from many different styles of martial arts and self-defense systems, including judo, kickboxing, karate, wrestling, Brazilian jujitsu, and other weapons-based systems. By utilizing the very best techniques of these other arts and systems, Krav Maga is able to defend effectively against a wide range of attacks.

Unlike other self-defense systems, however, Krav Maga is not a sport. The goal of Krav Maga is simply to allow all types of people to defend themselves using only what's at hand in all types of attack situations, with an awareness that no two situations are exactly the same. While we encourage any person to avoid confrontations, sometimes this simply isn't possible. Krav Maga gives you a solid foundation of both physical and mental training so you can be more aware of your surroundings, properly assess them, and react with appropriate techniques when running away just isn't an option.

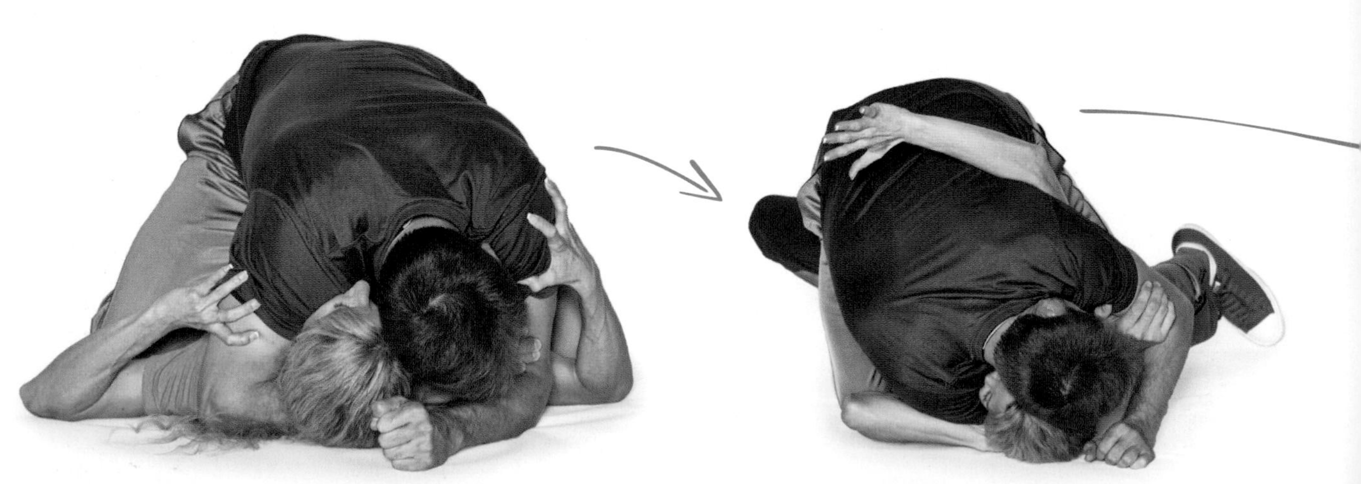

The Purpose of Krav Maga

The purpose of Krav Maga is to "walk in peace." To truly get what self-defense is, you must understand the deeper meaning of this quote. In order to walk in peace, you must have confidence, technical ability, situational awareness, and emotional strength.

As you learn to practice Krav Maga, you'll be challenged physically, mentally, and spiritually to achieve higher levels of performance. The first step in your journey toward walking in peace with Krav Maga is developing your physical skill sets. This is your ability to address common attacks using the Krav Maga principles. Once you do that, you'll learn to face the mental and spiritual challenges of the system—such as strategy, tactics, and situational awareness training—which will lead to greater emotional strength and fortitude.

But how does all this help you walk in peace? With Krav Maga, you gain the ultimate confidence from knowing you have developed your skill sets and organized your life in such a way that you can avoid most situations in which you or others around you could be harmed. There can be no peace without confidence in your abilities. As the old saying goes, "If you want peace, prepare for war"—preparedness is the path to peace. Krav Maga training and principles give you the vehicle, strategy, and tactics to develop the necessary skill sets for this physical, emotional, and spiritual growth.

FAKE IT UNTIL YOU MAKE IT

A key element to walking in peace is confidence. Have good posture and walk with your head up while scanning your environment. Human predators key off weak physical signals.

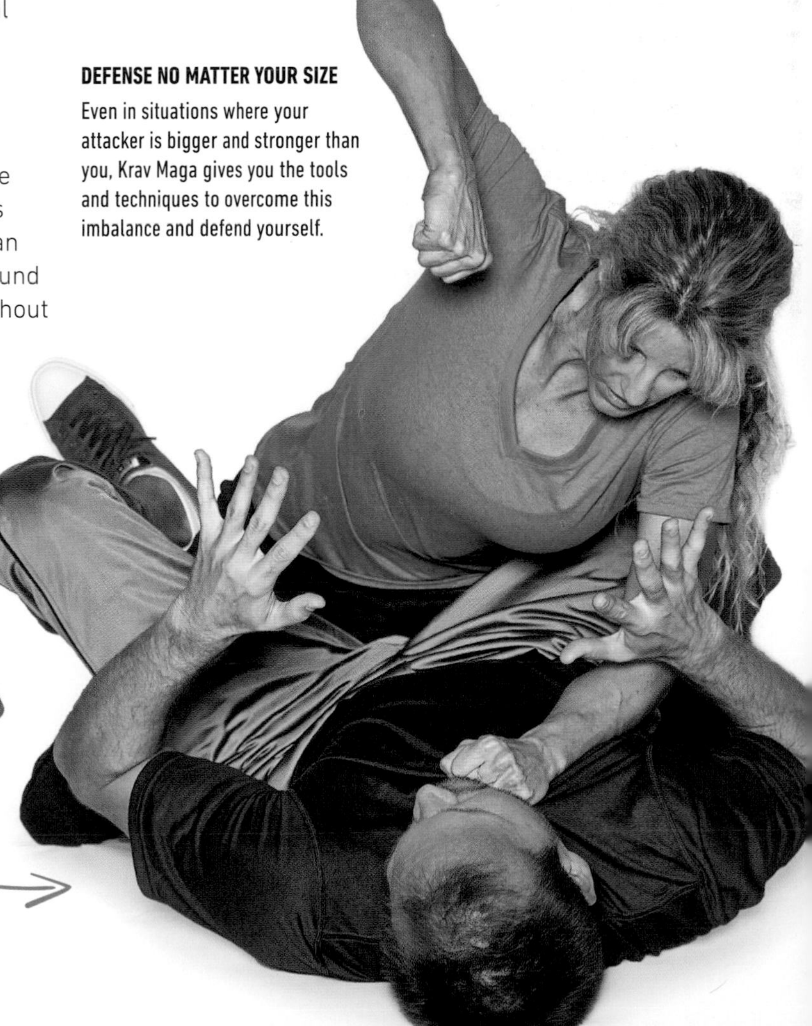

DEFENSE NO MATTER YOUR SIZE
Even in situations where your attacker is bigger and stronger than you, Krav Maga gives you the tools and techniques to overcome this imbalance and defend yourself.

THE ORIGIN OF KRAV MAGA

Krav Maga was founded by a man named Imi Lichtenfeld, a gifted athlete who learned his techniques through street fighting.

Imi Lichtenfeld

In his native Slovakia, Imi participated in wrestling, gymnastics, and boxing, and excelled at each of them. He won the Slovakian Youth Wrestling Championship in 1928, and in 1929, he went on to win the adult wrestling championship. If that wasn't enough, he also went on to win the national boxing championship and the international gymnastics championship. But his most notable contribution is developing Krav Maga.

Street Fighting
As anti-Semitic riots threatened the Jewish population in his home city of Bratislava, Imi led a group in protecting others from the terror taking place on the streets. It was this real-world fighting experience that helped Imi realize there was a huge difference between sport fighting and street fighting.

Training Israeli Soldiers
After being forced to leave his homeland in 1940, Imi settled in Palestine and joined a paramilitary organization called the *Haganah,* an organizational part of the Jewish community that fought to create the independent state of Israel. During this time, he began teaching soldiers basic self-defense techniques.

However, it was only after the state of Israel was formed in 1948 that Krav Maga was created. The Israeli government asked Imi to develop a simple-yet-effective fighting system for its Israel Defense Forces. After accepting this challenge and creating the self-defense system, Imi was awarded the title of the military school's chief instructor for physical training and Krav Maga. Over the decades that followed, Imi's techniques were constantly tested in the real world.

Timeline

1910
Imi Lichtenfeld is born.

1948
Imi is asked by Israel's government to train the Israel Defense Forces in Krav Maga.

1978
Imi and several of his students in Israel create the nonprofit Krav Maga Association, aimed at promoting the teachings of Krav Maga in Israel and throughout the world.

1930S
Imi develops Krav Maga while fighting in the streets of Bratislava.

1964
Imi retires from service and puts his time toward adapting Krav Maga for everyday civilian life.

1981
The Krav Maga Association and the Israeli Ministry of Education hold the first instructors' course at the Wingate Institute for Physical Education. U.S. student attendance of this course leads to the start of Krav Maga being disseminated in the West.

NOW
From Los Angeles, California; to New York, New York; to Miami, Florida, Krav Maga continues to grow in the West and is touted as one of the fastest-growing self-defense systems.

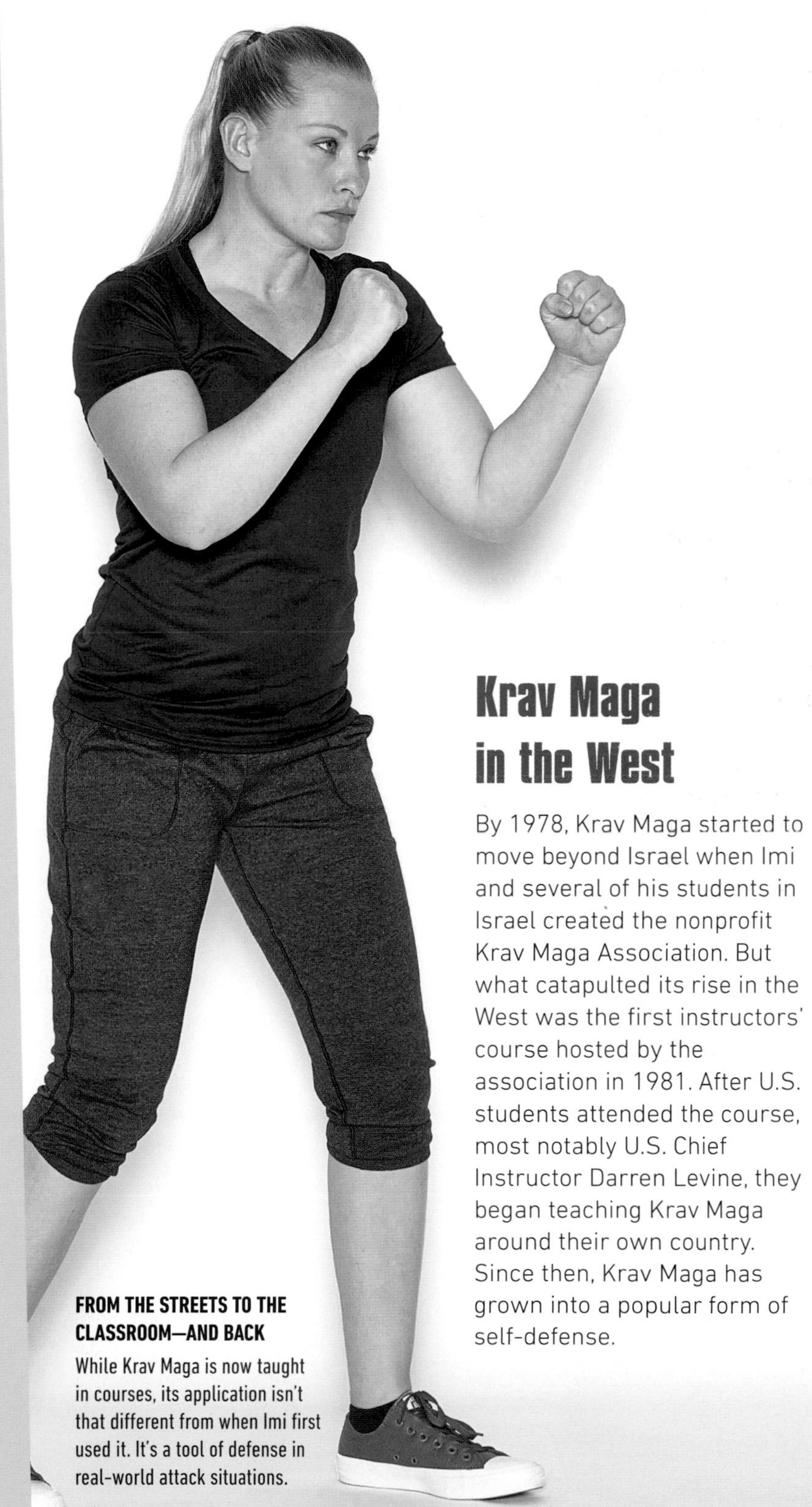

FROM THE STREETS TO THE CLASSROOM—AND BACK
While Krav Maga is now taught in courses, its application isn't that different from when Imi first used it. It's a tool of defense in real-world attack situations.

Krav Maga in the West

By 1978, Krav Maga started to move beyond Israel when Imi and several of his students in Israel created the nonprofit Krav Maga Association. But what catapulted its rise in the West was the first instructors' course hosted by the association in 1981. After U.S. students attended the course, most notably U.S. Chief Instructor Darren Levine, they began teaching Krav Maga around their own country. Since then, Krav Maga has grown into a popular form of self-defense.

HOW KRAV MAGA DIFFERS FROM OTHER MARTIAL ARTS

Krav Maga differs from other martial arts in that it's a defensive tactics system (or methodology) for problem-solving self-defense and fighting situations.

The Primary Goal

When you read the name of Japanese martial arts, you'll notice they end in the suffix –*do,* such as karate–*do,* ju*do,* or ken*do*. *Do* means "the way" or "a way" to personal enlightenment, which expresses the main focus of martial arts. The primary goal of martial arts is achieving enlightenment, followed by a secondary goal of protecting yourself in attack situations. While the purpose of Krav Maga is to walk in peace, its primary goal is to provide you with a means to defend yourself from violent encounters.

REAL-WORLD DANGERS
Let's say someone very accomplished in martial arts is confronted with a real-life situation—for instance, an attacker jumps him or her in a parking lot as he or she is getting into the car. While this person may have the strength and skill for defense, what if the attacker pulls a gun? With no training for this in martial arts, there's no expectation of it and no defense against it—which could lead to deadly consequences.

Sport vs. Real-World Application

Unlike the traditional forms of martial arts, Krav Maga isn't a sport. To understand this, you must understand the difference between a sport match and a violent real-life encounter. Sport matches have a governing body, rules, and sometimes weight classes. Two challengers are entering into a known event at a specific time in a known place and have specific limitations on allowable weapons and techniques, and referees, coaches, and medical staff are present. However, tense, violent street encounters are uncertain and rapidly evolving; the attacker (or attackers) chooses the time, place, and weapons. In addition, you aren't aware of your impending violent encounter on the street. Krav Maga prepares you for these real-world surprise situations where you have to think fast or risk putting yourself at a disadvantage.

Traditional vs. Open System

Another way Krav Maga is different from other martial arts is through what we call an *open system*. An open system allows defenses to change as attacks change or as defenders find a better way to solve a problem. The key to this strategy is staying true to Krav Maga and universal principles such as Hick's law (discussed later in the book), which mainly focus on adapting to the current situation and stressors. By sticking to these universal principles, Krav Maga remains a highly effective and relevant defense system.

Other martial arts tend to be locked into tradition and therefore unable to evolve. Training is based around a regimented structure, with very little modern retooling. However, Krav Maga incorporates modern training methodologies, training under stress, and training with a noncompliant partner to move you through the different levels of technique understanding. This pressure testing ensures you have a higher rate of success compared to other martial arts when you're involved in a sudden, dynamic violent encounter.

KRAV MAGA VS. MARTIAL ARTS

	KRAV MAGA	MARTIAL ARTS
Origin	• Israel Defense Forces • Evolved from street fighting	• Warrior arts in Japan, Korea, and China • Evolved from methods of self-development
Fighting Techniques	• Principle based • Founded on instinctive reactions • Allows the smallest defender to defend against the largest attacker	• Technique based • Primarily attribute based (for instance, focusing on speed, strength, or agility) • Learned by repetition
Purpose	• Self-defense • Fighting • Weapons defense	• Personal enlightenment • Sport • Secondary self-defense use

BENEFITS OF KRAV MAGA

Beyond the ability to defend yourself, learning Krav Maga can help you in many different ways. The following are just a few of the key benefits you get from this system.

Low Cost

Krav Maga helps you effectively neutralize threats by using your environment and weapons of opportunity to your advantage. Because Krav Maga is focused on these real-world scenarios where you may only have yourself as a form of defense, you don't have to invest much money in it. Although training pads and other equipment (discussed more in Part 4) are helpful to have for training purposes, they aren't necessarily required. All you really need is yourself (and this book, of course)!

CHOOSE YOUR WEAPON

When training, you can use household items as improvised weapons of opportunity. For instance, a rolled-up newspaper can extend your reach, as well as be used for defense and counterattacks.

Increased Mental Fitness

Krav Maga is also a great way to relieve everyday stress, as multiple studies have shown that increasing your physical fitness can have life-changing effects on stress levels. With punches, kicks, elbows, and so on, this self-defense system lets you use physical action to release any pent-up emotions, such as anger, in a safe and legal way. And if you're participating in Krav Maga in a group or class environment, you can expand your social circle and make lasting friendships, further improving your mental well-being.

Krav Maga sharpens your mind by allowing you to become more attuned to potential threats in your environment. This mind-set is born through learning to filter out key sensory information from your surroundings. For example, by practicing multiple-attacker situations in a controlled environment or training from a position of disadvantage, you'll be able to better control your emotions, which will allow you to slow down, think, and analyze the situation. Thus, you'll become more aware of your surroundings and make more informed decisions so you can react appropriately.

Improved Physical Fitness

Krav Maga improves your physical fitness by increasing your heart rate. In a very similar way to interval training, Krav Maga adds speed to self-defense techniques with multiple fast-paced repetitions, utilizes your strength by moving around people larger than you are, and implements stress into situations in a controlled, safe environment (whether at home or in a class). Over time, these adjustments will lead you to see drastic improvements in your physical abilities, all while you're gaining muscle and losing fat. Plus, working at a higher intensity trains your body to come to a high state of readiness in the shortest possible amount of time.

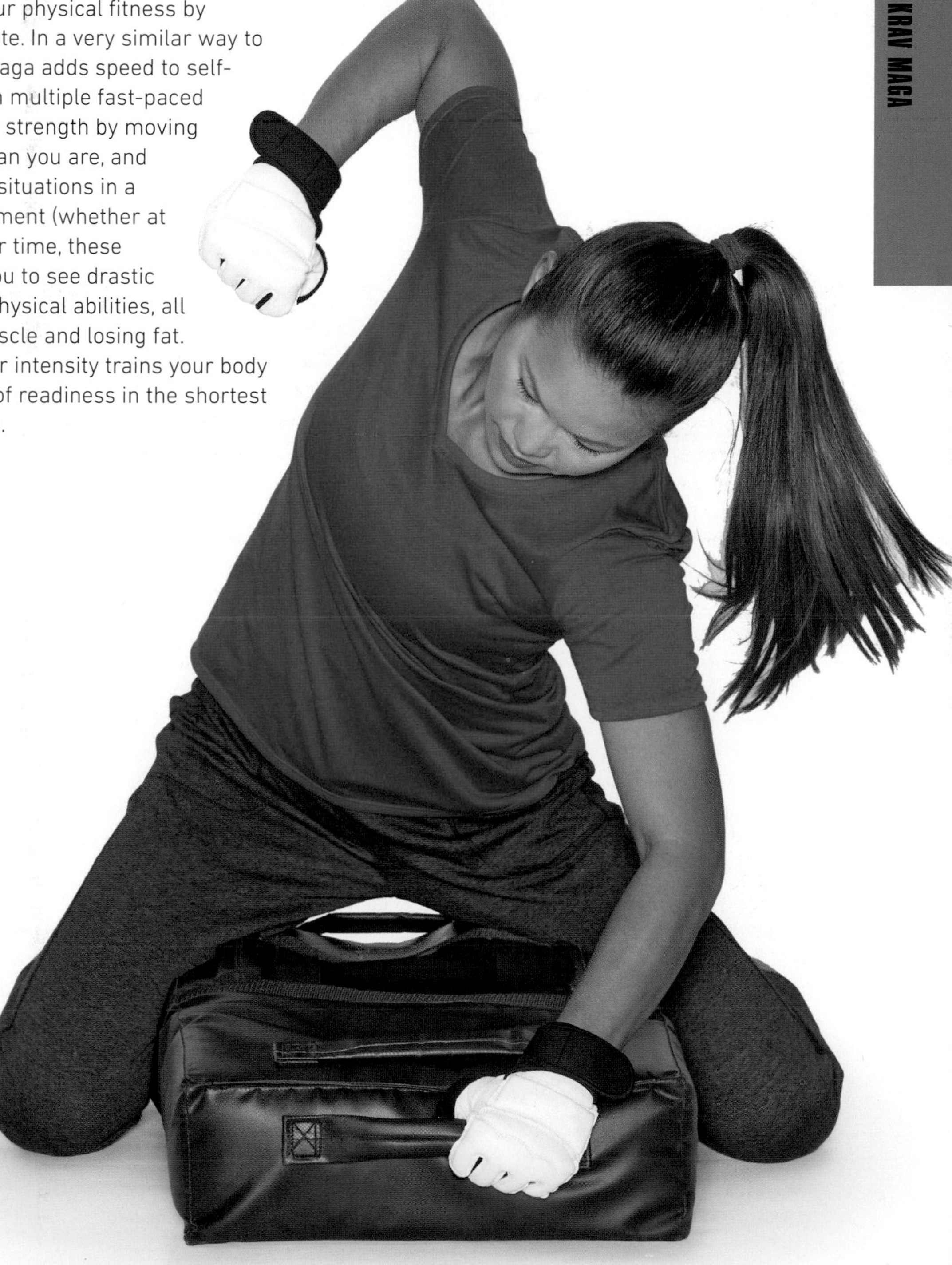

GROUND AND POUND DRILL

The ground and pound drill, discussed later in this book, is a great cardio workout that increases your strength and conditioning.

TYPES OF PEOPLE WHO PRACTICE KRAV MAGA

So who can do Krav Maga? While it may have started as a training tool for the Israel Defense Forces, Krav Maga can be practiced by all walks of life. From law enforcement, to first responders, to civilians, people are using the principles of this form of self-defense to protect themselves.

Law Enforcement/Security

Many U.S. law enforcement and security agencies are using Krav Maga due to its proven results in keeping officers safe. These agencies have limited budgets and timeframes in which to train officers, so Krav Maga's ability to bring an officer to a high state of readiness in a short time makes it an ideal defensive tactics system. Many officers continually train to maintain the Krav Maga skill set to ensure they arrive home safely. Another benefit of Krav Maga in law enforcement is how it offers additional, less lethal options for getting a situation under control, something that has been adopted by many departments as part of their "Use of Force" policies.

First Responders

Because they're often responding to calls in which they have to deal with both the task at hand and the potential danger of an unsecured scene (where attackers may be lurking), many fire investigators, firefighters, and paramedics have adopted Krav Maga. Krav Maga enables these responders to train quickly to get to a high state of readiness, allowing them to be better prepared to attend to fires or victims without fearing for their survival in a possible attack. By incorporating Krav Maga into their overall training, first responders essentially give themselves extra insurance that they're protecting both themselves and others in their care.

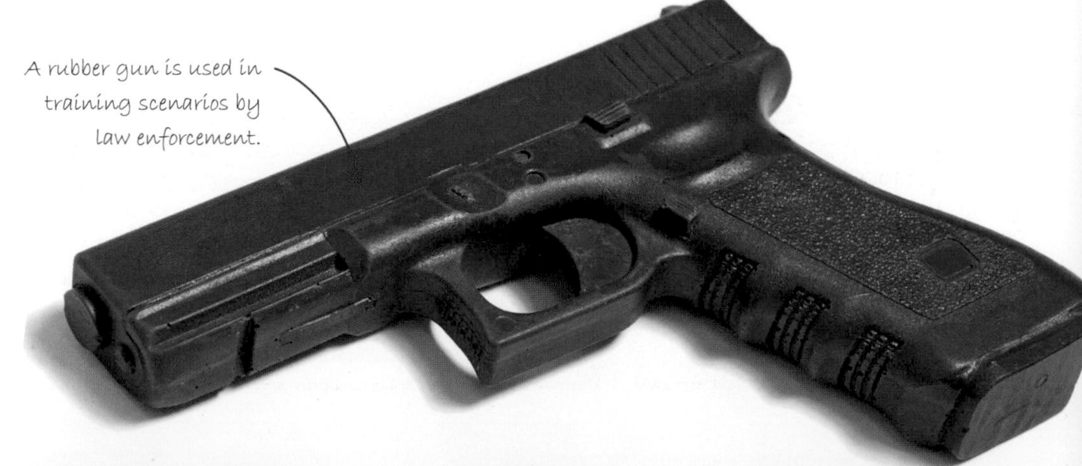

A rubber gun is used in training scenarios by law enforcement.

Civilians Who Want to Defend Themselves

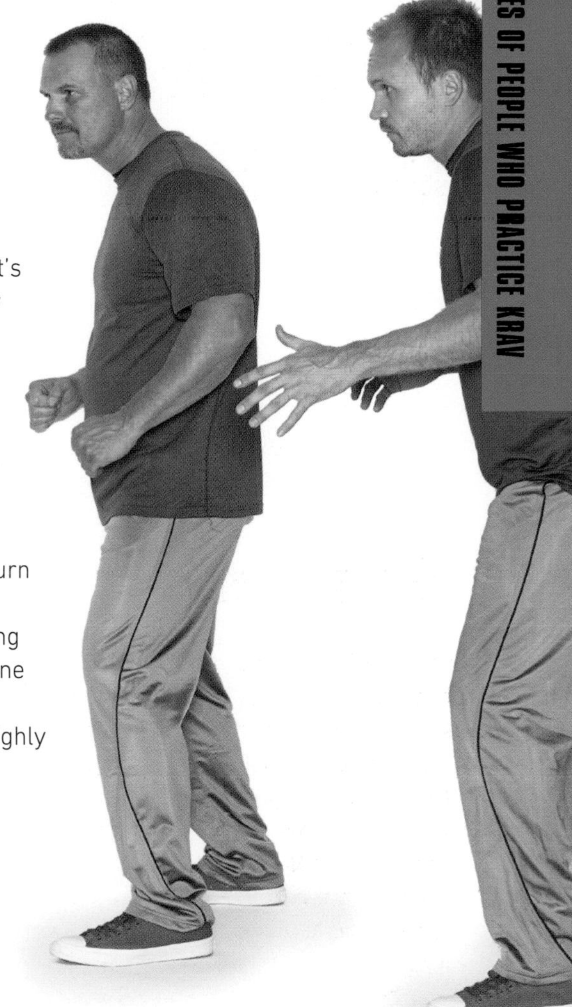

Krav Maga isn't limited to those in law enforcement or other emergency responder positions. It's also a great choice for the everyday person. From ages 8 to 80, regular people have been taught to protect themselves using the principles of Krav Maga. As for fitness level, everyone from the most physically fit to those who don't work out can use it effectively. Due to its fast learning curve and principle-based teaching, Krav Maga provides a great return on training-time investment. The highly effective self-defense and problem-solving strategies Krav Maga teaches allow anyone to ably defend their lives and the lives of their loved ones without having to be a highly trained fighter.

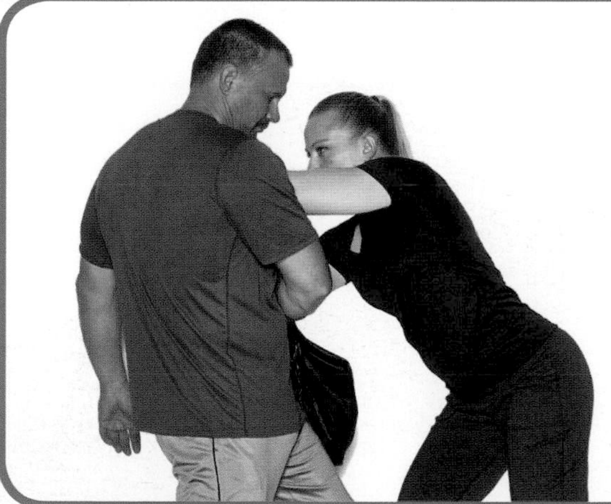

KRAV MAGA FOR WOMEN

While Krav Maga can be used by anyone, women will find it particularly effective as a self-defense technique. Unlike other self-defense strategies, Krav Maga allows even the smallest body types to gain an advantage over the largest body types. This can make Krav Maga training feel truly empowering to women, allowing them to develop self-confidence from knowing they can defend themselves against any attack.

LEVELS

There are many different grading systems in the world of Krav Maga. However, we focus on two main ones: the belt grading system and the patch grading system.

Belt and Patch Systems

Krav Maga Worldwide, the Israeli Krav Maga Association, and Krav Maga K.A.M.I. use Imi Lichtenfeld's original colored belt grading system. His belt system is based upon the judo ranking of, in ascending order, white, yellow, orange, green, blue, brown, and black. The black belt grade level has many different sublevels that are all by invitation only. Some of these organizations have different time requirements, as well as technique requirements, they have adapted over the years in order to progress through the belt system.

The patch grading system, developed by Imi after the belt system in the late 1980s, is used by organizations such as the International Krav Maga Federation, Krav Maga Global, and International Krav Maga. It has levels divided into three groups: practitioner (P), graduate (G), and expert (E). Students start with the P levels and then work their way up to the G levels, at which many of the students are Krav Maga veterans and instructors. Like the black belt, very few achieve the level of expert—they're all people who have dedicated their lives to Krav Maga training and instruction.

ARE THERE ACTUAL BELTS AND PATCHES?

Even within the schools that teach these systems, there are slight differences. Some may use actual belts or patches that are earned and then handed out, while others may test their students through the levels but not actually dispense belts or patches to students.

BASIC REQUIREMENTS

These descriptions give you a general idea of what you need to know to advance. However, the specific requirements can differ depending on the organization.

Patch and Belt Level Progressions

PATCH	BELT	DESCRIPTION
P1	White	Where the journey starts
P2 and P3	Yellow	Basic combatives and choke defenses
P4 and P5	Orange	Intermediate combatives, bear hugs, ground fighting, and basic fighting skills
P6 and G1	Green	Intermediate combatives, intermediate ground fighting, and intermediate fighting
G2 and G3	Blue	Advanced combatives, gun defenses, stick defenses, advanced fighting skills, and advanced ground fighting
G4 and G5	Brown	Advanced combatives, knife defenses, long gun defenses, and advanced ground fighting
E1, E2, E3, E4, and E5	Black	Expert third-party protection, hostage scenarios, and multiple-attacker defenses

FINDING A KRAV MAGA INSTRUCTOR

One of the most important aspects in improving your training is finding a trusted Krav Maga practitioner to learn from, so you can take your self-defense learning beyond this book.

Doing Your Research

Finding a Krav Maga school means doing your research. You'll ensure you get the best training in Krav Maga if you verify the school and instructor. To start, look into a particular school's general reputation in the community. You can find this information through online reviews or through word of mouth. Once you've verified the school you're looking into is highly regarded, ensure the main focus of the school is Krav Maga. This means the school should offer more than just a few classes per week. You want a school whose priority is Krav Maga training.

In terms of instructors of Krav Maga classes, they should be credentialed through one of the four main Krav Maga certifying bodies, as well as have an ongoing continuing education program provided by the school for them. A quality school and great instructor may also have connections to local police forces. By sticking with certified instructors, you can be confident they have the intense training necessary to show you what Krav Maga is really about. In addition, the instructors should also have a basic level of fitness certification, as they will guide you in performing fitness-related activities throughout your training process.

Krav Maga Certifications

In the past few years, over 200 new Krav Maga organizations have been created. To help you whittle down your options, it's always best to stick with the organizations that have been around the longest and adhere to teaching the Krav Maga principles. These organizations have the most strict instructor standards and have consistently been proven to produce the most reputable instructors.

You can trust any Krav Maga school that falls under one of the four main certifying bodies:

- Krav Maga Worldwide, led by U.S. Chief Instructor Darren Levine
- Israeli Krav Maga Association, led by Haim Gidon
- Krav Maga Global, led by Eyal Yanilov
- Krav Maga K.A.M.I. (Israeli Krav Magen Association), led by Avi Avisidon

Checking It Out

When it comes to picking a school and instructor, nothing beats the "eyeball test." Personally go inside and check out the Krav Maga location you're interested in to ensure that the atmosphere is appropriate for you and that it has a sufficient number of classes that fit your schedule. And if you have any questions, you can receive first-hand knowledge from one of the employees or even some of the students.

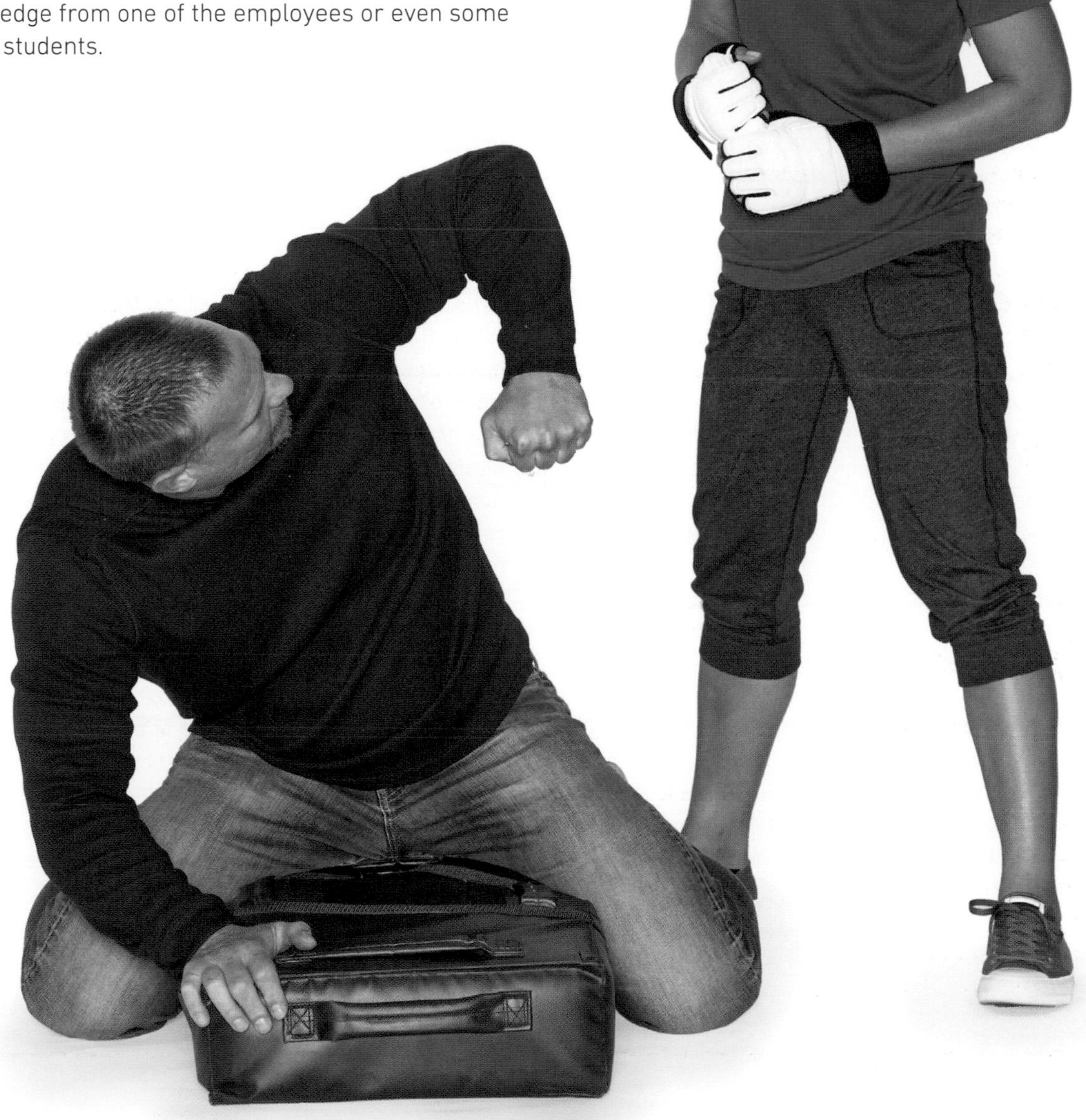

KRAV MAGA FAQS

The following are some of the most frequently asked questions we've encountered concerning Krav Maga.

What is Krav Maga?
Krav Maga, Hebrew for "contact combat," is a no-nonsense self-defense and fighting system developed by Imi Lichtenfeld. It's the same system used by the Israel Defense Forces, law enforcement agencies, first responders, and civilians looking to defend themselves around the world. Krav Maga focuses on real-world situations, and its counterattacks are brutally effective, efficient, and easy to learn.

What sorts of situations does Krav Maga prepare you for?
Krav Maga training includes ways you can defend yourself and escape from a variety of situations. Just a few things you'll learn are how to defend yourself when on the ground, block attacks, throw punches, escape a chokehold, and defend against weapon attacks (from knives, baseball bats, guns, and so on).

How much does Krav Maga cost to do?
Krav Maga is a very low-cost system that was developed to be performed on the streets in real-world clothing, so you don't need any fancy outfits or expensive equipment. As for the venue, you can train in a club, outside in a park, or in your home. However, you should always train with a certified instructor who has the knowledge and teaching experience to help you learn the principles of Krav Maga.

Do I need martial arts self-defense experience to start?
Absolutely not. Krav Maga was specifically developed to utilize the body's natural instincts to react quickly and efficiently to threats or attacks. A good Krav Maga instructor can educate you so you progress from having no knowledge and zero experience to having self-confidence, more awareness, and the ability to defend yourself.

Is there an age requirement for learning Krav Maga?
Because Krav Maga can be used no matter your fitness level, people of almost any age can learn to practice it. Programs are available for children as young as 3 to 4 years old. These are specially tailored to their physical and emotional needs, with more games than defense techniques. Classes then transition away from game-based learning to more focused training as students get older.

How long does it take to learn Krav Maga?
Not long and forever. If you're simply wondering how long it will take until you can defend yourself, you'll pick up some necessary defense abilities after your first class or private lesson (with a certified instructor). In addition, you'll also have more confidence in your abilities after reading this book. The "forever" part comes into play as simple maintenance; you should always be learning and refining your techniques.

How long does it take to move up in patches or belts?
While each Krav Maga system varies slightly, the ranges generally fall between the following if you're training with a certified instructor an absolute minimum of twice per week:

- White (P1): 3 to 4 months
- Yellow (P2 and P3): 4 to 6 months
- Orange (P4 and P5): 6 to 8 months
- Green (P6 and G1): 8 to 10 months
- Blue (G2 and G3): 8 to 10 months
- Brown (G4 and G5): 12 to 14 months
- Black (E1, E2, E3, E4, and E5): Many-year or lifelong commitment

You'll have to abide by your school's choice of structure. Generally, you must take a minimum number of classes over a certain period of time. In addition, you'll have to get a test form signed off by a certified instructor in order to test to the next level.

Do I have to follow the levels in order?
Yes! There is a specific curriculum taught in each level of Krav Maga. These levels build upon each other and are essential to learning the new techniques that each new level brings in. While you can progress at your own pace, you must progress from one level to the next through testing before moving on.

How do I get the most out of Krav Maga training?
To continually have forward growth in your development, you should follow a regimented training schedule that includes the following aspects: training in classes with an instructor, general fitness training, specific fitness training, solo training, partner training, and mental training (situational awareness, strategy, and tactics). Each aspect will be important to develop your individual attributes. Having a good instructor or mentor who can evaluate and develop your skill sets will save you a tremendous amount of time and effort.

How can I become a Krav Maga instructor?
Each Krav Maga system differs in their requirements, so it's best to contact your local certified Krav Maga school (which you can find in the discussion of certified instructors earlier in this book). However, some basics still apply. Candidates must have the following:

- A minimum number of classes, time invested, and patches or belts achieved
- Adequate knowledge of all techniques up to that level being tested
- Above-average fitness and conditioning
- A willingness to keep learning
- Good moral character
- Successful completion of the certification process

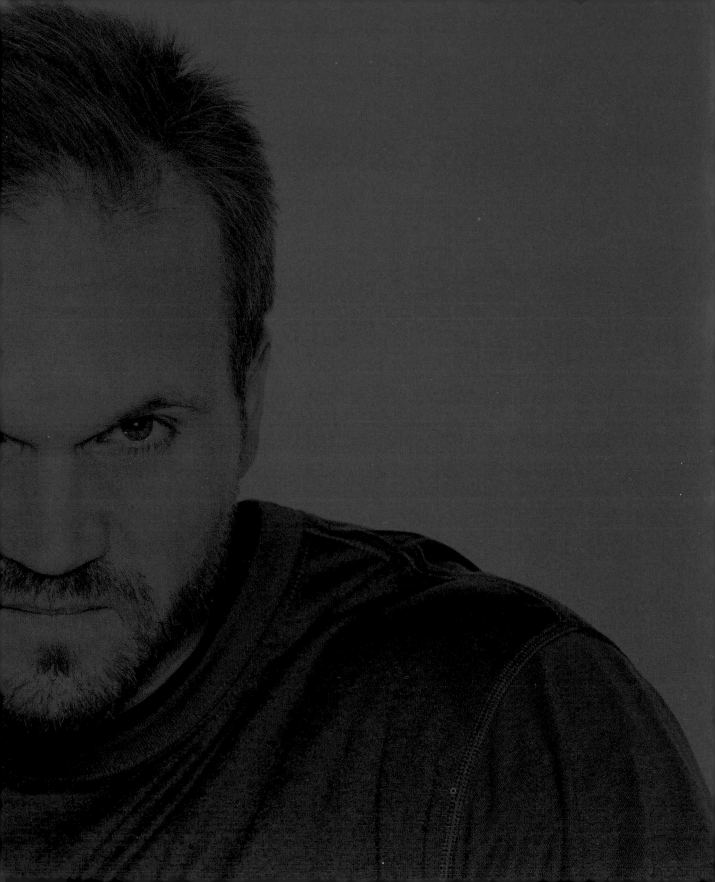

PART 2

GETTING INTO THE RIGHT MIND-SET

HAVING SITUATIONAL AWARENESS

One of the first ways to get into the Krav Maga mind-set is to have good situational awareness. After all, if you can't see the threat, you can't avoid it or defend yourself from it.

What Is Situational Awareness?

The term *situational awareness* simply refers to your ability to recognize potential threats to yourself or your family. For instance, when you're walking home alone or in a dark parking lot, you should be on alert for any potential danger.

However, you aren't expected to be at a heightened state of alertness all the time or for extended periods of time—that would be exhausting. So how do you know when to increase your alertness? You should be looking for anything different from the baseline or normal state of an environment. There's a baseline for your office, your neighborhood, and for a nightclub, all of which are very different. For instance, your office may be a quiet cube farm in which you have a handful of workers who normally don't interact much—that's its baseline. Once you can recognize your environment's baseline, you can easily see what doesn't fit.

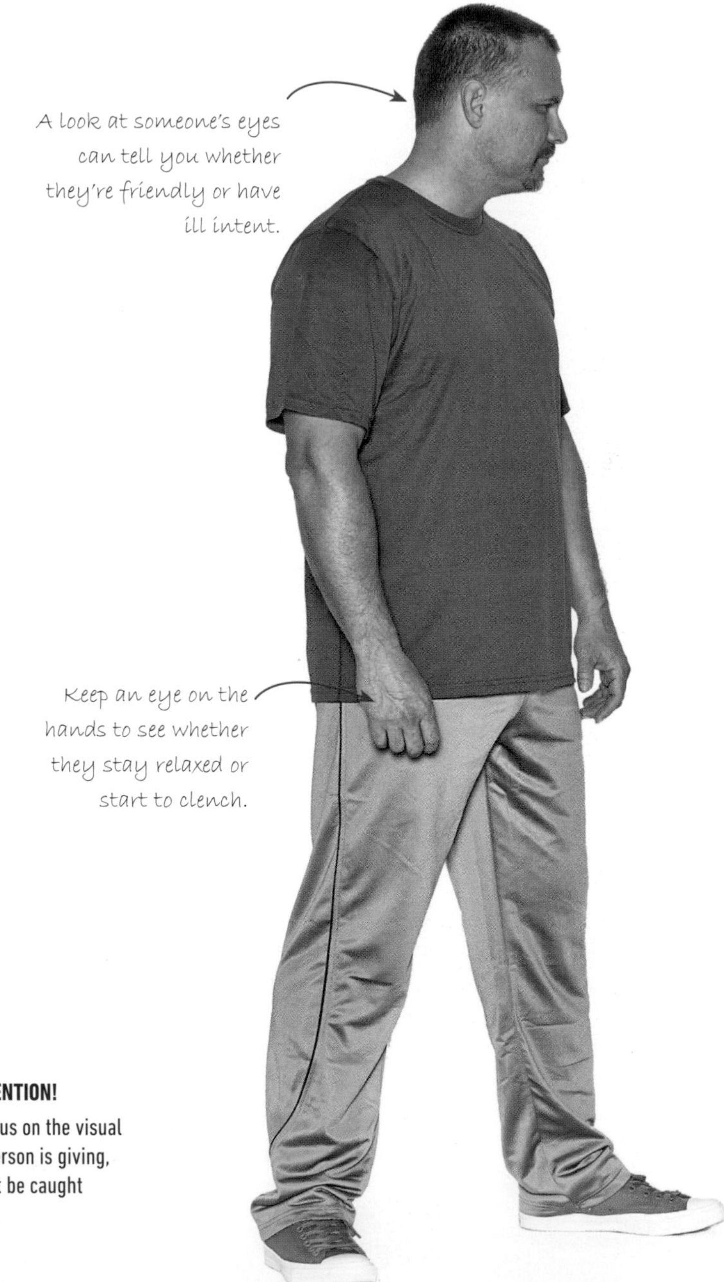

A look at someone's eyes can tell you whether they're friendly or have ill intent.

Keep an eye on the hands to see whether they stay relaxed or start to clench.

PAY ATTENTION!

If you focus on the visual cues a person is giving, you won't be caught unaware.

TRUST YOUR GUT

Beyond what you can pick up with your physical senses, you've been given a great survival tool of intuition or gut feeling. So if you get a gut feeling about a situation, whether good or bad, trust it.

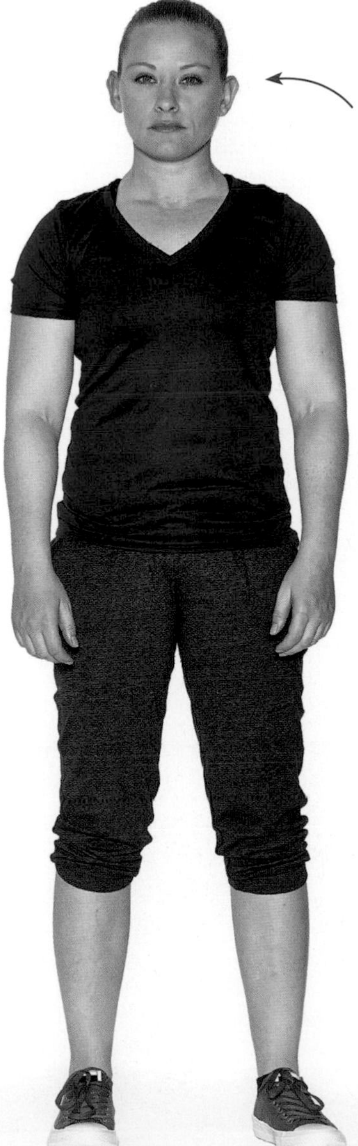

If caught in the Passive Stance (discussed more later), you're more vulnerable to attack.

Visual Cues

When you recognize the anomaly in your environment, you must question whether it's suspect or sinister. Based on how you answer that question, you can then take the appropriate action of either further investigating or simply walking away.

Avoiding the problem before it happens is always a great choice. However, if an individual is approaching you and you're unable to get away, you can use the following visual cues to verify that person's intention before he or she enters your personal space (roughly 15 to 20 feet; 4.5 to 6m).

- **Check the eyes for intention.** Does the person smile? Or does the person look away or narrow his or her eyes?
- **Check the hands.** Is the person holding anything? Are the hands open and relaxed or clinched in fists?
- **Look at the waistband and pockets.** Do you see a weapon, a knife clip, or any bulges where a weapon could be hidden?

By raising your awareness levels using visual cues, you begin your journey of changing your personal protection mind-set.

Cooper's Color Codes

One of the most recognized ways of defining levels of situational awareness is Cooper's color codes. Developed by Jeff Cooper, a U.S. Marine, this guide breaks down awareness into different levels and what the response to a situation would be based on that. Because you won't always be ready for a potential threat, Cooper's color codes provides information on which level is ideal for any given time. The bar here shows a modified color code to illustrate the differences between the levels.

CONDITION WHITE

UNAWARE OR UNPREPARED

Another way to say this is you're "tuned out" or "zoned out." This is your typical state when you're at home and have your doors locked and the alarm on. If you're attacked in condition white, you'll most likely have an "I can't believe this is happening to me" moment.

CONDITION YELLOW

PREPARED, ALERT, AND RELAXED WITH GOOD SITUATIONAL AWARENESS

In this level, your eyes are openly looking for the baseline in your environment. You're aware of each person coming into your personal space while maintaining a relaxed frame of mind. You're typically in this state when you're in familiar but less-secure environments, such as at work.

CONDITION ORANGE

ALERT TO POTENTIAL AND PROBABLE DANGER

You're ready to take action. In this condition level, you've recognized an anomaly and determined you need to narrow your focus to further identify the threat. This occurs in situations in which you notice your baseline for an environment has been disrupted.

CONDITION RED

ACTION MODE

You're focused on addressing the immediate danger. In this condition, an attack has happened or is imminent.

CONDITION BLACK

PANIC AND/OR BREAKDOWN OF PHYSICAL AND PSYCHOLOGICAL PERFORMANCE

You're either in fight-or-flight or in freeze mode. If you're fully experiencing the latter, you've shut down—this is panic-induced paralysis, which can happen in highly stressful situations such as an attack.

OODA Loop

Another useful tool to help you understand situational awareness is the OODA (observe, orient, decide, and act) loop. Developed by military strategist and U.S. Air Force Colonel John Boyd for combat operations, this approach is used today to represent how people make tough decisions in any endeavor. For instance, if you're surprised by an attack, you're technically behind the OODA loop compared to your attacker, who has already observed, oriented his or her attack, and decided to take action. Because you weren't ready when you were attacked, you have to catch up by running through your own OODA loop and then responding.

In most deadly encounters, you'll start behind in this reaction process, which is why Krav Maga techniques are based on instinctive reactions to reality-based threats. The faster you can act through the OODA loop, the shorter your reaction time and the higher state of readiness you can achieve to react appropriately to that given situation. While your instinct will always cause you to have a flinch response of some kind, ideally, you'll have trained enough to decide and react with a general defense in order to catch up in the fight. This, combined with counterattacking aggressively, will give you the needed window of opportunity to defend yourself.

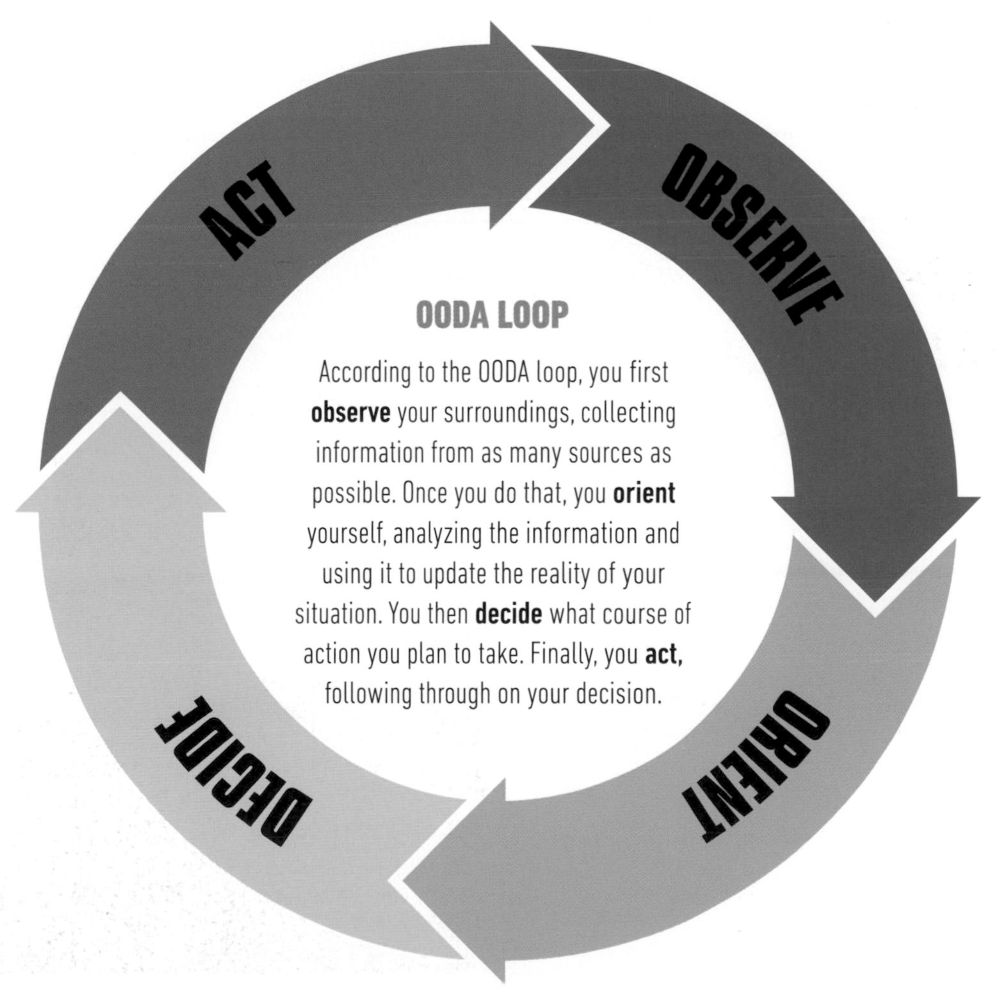

OODA LOOP

According to the OODA loop, you first **observe** your surroundings, collecting information from as many sources as possible. Once you do that, you **orient** yourself, analyzing the information and using it to update the reality of your situation. You then **decide** what course of action you plan to take. Finally, you **act,** following through on your decision.

ATTACK CYCLE

Increasing your situational awareness is only the beginning. Knowing the cycles of an attack will help you better understand how an attack develops, what happens during an attack, and how to deal with the aftermath.

The Four Parts of the Cycle

No matter the type and level of attack, the process follows the same cycle: nonconflict, preconflict, conflict aware, and postconflict.

Nonconflict
This is the normal or baseline state. In this part of the cycle, an attacker hasn't come into contact with you or made any sort of attack plan. Ideally, you want your interactions with others to stay in this part of the cycle.

Preconflict
Before a conflict, the attacker may survey an area to determine the method, place, time, and victim (or victims) for an attack. In a personal self-defense situation, this surveillance may be just a few seconds or minutes.

Strong situational awareness is very important at this time to help you identify any shady characters who are surveying you. If you're visibly aware, your potential attacker may notice this and move on to another less aware target (known as a *soft target*).

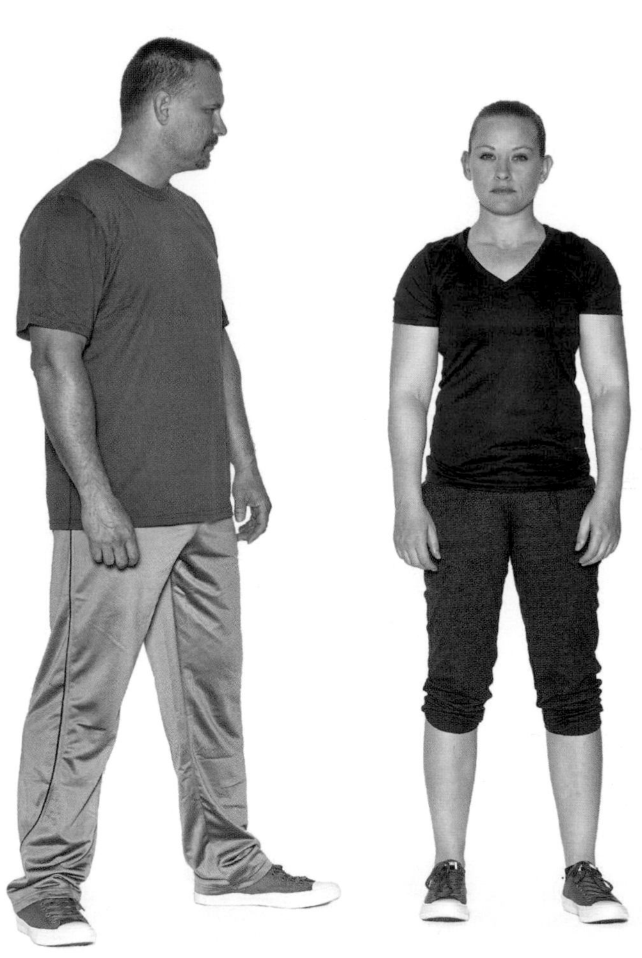

NONCONFLICT OR PRECONFLICT?
While this could simply be a nonconfrontational look, it could also indicate potential danger. This makes using situational awareness critical so you know the difference.

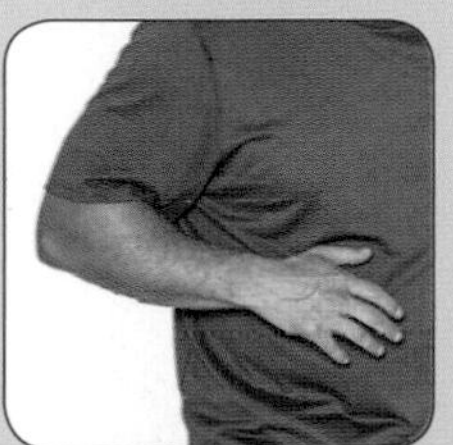
BODY BLADING

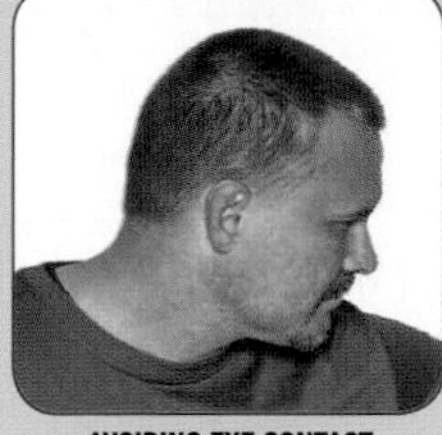
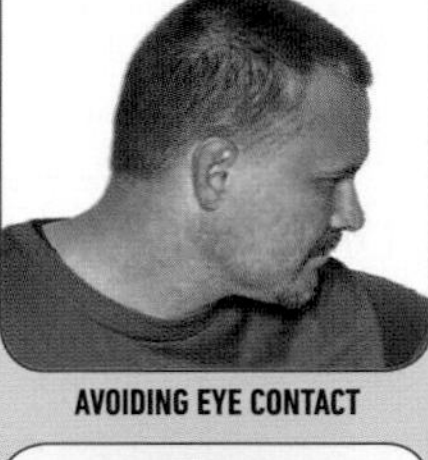
AVOIDING EYE CONTACT

FIST CLENCHING

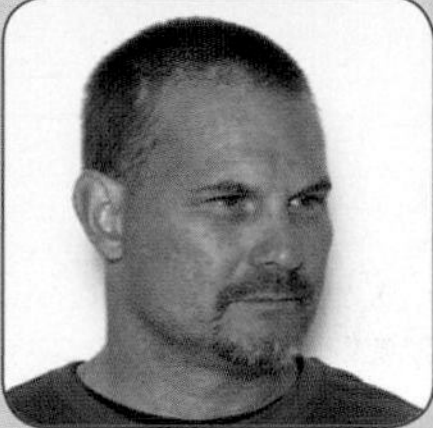
THOUSAND-YARD STARE

PREASSAULT INDICATORS

Certain physical responses indicate a looming an attack. By recognizing these indicators, you can interrupt the attacker's OODA loop by asking an out-of-context question, such as "Do you have peanut butter?" to help defuse the situation.

- Body blading (for instance, getting into a Fighting Stance)
- Fist clenching
- Trembling
- Rapid or shallow breathing
- Avoiding eye contact
- Hiding the face
- Target lock (such as staring or focusing on a specific area)
- Thousand-yard stare (looking through you)

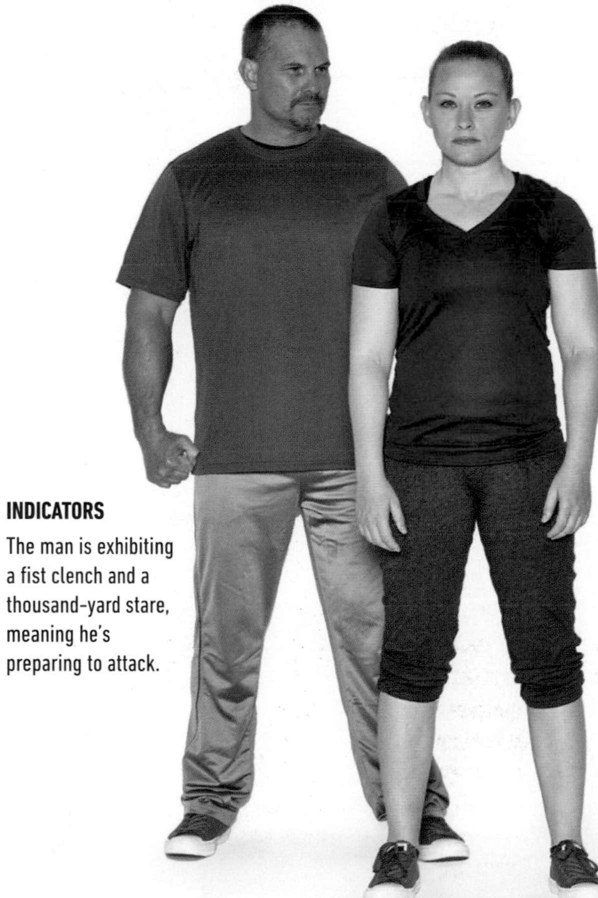
INDICATORS
The man is exhibiting a fist clench and a thousand-yard stare, meaning he's preparing to attack.

Conflict Aware

If the attacker chooses to make you the target, he or she will begin to show *preassault indicators*. These involuntary physiological responses can clue you in to the fact that this person plans to attack you. If you can't avoid the assault, you must continue to try to interrupt the attacker's OODA loop and upset his or her balance with aggressive counterattacks

While this is all going on, you'll experience a range of physiological responses, increased adrenaline, and other hormone releases in reaction to the high stress. For this reason, you must constantly keep fighting until the attacker is incapacitated, disengaged, and no longer a threat.

Postconflict

After you've defended yourself and possibly called 911, you might still have emotional and physiological responses to the violent encounter, such as remorse or sadness, anger, or even hysteria (whether laughing or crying). Realize that these reactions are normal after violent attacks—don't judge yourself. You survived, and that's always most important.

YOUR BODY'S RESPONSE TO STRESS

While going through the high-stress situation of an attack, your body responds in various physiological and psychological ways. Understanding how you feel under stress will help your training in Krav Maga.

Physiological Responses to Stress

Your body's fight-or-flight response leads to certain changes in you that are meant to prepare you to either defend yourself or get away. Your autonomic nervous system—the primary system in control of your fight-or-flight response—regulates everything from your heart and respiration rates to your digestion, leading to changes when presented with an attack. Your sympathetic nervous system releases norepinephrine at this time as well, which prepares your brain and body for action by increasing alertness, quickly retrieving memories, and strengthening attention. Your adrenal gland simultaneously releases epinephrine into your body, giving you a boost of energy and signaling the release of other hormones, such as adrenaline (which increases your heart and breathing rates and inhibits digestion). All of these automatic responses enable you to function in a highly alert state when confronted.

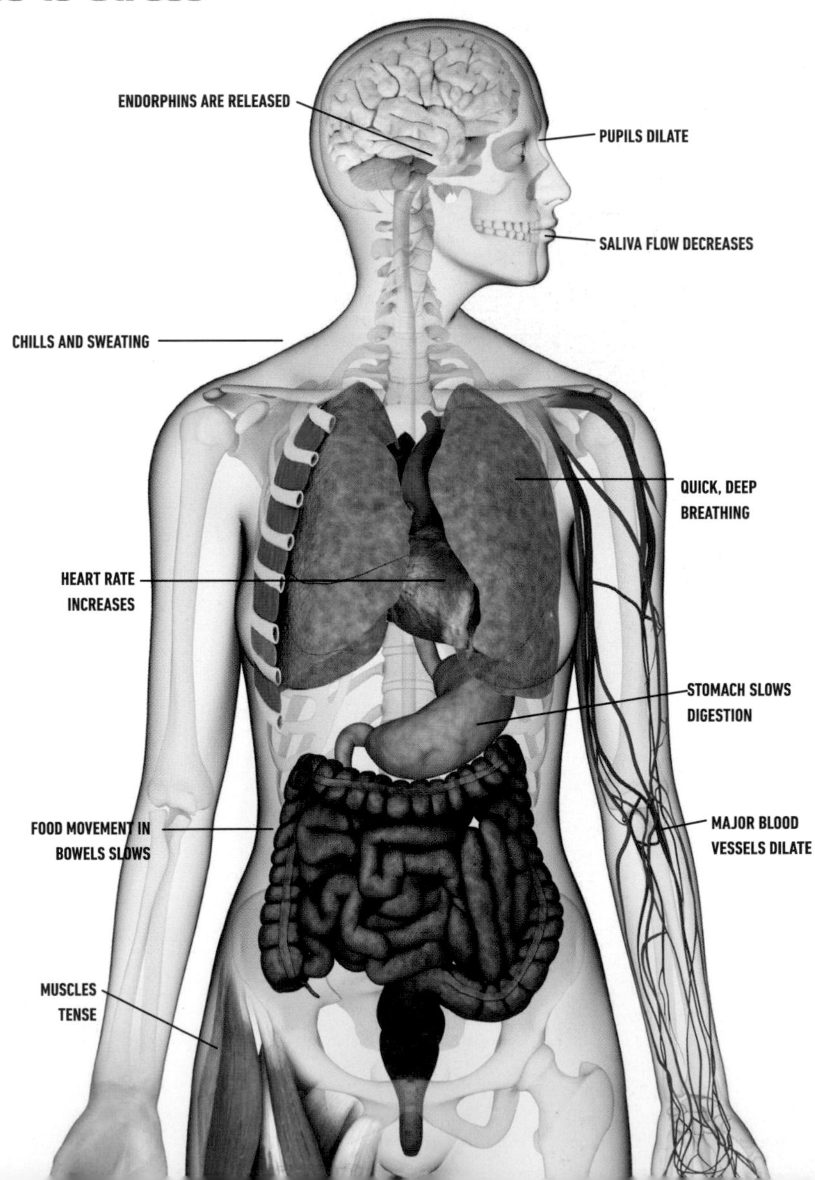

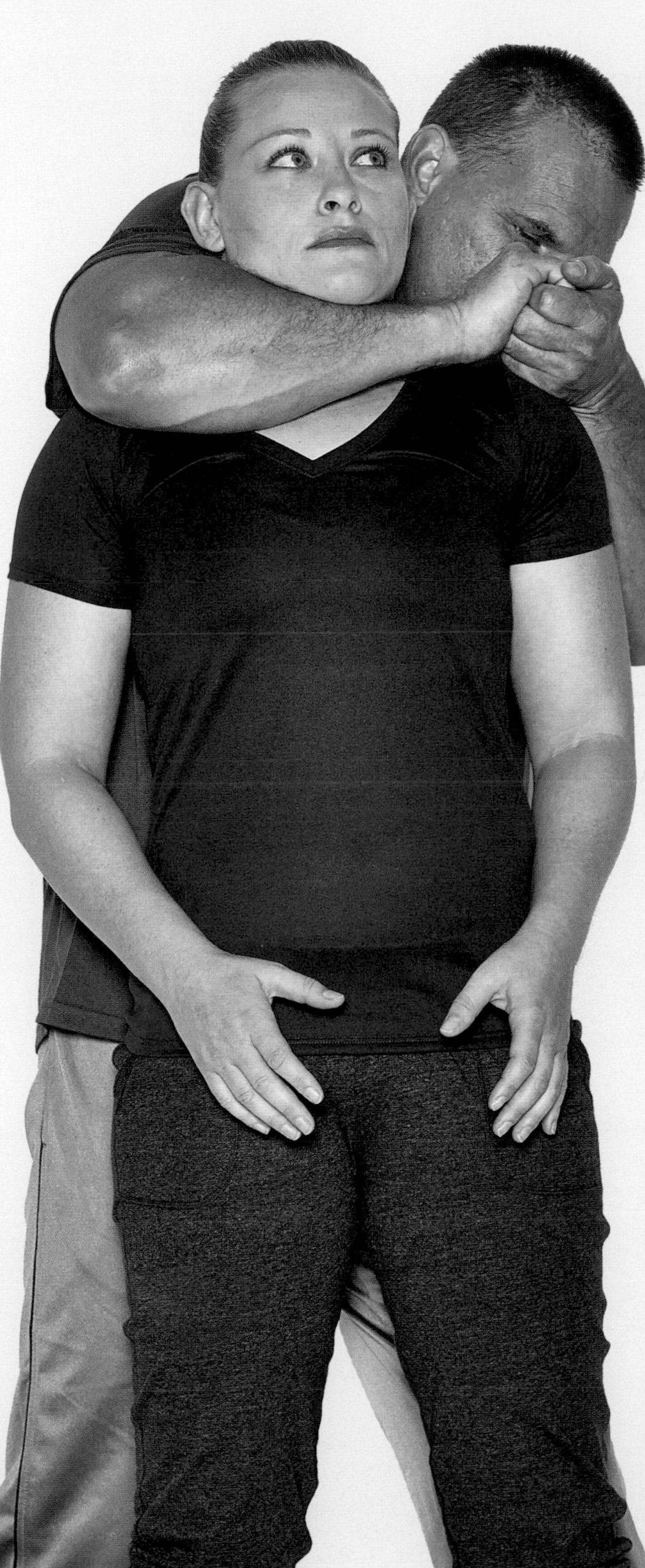

Psychological Responses to Stress and Reaction Time

When put in a highly stressful situation, such as an attack, you also have a number of psychological responses. This is due to vasoconstriction, or the tightening of blood vessels, which reduces oxygen flow to your brain. As a result, the rational thoughts you normally have are replaced with irrational thoughts and panic. Your ability to think clearly then diminishes, causing you further stress and panic.

You might also experience great distraction and poor judgment. Because stress can make you feel like the world is ending, you could become pessimistic about your approach to the situation at hand. Moodiness, feeling overwhelmed, and becoming highly tense are also quite common. During or after an attack, you may even remember events incorrectly, recalling details that never happened and forgetting ones that did.

All of these overwhelming psychological reactions lead you to perform at a slower pace, thus increasing your reaction time and decreasing the effectiveness of your response. This makes it very important to train yourself with Krav Maga to overcome your normal stress response. By training properly and using stress testing in a controlled environment, you learn acute situational awareness. Krav Maga training will better prepare you to react appropriately and in a more focused manner, so you can get home safely.

STOP PANIC IN ITS TRACKS

With Krav Maga, you can learn how to think and react more clearly, even when in a stressful attack situation.

UNDERSTANDING HUMAN PREDATORY BEHAVIOR

Once you understand your own reactions and motivations, you must look at the types of character-impaired personalities around you to understand what motivates them to perform their heinous acts.

Personality Subtypes of the Aggressive Personality

People who engage in human predatory behavior are categorized as aggressive personality types. What this means is that these people are, at their core, in a fight against anything that stands in the way of their desires. They are responsible for the victimization of those they come into contact with or choose as their next target. Because those with aggressive behavior are more uninhibited and feel entitled to fight, they have great potential to turn predatory. These aggressors might abhor the idea of denying their fighter instinct and lash out at others in physically and emotionally destructive ways. As a whole, these personalities tend to be remorseless, narcissistic, and dangerous. And while some aggressive types of people may not have a criminal record, they have the potential pose a threat to you and anyone they encounter. This threat could be anything from verbal abuse to physical violence.

So what types do you have to watch out for? There are four different subtypes of the aggressive personality: unbridled aggressive, channeled aggressive, covert aggressive, and sadistic aggressive.

UNBRIDLED AGGRESSIVE

These people oppose subjecting themselves to society's rules. They're frequently in conflict with the law due to a lack of impulse control and are often labeled as antisocial or narcissistic.

CHANNELED AGGRESSIVE

These people generally limit their aggressive ruthlessness to noncriminal acts, such as competing in sports or being relentlessly driven in the workplace.

THREE TIPS TO AVOID TROUBLE

While it's unrealistic to think you can avoid aggressive personalities, three simple things can help make it less likely you end up in a violent encounter.

1. Stay alert. As discussed earlier with situational awareness, knowing what's going on around you at all times makes it less likely that aggressives will target you.

2. Be unpredictable. You don't have to alter your life every day; you simply have to make sure you don't fall into habits that are very easy to track and therefore exploitable by others.

3. Keep a low profile. Fit the baseline of the area you're in. If you don't stick out, you won't draw unwanted attention from unsavory types.

COVERT AGGRESSIVE

These people hide their cruel behavior behind civility. For instance, when confronted about a bad behavior, they might cast themselves as the victim and make the confronter seem in the wrong.

SADISTIC AGGRESSIVE

These people lack concern and empathy and enjoy demeaning or injuring other people. Some even gain a sexual thrill from their destructive actions.

Dealing with Unbridled Aggressives

Krav Maga focuses on countering the aggressives who turn predatory—usually the unbridled aggressive criminals, called *psychopaths* or *sociopaths*. These people feel superior to "normal" people and therefore entitled to prey upon them. Unbridled aggressives understand norms of behavior and could choose to conform to societal standards but simply opt not to. This notion leads them to victimize those who deny predators exist among us, enabling them to catch others off guard.

If you encounter an unbridled aggressive, knowing how to respond can get you out of the situation before it gets violent. For instance, the unbridled aggressive will most likely start with verbal abuse to intimidate or goad you into responding so he or she can then escalate to physical violence. Because the unbridled aggressive's goal is to feel superior, often the best course of action is to walk away. Your walking away or backing down in their eyes satisfies their need, and he or she will most often let you go.

Look for the signs and always trust your gut feelings that alert you to the presence of aggressive personalities, or you might be tricked into a false sense of security that you won't be victimized.

THE IMPORTANCE OF AGGRESSION

A key mind-set of training to survive a violent attack is the ability to "flip the switch" and activate your will to survive. The form of aggression we're discussing here doesn't mean you're looking to a start a fight. It simply means you have the motivation to get the upper hand when attacked.

The Benefits of Aggression

Having an aggressive mind-set during an attack can benefit you in many ways, including the following:

You surprise your attacker. Your attacker expects you to submit or else you wouldn't be the victim of an attack. Unbridled aggression surprises him or her and upsets his or her OODA loop.

You can overcome being late in the fight. Responding with overwhelming force and violence enables you to overcome the surprise of an attack and can change the momentum of the fight. In a fight, you'll likely be behind your attacker when it comes to processing the attack, so an aggressive response turns the table, advances your own OODA loop, and resets your attacker's OODA loop.

You compensate for any disadvantages. Aggression makes up for any number of disadvantages you might have in a fight, such as lack of training, lesser strength, or deficiency in size. This compensation is commonly referred to as the *mama bear instinct*, as it's similar to how a mother bear is willing to lose her life in order to protect her cubs no matter the odds. You must be like the aggressive mama bear and make your will to survive a powerful force to contend with.

You tap into your will to live. There's no stronger drive in your DNA than your will to survive. Krav Maga students have endured the most brutal attacks but have kept fighting and survived. The moment you throw your aggressiveness switch, you won't stop until your attacker is no longer a threat.

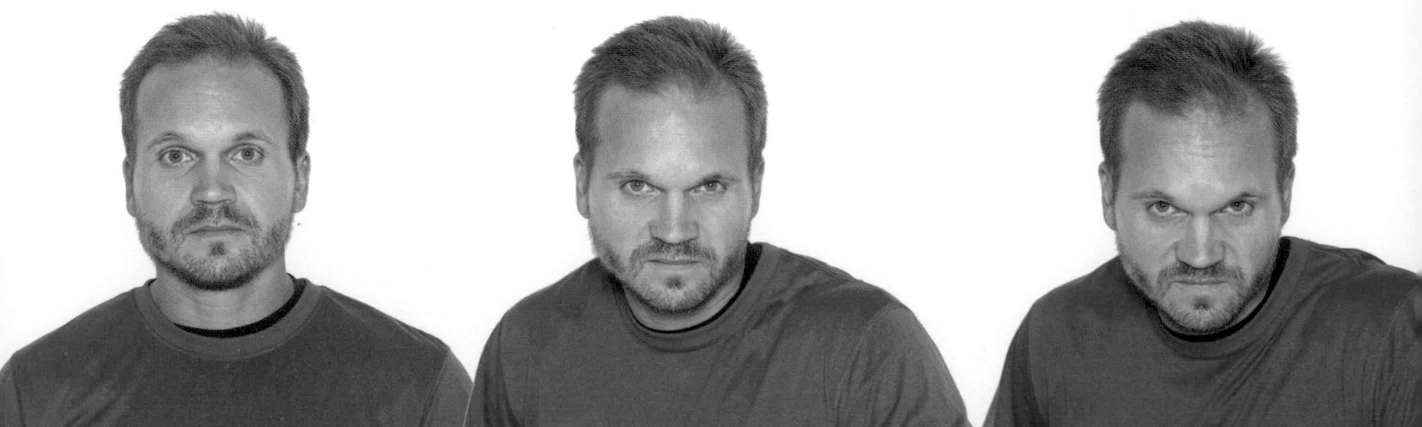

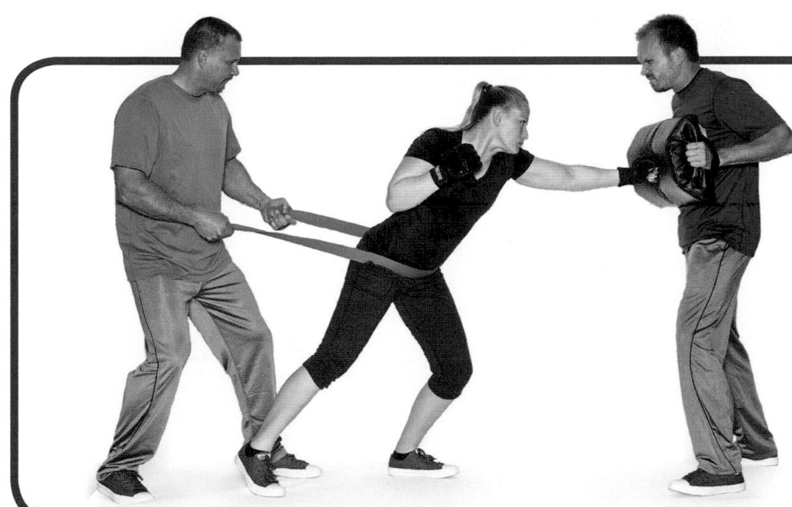

AGGRESSIVENESS TRAINING
Later in this book, you'll learn this training program, which helps bring out your aggressive side by shifting you around so you have to work harder to hit the target.

How to Become Aggressive

While you know how aggressiveness can benefit you, you may be wondering just how exactly to get into the mind-set. To tap into your natural will to live, ask yourself a few basic questions:

- What am I willing to do to save my life and/or the lives of my loved ones?
- What value do I place on my life and those around me?
- Am I willing to become another one of the attacker's victims?

After you've answered these questions, imagine the anger you'd feel if you or your loved ones were to die at the hands of an attacker. Anger at this idea should start to swell inside you, and in an attack, your mind should say "I'm going to survive this and get home to my family. If I have to go through this sociopath to do that, so be it!"

Through specific drills using Krav Maga, we encourage our students to develop this thought process of mounting aggression. This type of training teaches you to fight like your life depends on it. A switch is either all on or all off; when you're attacked, the survival instinct must be turned all the way on. Your animal instinct should show in the relentless aggression of your defenses and counterattacks until your attacker is no longer a threat and you've safely escaped.

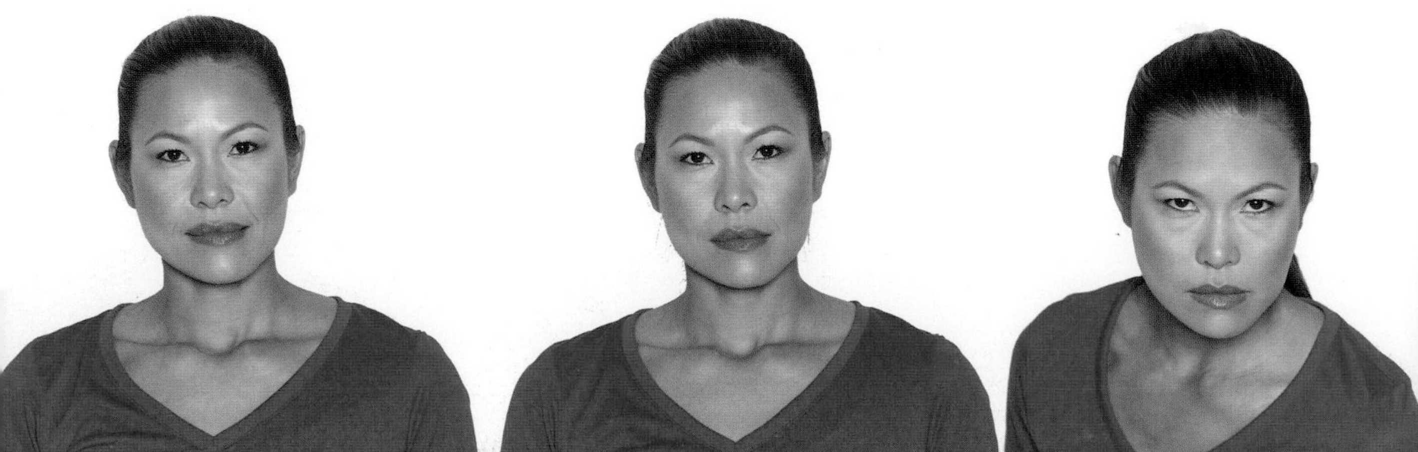

USE OF FORCE

In the reality-based self-defense community, we know that when it comes to defending your life, there are actually two fights. The first is the actual self-defense fight in which you protect yourself and get to safety. However, a second fight can start the moment the first fight ends—the legal fight.

Legal Use of Force

Before you begin to learn and practice Krav Maga, you should become familiar with the legal ramifications for when you take action. Under U.S. law, an individual will be held accountable for the amount of force used in any given situation, based on the specific facts of each case. Readers are advised to consult local legal experts, and to understand and refer to specifically applicable local laws, in order to determine the specific considerations governing their conduct. The following concepts represent *typical* U.S. laws and are presented merely as a general overview of the subject, as specific laws vary from state to state, and even by local jurisdiction. Not all of the presented concepts will pertain in every jurisdiction.

Jeopardy
The key concept—*I feared the loss of life*—known as jeopardy generally has to be present to justify the use of force, which must be proportionally reasonable.

Duty to retreat
This requires you to try to escape the situation before using deadly force. While most states have removed this concept from case law, you should still follow it when confronted with deadly force.

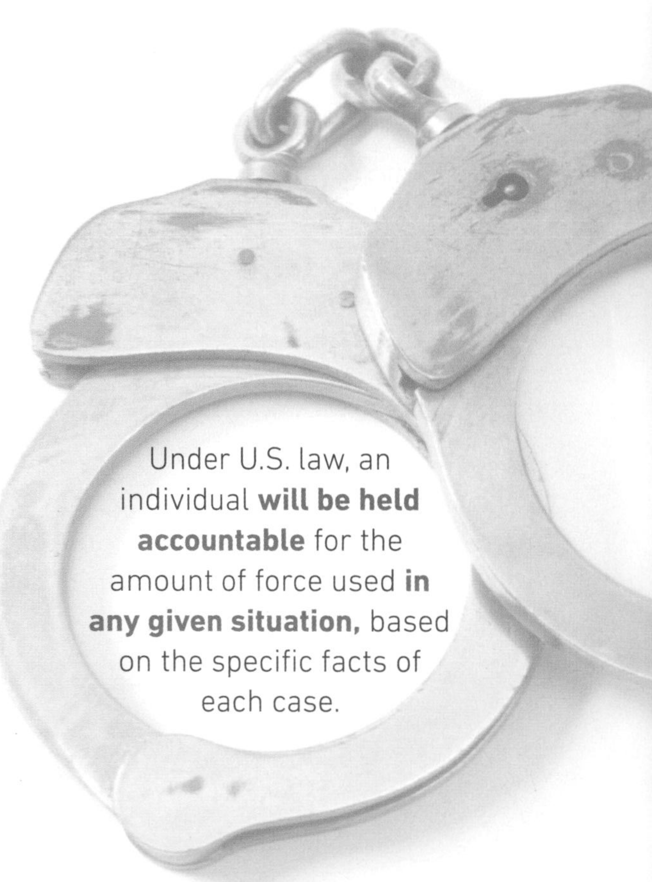

Under U.S. law, an individual **will be held accountable** for the amount of force used **in any given situation,** based on the specific facts of each case.

Doctrine
This concept allows you to defend your home and your life against intruders who enter your house unlawfully.

Self-defense
This justifies you, as a right, to prevent suffering force or violence through the use of sufficient counteracting force. To determine sufficient force, consider this: Is the threat imminent? Self-defense only justifies the use of force when it's used in response to an immediate threat. The threat you receive can simply be verbal, so long as it puts you in an immediate fear of physical harm or death. Once the fear of harm has ended, any use of force by you against the assailant would be considered retaliatory and not defensible.

Proportional response
This dictates the use of force must match the level of the threat. You can only employ as much force as is required to remove the threat. If the threat involves deadly force, that means you can use deadly force to counteract or stop the threat. If the threat were to involve minor force and you used force that caused grave bodily harm or death, you would be held criminally liable.

Stand your ground
This permits you to stand your ground and defend yourself. This removes your duty to retreat in nonlethal attacks. When states withdrew duty-to-retreat laws, many replaced them with stand-your-ground laws.

How to Act

After a life-or-death defense, you could be adrenalized, traumatized, and experiencing an abundance of feelings and emotions you may not necessarily want to share with bystanders, witnesses, law enforcement, and first responders. Review the sections on psychological and physiological effects of stress so you know what to potentially expect from yourself in these situations. Because any comments can and will be used against you in a court of law, it's important to collect yourself before making an official statement.

Making a Self-Defense Card
To help you provide the proper information and keep emotion out of the situation, you can create a card such as this one (for a situation where someone is acting in self defense and is in fear of his or her life), to keep in your wallet and present to law enforcement officials as required.

I just had to defend my life.
"If I have given this to you, it has been necessary to take actions to defend innocent life. I am willing to sign a criminal complaint against the perpetrator(s). I will point out witnesses and evidence. As you may have experienced yourself, this is a stressful and traumatic experience for me. Therefore, I wish to make no further statements until I have contacted an attorney and composed myself. I also do not consent to any searches. I will cooperate fully once I have consulted with an attorney. As a lawful citizen, I ask for the same courtesy that you would show a fellow officer who was involved in a similar situation. Thank you for your understanding."

NOTE: **THIS IS A SAMPLE CARD.**
Please consult your local laws and your attorney for help creating your personal self-defense card.

EMPLOYING KRAV MAGA PRINCIPLES

Krav Maga is based on certain principles that influence how it's taught to and used by students. The following can help you understand how Krav Maga works as a system of self-defense.

Krav Maga Foundations

A few principles make up the foundations of this self-defense system, underlying the reasons why you should learn these techniques.

The Number-One Principle: Getting Home Safe
To get home safe is both a principle of Krav Maga training and the supreme goal of all violent encounters. While you must assess the risk-to-benefit ratio of drills and exercises in training to avoid injury, in an actual violent encounter, you must use all of your physical and mental strength to respond aggressively and immediately. Never stop fighting until you and/or your loved ones can get home safe.

Smallest Defender and Biggest Attacker
Krav Maga assumes an effective technique succeeds even when the defender is smaller than the attacker. If a technique does not work for the smallest defender and biggest attacker (SDBA) principle, the Krav Maga system assumes it won't work for most people.

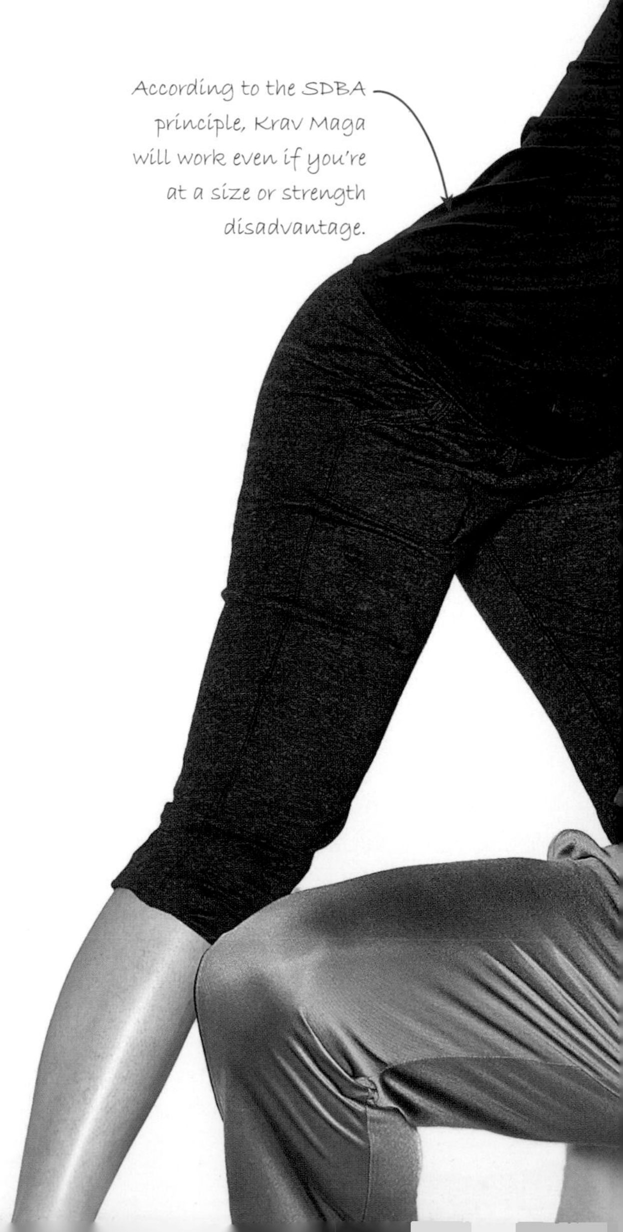

According to the SDBA principle, Krav Maga will work even if you're at a size or strength disadvantage.

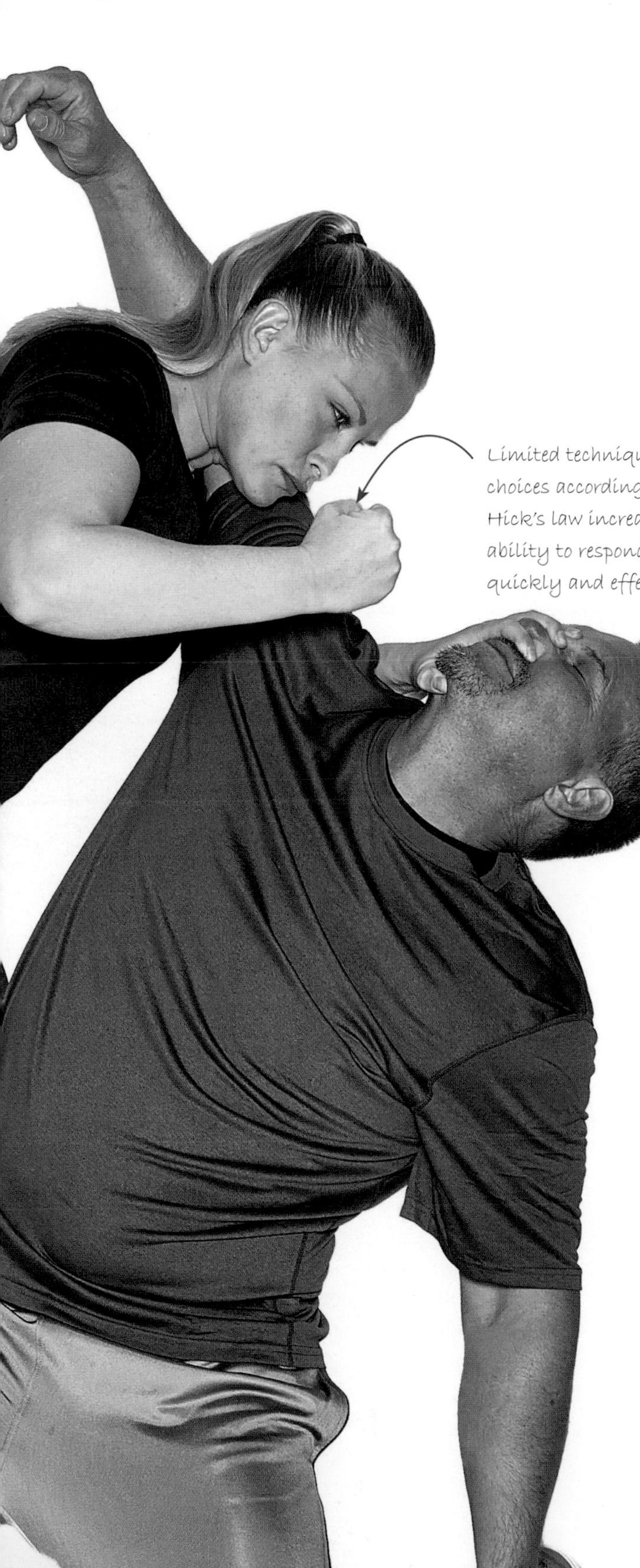

Limited technique choices according to Hick's law increase your ability to respond quickly and effectively.

ABSORB WHAT'S USEFUL

This concept from kung fu legend Bruce Lee simply means you should borrow from any method that will enhance your ability to defend your life. Krav Maga allows you to pull in what you need from wherever to best protect yourself.

Hick's Law

To help improve reaction times in a fight, Krav Maga applies the well-known, universal principle called *Hick's law* or the *Hick-Hyman law*. The theory explains that the time it takes a person to make a decision is directly related to the number of choices available in the scenario. So when there are more options available to a person in a particular situation, the person's reaction time increases.

In combat, a longer reaction time is bad, as it could give your attacker the time needed to make a strong attack. Therefore, Krav Maga limits the options available to you by simplifying the system; one self-defense technique can cover a variety of attacks. So to apply Hick's law, the limited technique choices decrease your reaction times and increase your chances of making effective and quick counterattacks.

Action and Reaction

These Krav Maga principles focus on what makes the self-defense techniques so effective, as well as what basic actions you should take in an attack.

AWARENESS AND RESOURCEFULNESS

With Krav Maga, you learn to stay safe by being situationally aware. Awareness means knowing your environment and not trading one danger for another. For example, don't run blindly from an attack into an unknown area, such as an alley, only to find that there's no exit (called a *fatal funnel*). This awareness can help you be resourceful, allowing you to improvise weapons or shields with nearby materials, such as throwing your keys at an attacker's face to distract him or her.

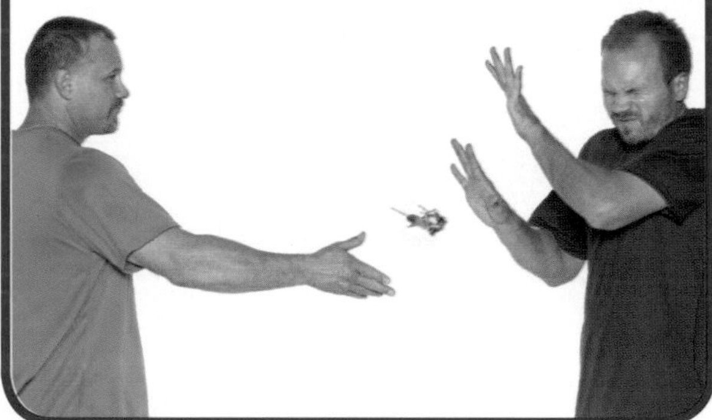

Dealing with the Immediate Danger

Say you're being accosted by two attackers; one is armed with a stick, while the other is armed with a knife. Deciding whom you defend yourself against can be a complex problem. Which attacker is closest? Bigger? Stronger? Which attacker has the more lethal weapon? Do you have any escape routes? What is the environment like? Is there an item you can use as a weapon to gain the advantage? If you defend and strike first, can you use that weapon against the attacker's weapon?

You can simplify your thought process by dealing with the immediate danger first. Through consistent physical and mental training with Krav Maga, you can run through such scenarios in order to learn how to react appropriately. Because each scenario is slightly different, Krav Maga helps you role-play to decide which danger could cause you the most harm (such as an attacker's hands around your throat) or which danger is closest to you (such as in a multiple-attacker situation). Through trial and error in a safe environment, you can gain the instinct to size up a situation quickly and figure out what the most immediate threat is, how to react to it, and then how to make your escape. By dealing with the immediate danger first, you ultimately give yourself a better opportunity to meet the requirements of the first principle: get home safe.

Direct and Decisive Action

You must commit to decisive action when defending your life. For example, an Eye Strike is simple, direct, and effective, and can quickly end a fight. While you should never rely on just one strike, you want to focus on using techniques you're confident with in order to end a fight as soon as possible.

Closest Weapon, Closest Target

In this concept, when an attacker advances to attack you, he or she moves into your attacking range. Interrupt the attack by using Krav Maga to strike the closest limb or vulnerable area. For example, Stomp Kick the attacker's lead knee when he or she steps toward you to economize space and energy.

Exploitation of Vulnerable Anatomy
Krav Maga teaches you to attack an aggressor's most vulnerable areas, such as the groin, eyes, throat, jaw, and joints. If your attacker can't stand, see, or breathe, he or she can't fight and harm you.

Table Principle
A Brazilian jujitzu theory, Krav Maga uses this idea to throw an attacker off balance in many ground defenses. By removing two legs from a table (in this case, trapping two of an attacker's limbs), it will have no base and fall over.

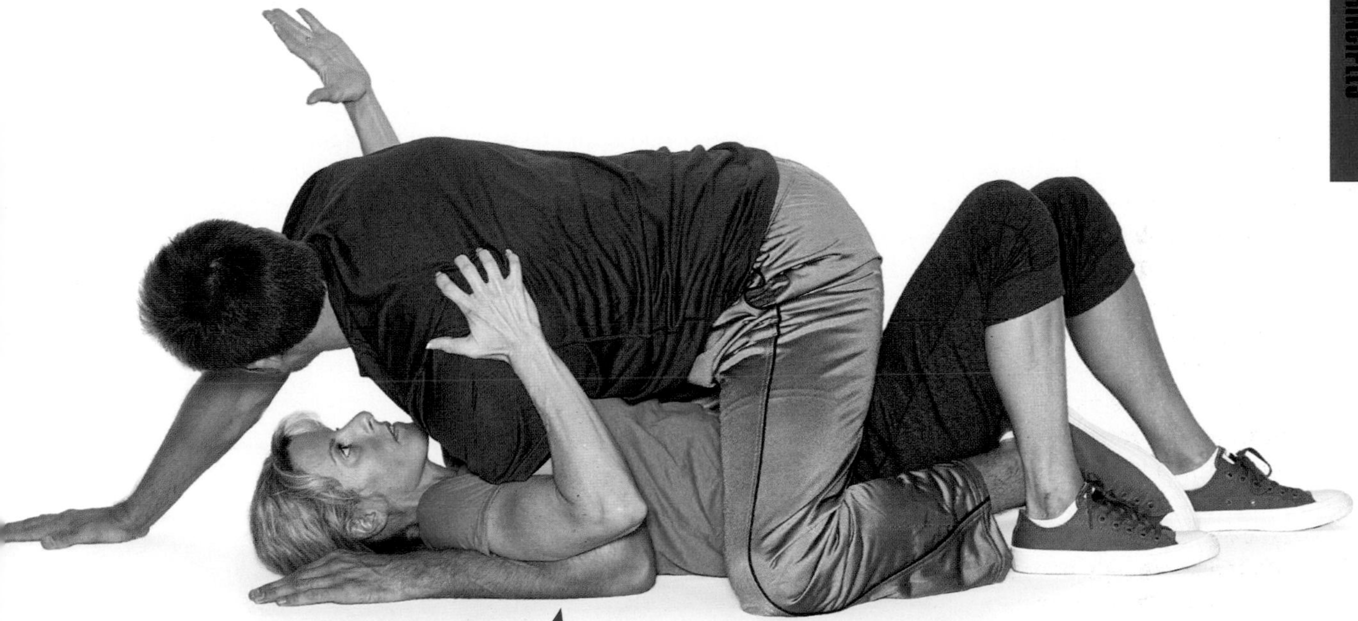

By trapping an arm and leg via the table principle, an attacker can't retain balance.

EFFICIENCY

In a life-or-death defense, you must be efficient in your movements. Because you don't have an endless supply of energy, Krav Maga teaches you to always use the simplest and most effective defenses available. This enables you to economize your energy so you can fight longer.

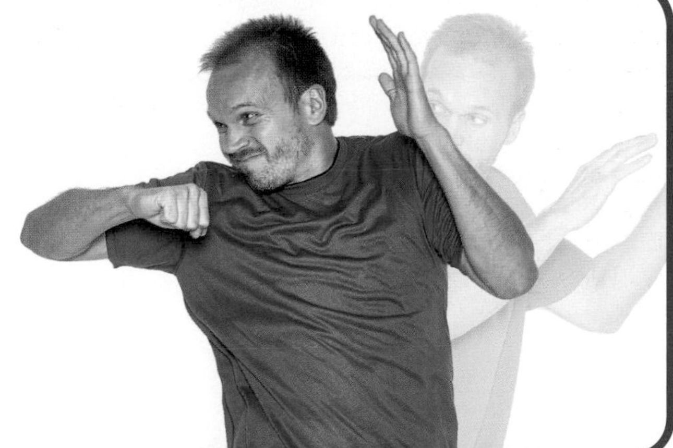

Continuous Motion
This is known by the military as *pressing the initiative*. After the initial contact, Krav Maga teaches you to continue to press your attacker with uninterrupted defenses and attacks to prevent him or her from reacting.

Instinctive Reactions
Krav Maga models defenses on the body's instinctive reactions to an attack so the techniques are easy to learn and retain. For example, your reaction to being choked is to bring your hand up to your throat. Accordingly, the plucking technique used to remove a chokehold is modeled after this reflexive response.

Simultaneous Defense and Counterattack
Krav Maga trains you to defend and counterattack simultaneously. The object of this is to interrupt your attacker's continuous use of motion.

Over Speed
Krav Maga emphasizes always exceeding the attacker's speed when defending yourself. For example, in defenses against hair grabs, hoodie pulls, or purse and backpack grabs, if the attacker pulls you at 1 mph, you must burst in the same direction at 3 mph. Doing so confuses the attacker, as he or she expects you to resist the pull, not to go with it explosively. You'll be able to knock the attacker off balance and have more chances to counterattack.

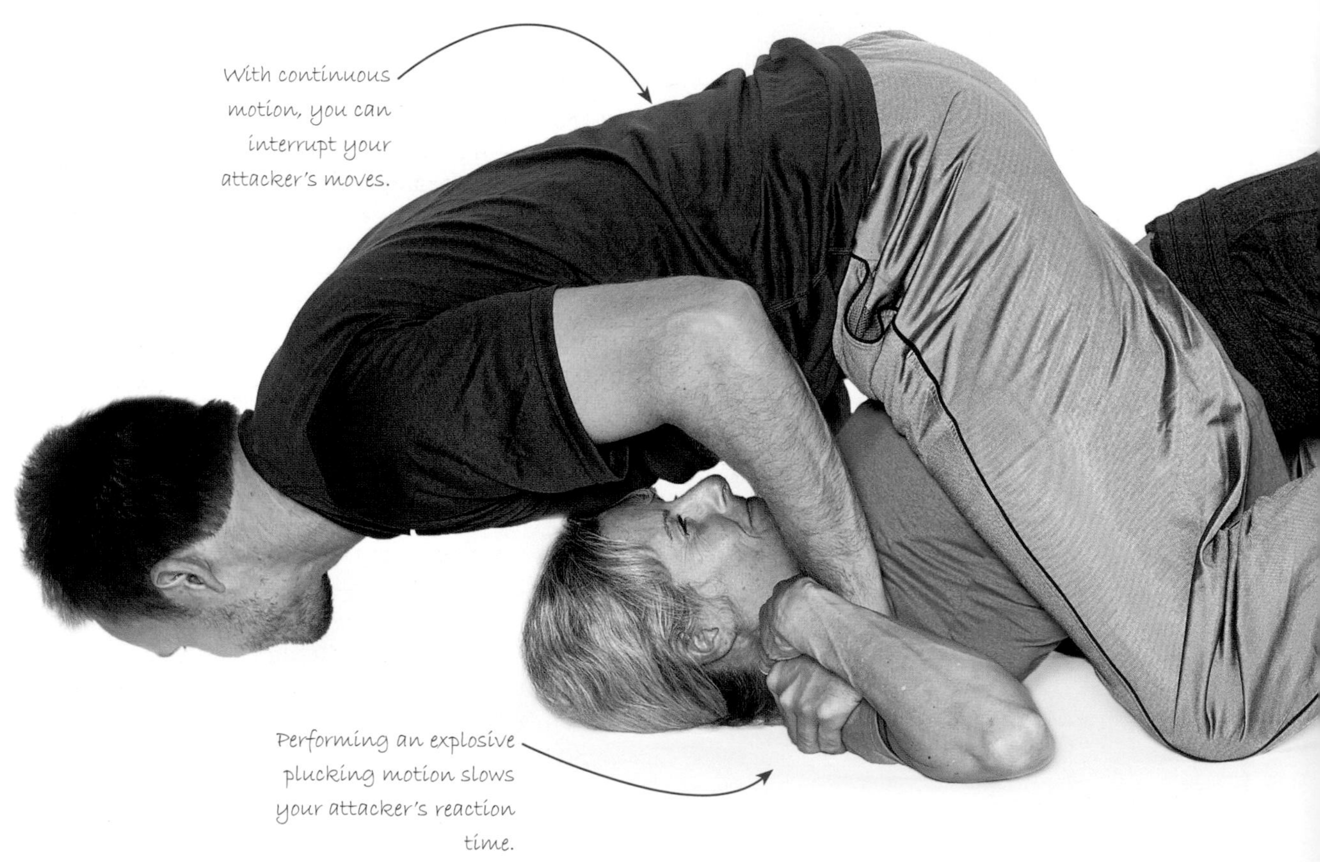

With continuous motion, you can interrupt your attacker's moves.

Performing an explosive plucking motion slows your attacker's reaction time.

PLUCKING

When you make an explosive pluck to an attacker's hands, the message that force has been applied doesn't travel fast enough to the attacker's brain for him or her to react and re-attack, giving you the advantage.

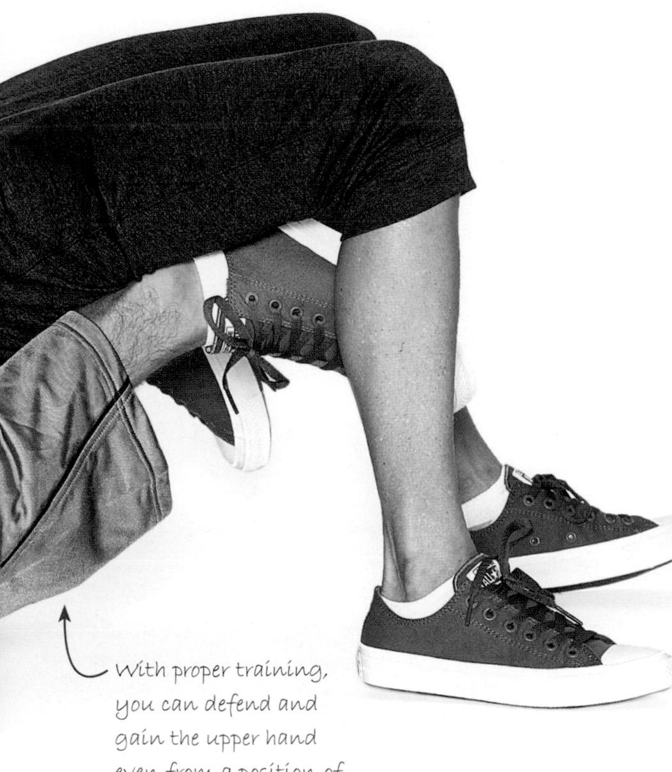

With proper training, you can defend and gain the upper hand even from a position of disadvantage.

Training

The training aspect of Krav Maga can't be understated as a preparation tool. The method behind Krav Maga training is reflected in these principles.

Progressive Training Methodology
In Krav Maga, instructors use a building-block process to train students. Training begins with simple, static repetitions and then builds upon this base with more dynamic training. With a trainer or partner, you can progressively break down the techniques to improve your understanding of the movements and to decrease your reaction time. You can then gradually add stress to your training to prepare for real violent attacks.

Clock Theory
Many fighting styles, including Krav Maga, use the clock theory to simplify training instruction by referring to directions as the numbers found on a clock face. For example, an instructor can say to a student, "Step to 2 o'clock to avoid a straight stab while making an inside defense."

Angles of Attack
This descriptive theory refers to how Krav Maga instructors explain the angle of a given attack in reference to the defender—for example, "A number-one attack defended by Outside Defense 1."

Training from a Position of Disadvantage
A key training concept for Krav Maga is to assume the worst-case scenario and simulate being caught off guard. Train from realistic positions of disadvantage and build your defenses so you can always succeed when at a handicap. For example, close your eyes, turn off the lights, or play loud music while training. This will build your confidence and improve your ability to react appropriately in real-world situations.

DEALING WITH THE AFTERMATH OF A FIGHT

While you may think the fight itself is the most important aspect of self-defense training, the aftermath is just as complex and fraught with emotions. It's critical to know what actions to take after the fight has ended.

What You Should Do

When you've defended yourself, you can expect to experience a number of physiological and physiological effects, as we discussed previously. So you may feel anything ranging from guilt or concern for your attacker to a callous "to heck with them." No matter your mental state, you should first move to a safe place, away from your attacker, and call the authorities and your lawyer (in case you need legal representation).

Once you've done that, do an overall health check of yourself. You need to perform a "wet check," which basically means you pat yourself down for any wet spots or noticeable injuries. This will determine if you're leaking any bodily fluids and or have injured yourself in some other way, such as a broken bone or large contusion. If you do have an injury, you should begin self-care, if possible. Keep a small emergency first-aid kit on your person or in your car so you'll be prepared to administer to yourself at any time. However, if you don't have your own kit, you can ask a bystander to get some help for you.

When paramedics and the police arrive on the scene, it's important to make sure everything is documented. For instance, it's always a good idea to ask to see paramedics so they can not only give you the aftercare you may need, but also document the injuries from the initial attack, even if it's just a few scratches. You should also ensure the officers who appear on the scene document and report your information. Be aware you may be taken into custody until they can figure out what happened and interview witnesses, if there are any. If you don't have a lawyer, you can ask for a public defender at this time.

When talking to the police and paramedics, keep your comments to just the facts—your injuries and the person who attacked you. Your emotions from the fight can affect your judgment and potentially lead you to make inaccurate or overly heated statements, so simply stick to what's obvious until you're more clear-headed and have talked to your lawyer or public defender.

The Eight Basic Aftermath Steps

1 Ensure the attacker is no longer a threat and that there are no immediate threats in the area.

2 Get to a safe distance and call for help.

3 Call a lawyer, if you have one.

4 Perform a wet check and begin self-care, if needed.

5 When the police or first responders arrive, give them your self-defense card (discussed previously) and/or don't say anything other than "I will fully cooperate when my lawyer is present."

6 Ask to be taken to the hospital to be examined.

7 Call family members and tell them what happened.

8 When talking to the police and first responders, keep your comments to your medical condition and the description of the attacker. Don't go into what happened.

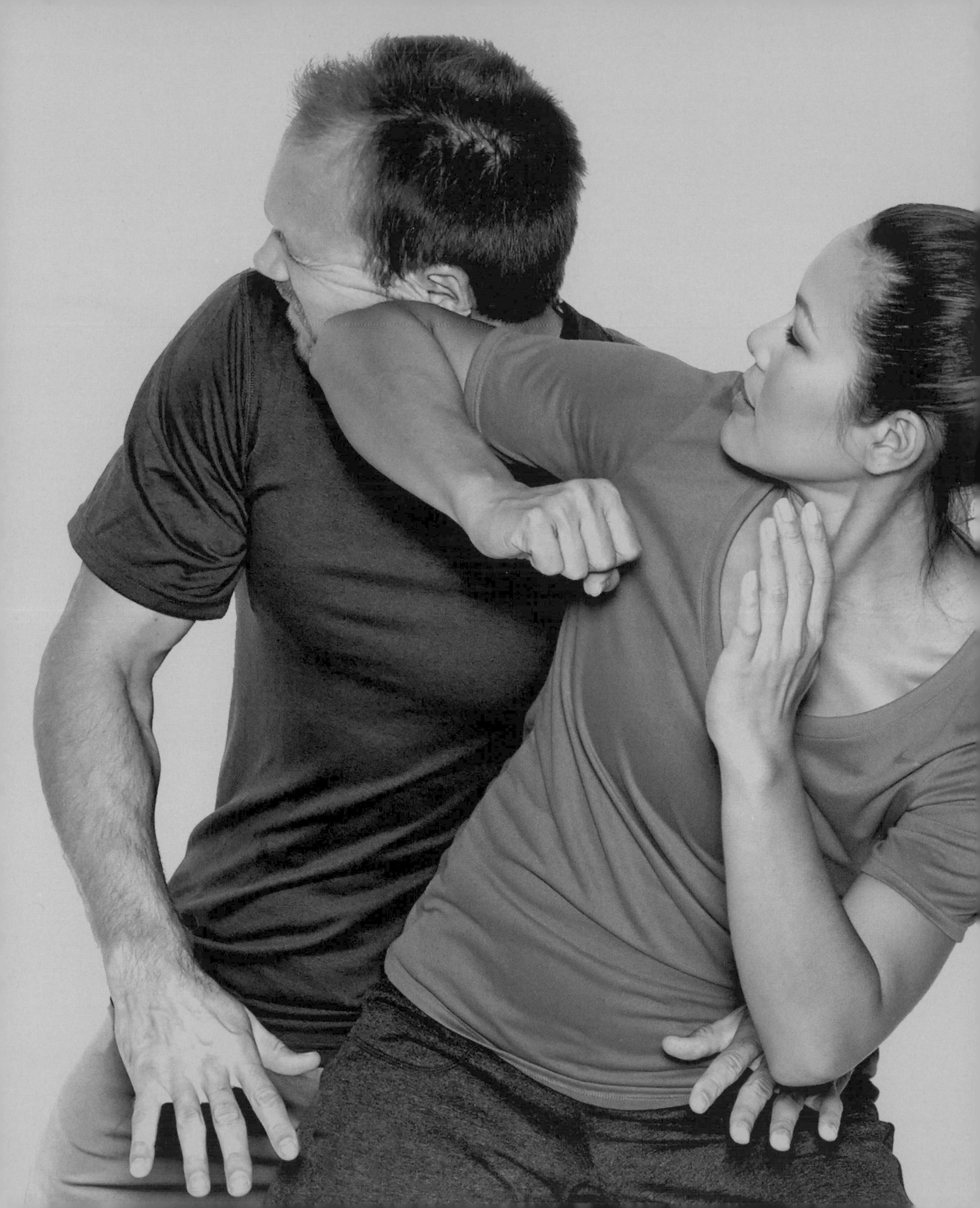

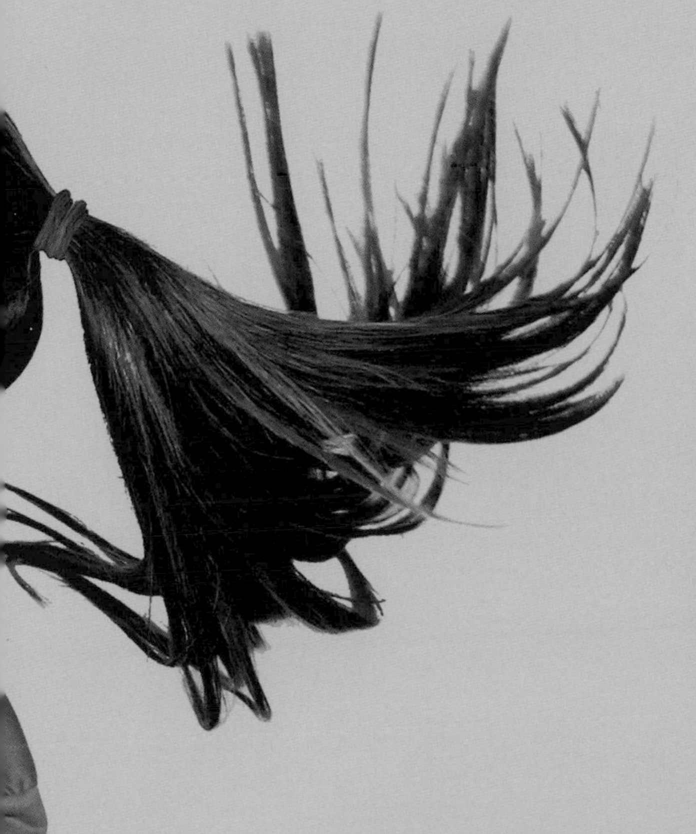

PART 3

KRAV MAGA TECHNIQUES

FUNDAMENTALS

The fundamentals of Krav Maga go beyond strikes, blocks, and kicks. Knowing how to position yourself, move, and even break your fall can increase your chances of success in a fight. This section takes you through these basic techniques.

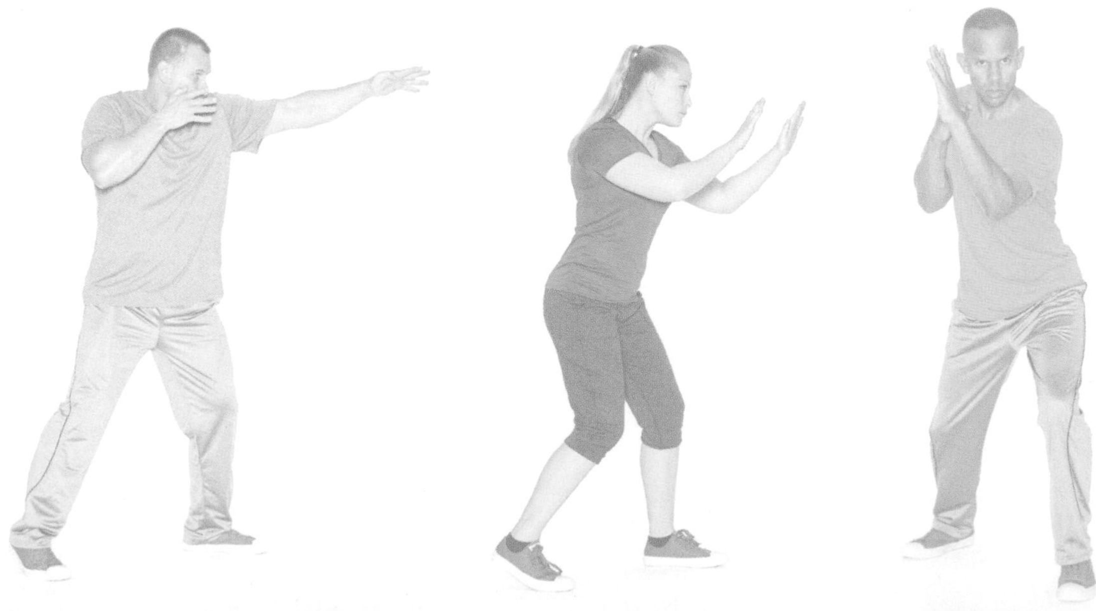

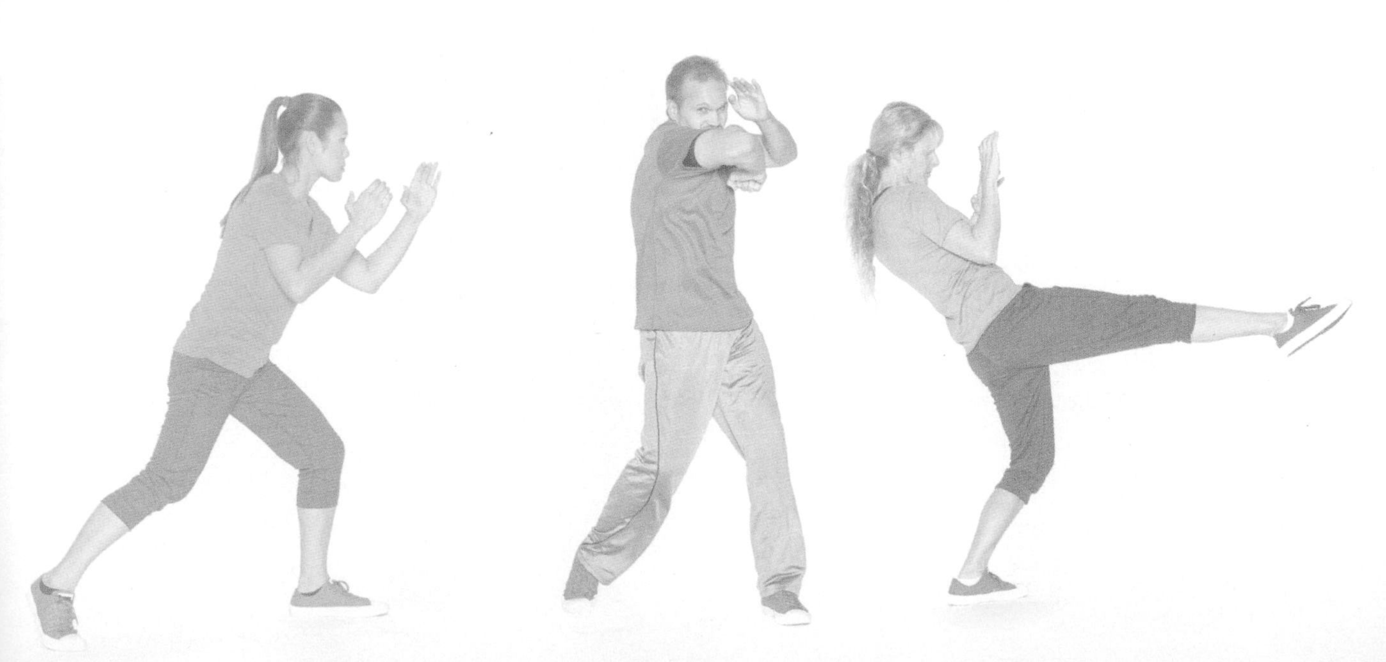

POSITIONS

Three basic positions teach you how to transition from a relaxed stance (which you're most likely to be in when confronted), to a defensive stance, to a position of control.

Passive Stance

It's likely you'll have to perform combatives and self-defense techniques when you're unprepared. This stance is used for training purposes to simulate being caught off guard when attacked.

POSITION NOTE

The width of your feet can affect the balance and power of your stance. Too wide, and you'll decrease the power of your legs; too narrow, and you'll more than likely barrel forward out of the stance with little control.

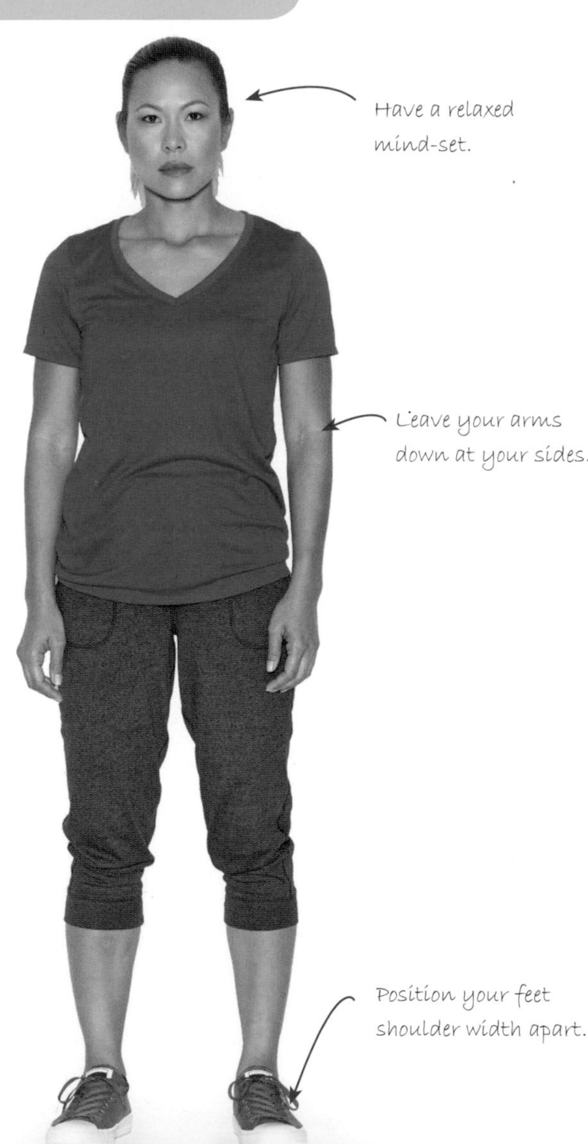

Have a relaxed mind-set.
Leave your arms down at your sides.
Position your feet shoulder width apart.

Fighting Stance

You move into this stance to prepare for confrontation. All of your defenses and counterattacks are performed from this position, with your hands up and palms toward your attacker to create a barrier.

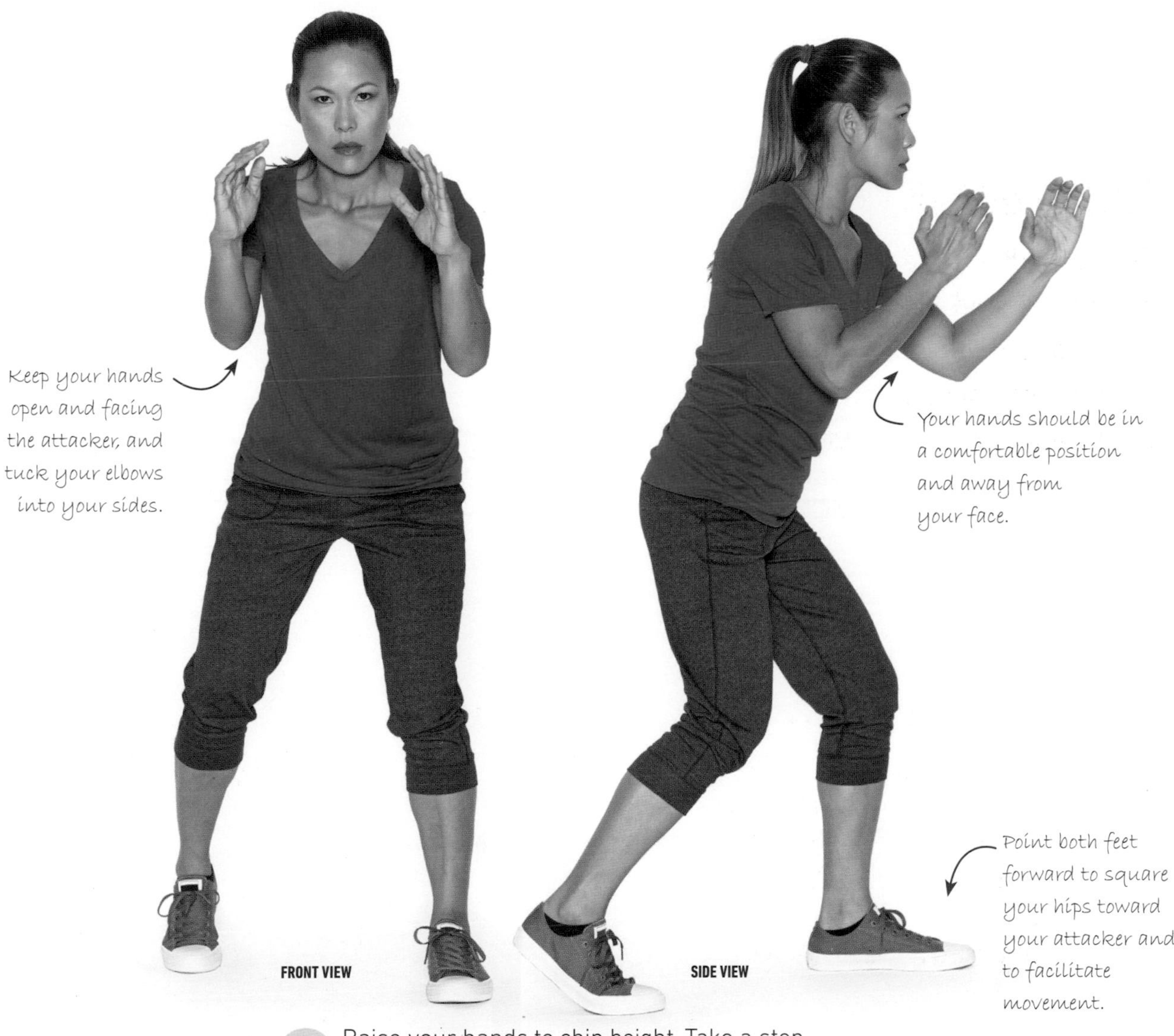

Keep your hands open and facing the attacker, and tuck your elbows into your sides.
Your hands should be in a comfortable position and away from your face.
Point both feet forward to square your hips toward your attacker and to facilitate movement.
FRONT VIEW
SIDE VIEW

1. Raise your hands to chin height. Take a step forward with your nondominant foot, shifting your weight forward on the balls of your feet and raising your opposite heel.

Control Position

You obtain the Control Position at a point when you have shifted the momentum of the fight in your favor. This position enables you a controlled moment to assess the condition of the attacker and your surroundings.

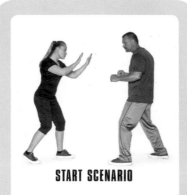

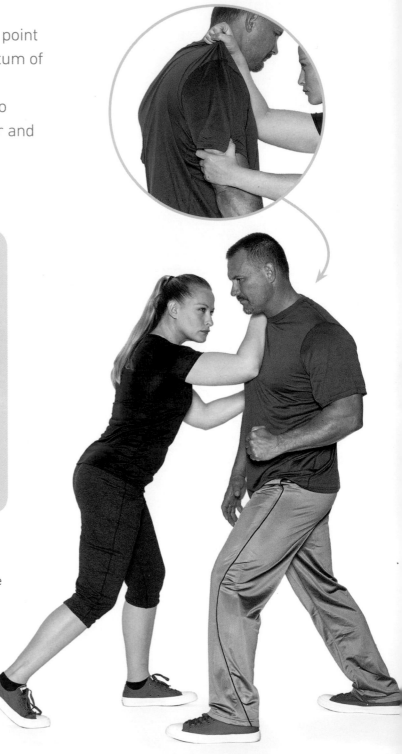

START SCENARIO

Stand in Fighting Stance facing your attacker.

1 From Fighting Stance, grab your attacker's arm with one hand above the elbow and the other hand on the shoulder on the same side.

WARNING

When grabbing your attacker, make sure you grip skin, not clothing. While grabbing clothing may allow you to gain a hold, the clothing could easily rip and allow your attacker to get the upper hand.

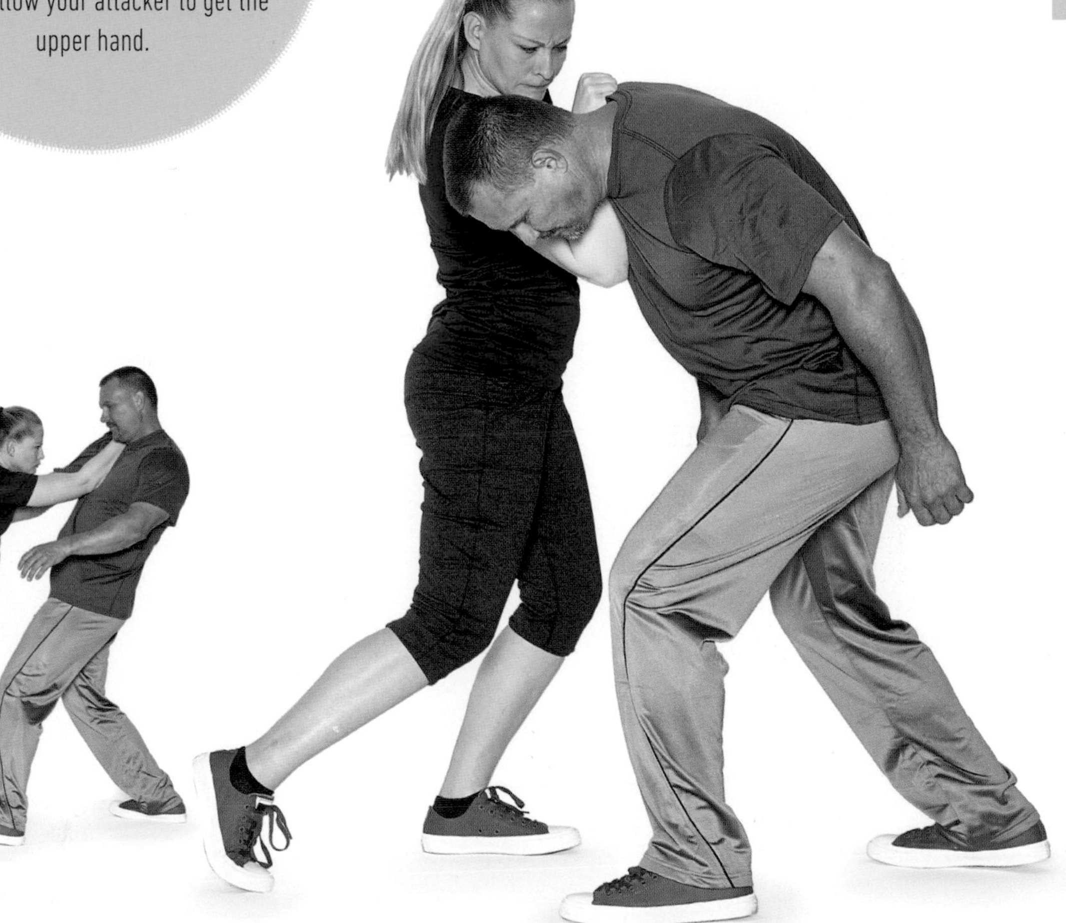

2 Disrupt your attacker's balance by sharply driving him or her forward and backward.

3 Based on the circumstances, decide whether you want to disengage or continue counterattacking.

MOVEMENTS FROM FIGHTING STANCE

Now that you know the basic stances, it's time to learn how to move out of them. These steps are generally your first line of defense in dodging attacks and positioning yourself to counterattack.

Forward Movement

The Forward Movement puts your body in range of your attacker to effectively deliver counterattacks.

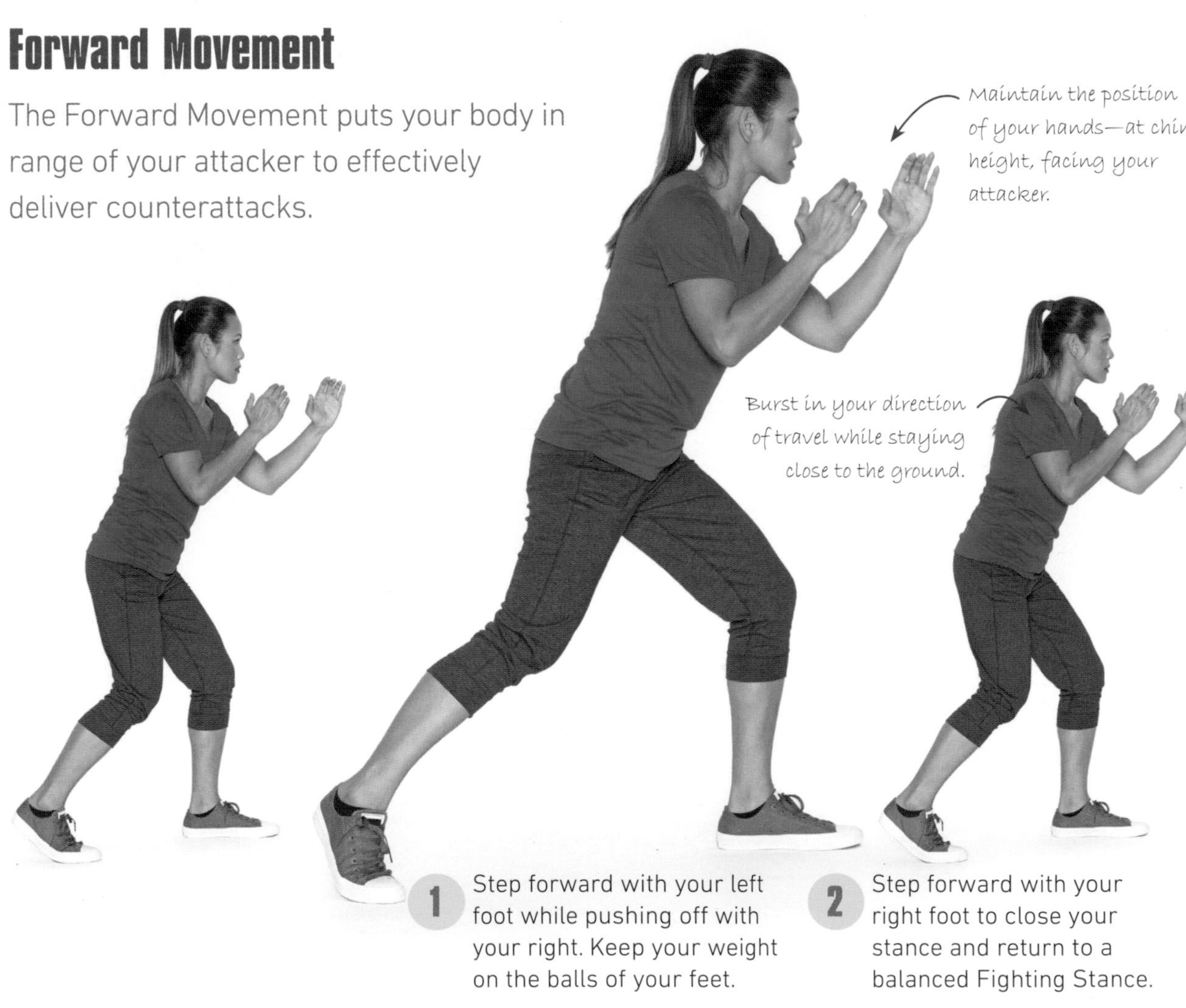
Maintain the position of your hands—at chin height, facing your attacker.
Burst in your direction of travel while staying close to the ground.

1. Step forward with your left foot while pushing off with your right. Keep your weight on the balls of your feet.
2. Step forward with your right foot to close your stance and return to a balanced Fighting Stance.

Backward Movement

For times when you're too close to deliver a defense, the Backward Movement provides you more space in which to work.

1 Step backward with your right foot while pushing off with your left foot. Burst in your direction of travel while staying close to the ground.

2 Step backward with your left foot to close your stance and return to a balanced Fighting Stance.

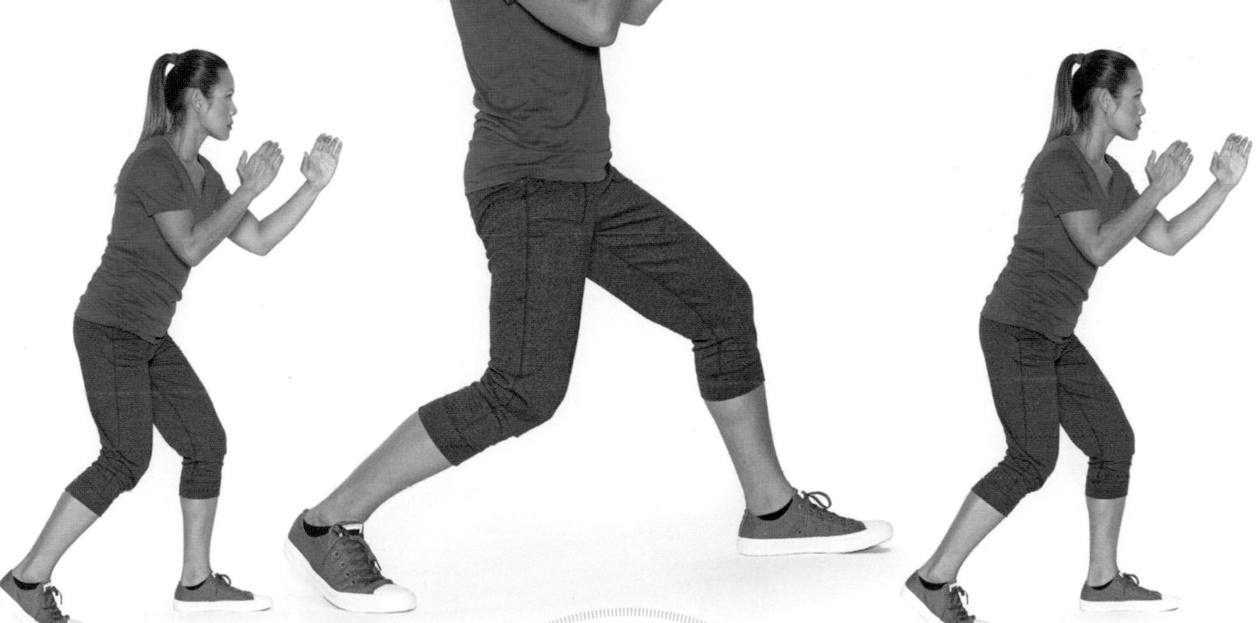

POSITION NOTE

When moving back, make sure you don't let your weight and balance shift back, as doing so will limit your ability to move off-angle. Remember, don't move back multiple steps without changing angles or moving laterally to get out of the line of attack.

Left Movement

The Left Movement puts your body into a position of advantage to effectively defend or counterattack by shifting to the left.

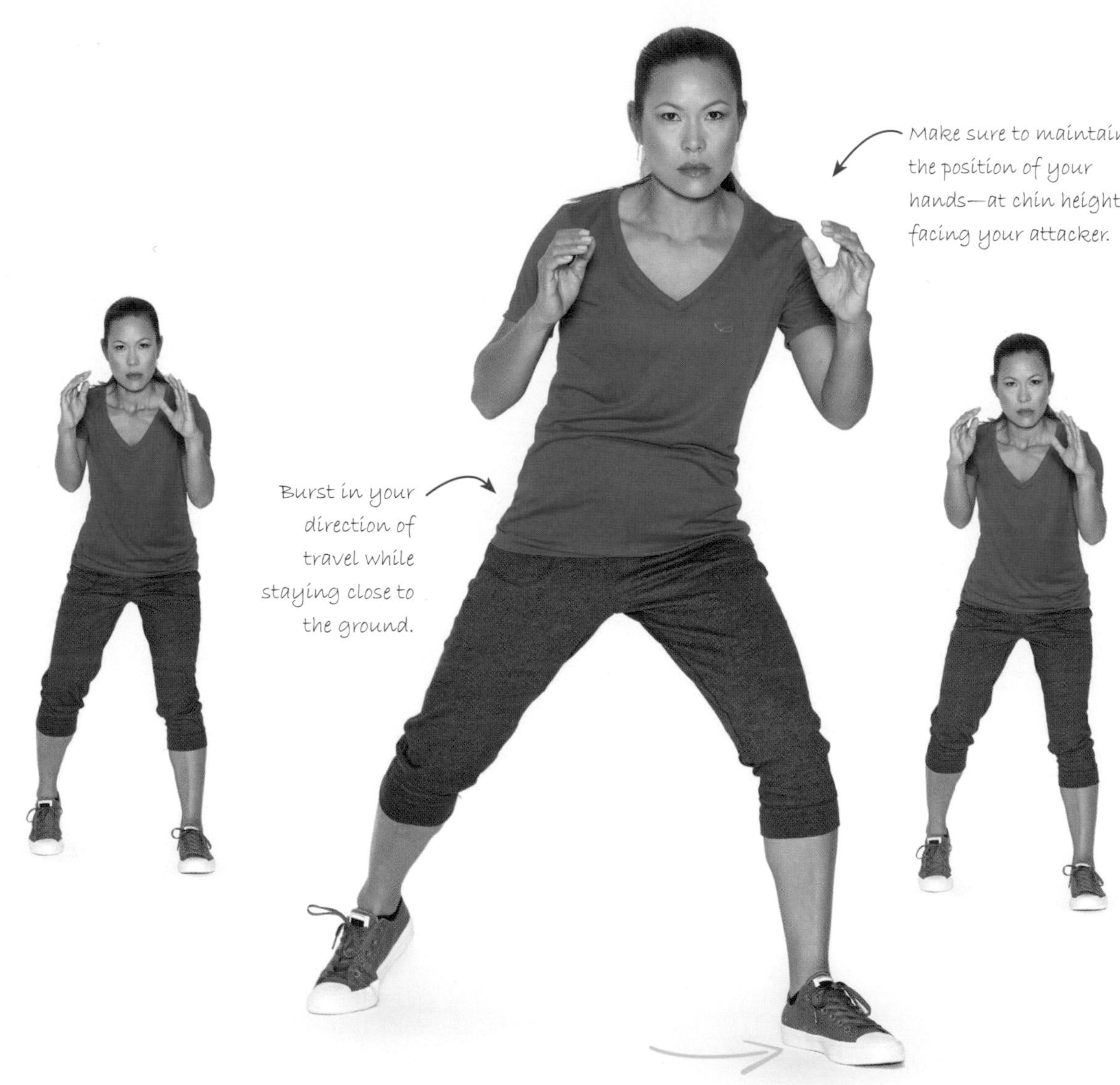
Make sure to maintain the position of your hands—at chin height, facing your attacker.
Burst in your direction of travel while staying close to the ground.

1. Step out with your left foot while pushing off with your right foot.
2. Step in with your right foot to close your stance and return to a balanced Fighting Stance.

Right Movement

The Right Movement puts your body into a position of advantage to effectively defend or counterattack by shifting to the right.

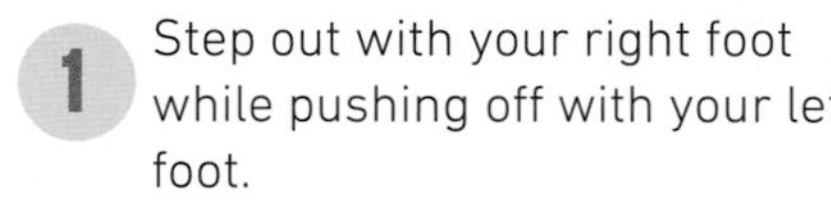

1 Step out with your right foot while pushing off with your left foot.

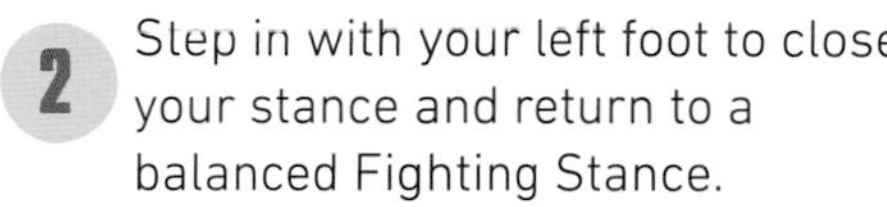

2 Step in with your left foot to close your stance and return to a balanced Fighting Stance.

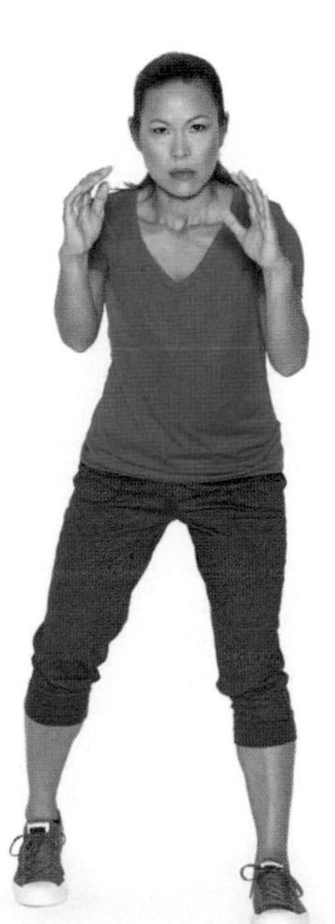

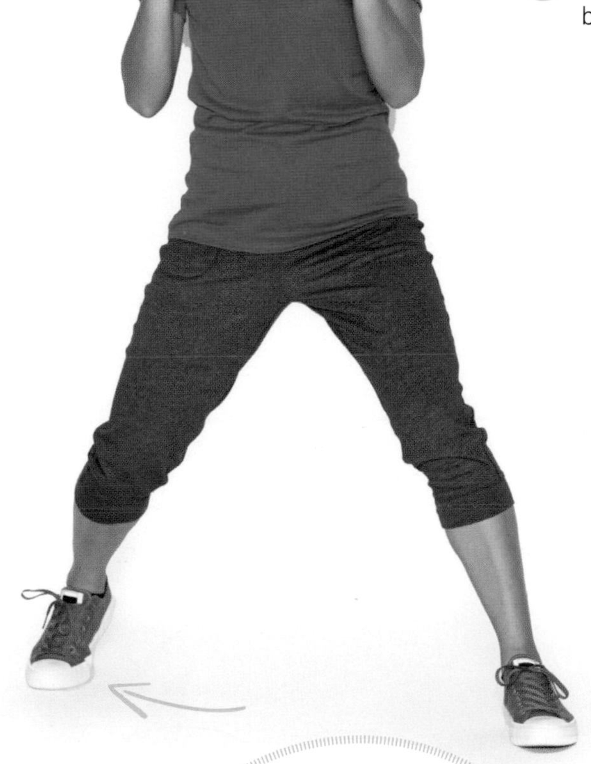

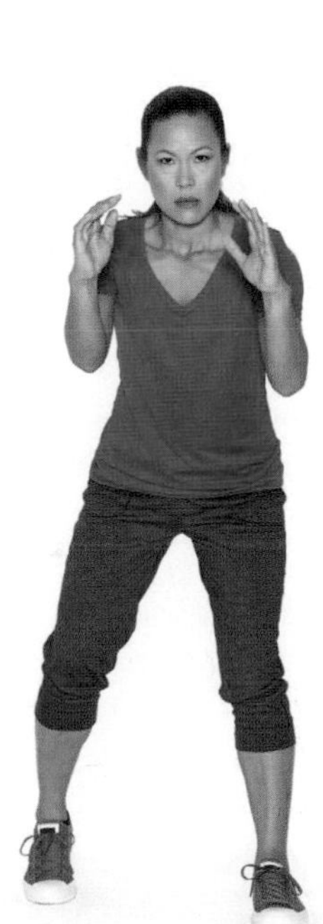

DEFENSE TIP

Maintain your weight in the balls of your feet. This keeps your body weight forward, allowing you to have more balance as you move. You can then quickly burst forward, backward, or side to side in order to respond to an oncoming attack.

MOVEMENTS FROM THE GROUND

Moving on your feet is easy enough. But what happens if you're on the ground—a position of disadvantage? You can bring yourself back into a position of advantage using basic techniques.

Back Position

If you find yourself on the ground on your back, your goal is to get up as quickly as possible. The Back Position enables you to fend off an attacker while striking and moving around on the ground.

POSITION NOTE

Keep the foot that remains on the ground (called your **base foot**) close to your rear. This will give you the power to push your hips up to kick or to push off of the ground.

1. While on your back, tuck your chin into your chest and round your shoulders off of the ground. Tuck one leg into your chest (known as *chambering*) and pull back your toes to expose your heel.

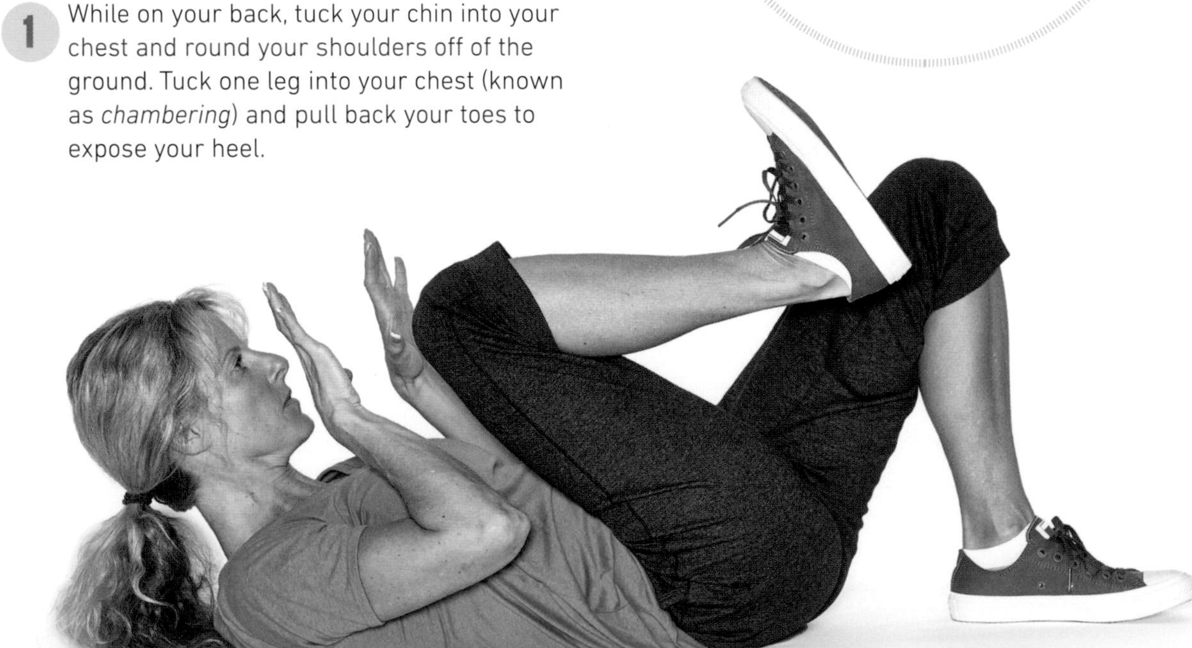

Side Position

After your attacker has moved away and you feel comfortable preparing to get up off the ground, you will transition to the Side Position.

DEFENSE TIP

The Side Position is the first step to getting off the ground. However, if your attacker closes the distance between you too quickly for you to get up, simply lie back down into the Back Position. Be ready to deliver strikes with the goal of creating distance and getting off the ground.

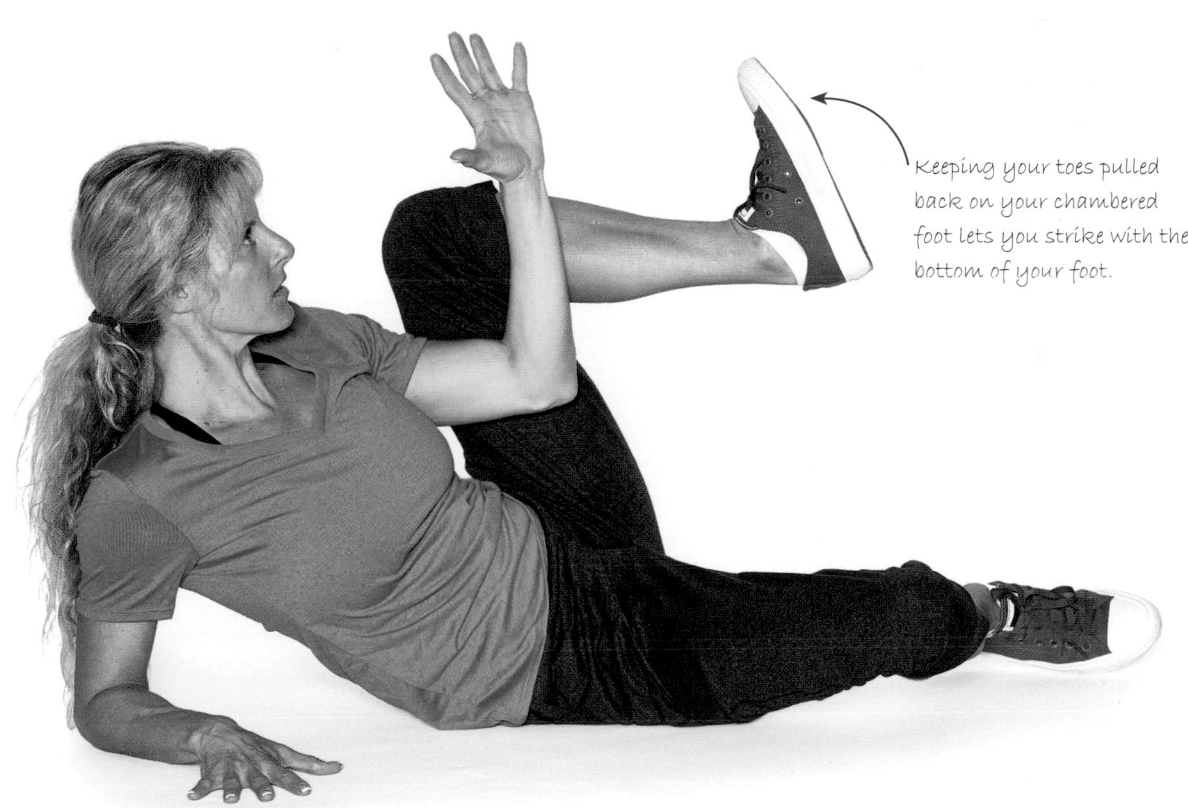

Keeping your toes pulled back on your chambered foot lets you strike with the bottom of your foot.

1 From your back, roll onto one side. Place your weight on your forearm, hand, hip, and leg while keeping your top leg chambered.

2 Hold your upper arm inside your chambered leg, bringing your hand in front of your face to protect yourself.

Getting Up from the Ground

Your goal is to get up as quickly and safely as possible. Once your attacker is at a safe distance, this technique allows you to stand up without exposing your vital areas—like your head.

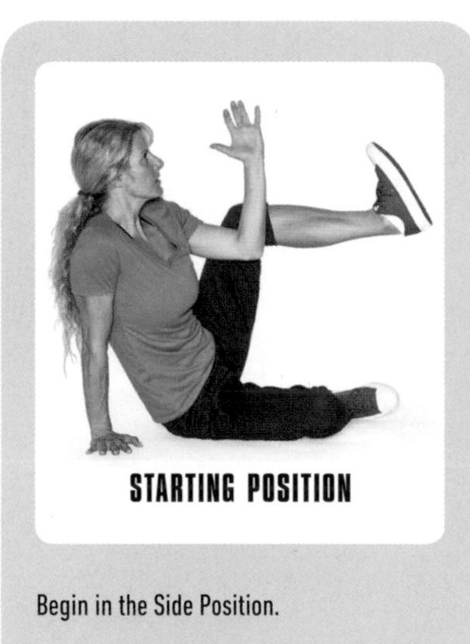

Begin in the Side Position.

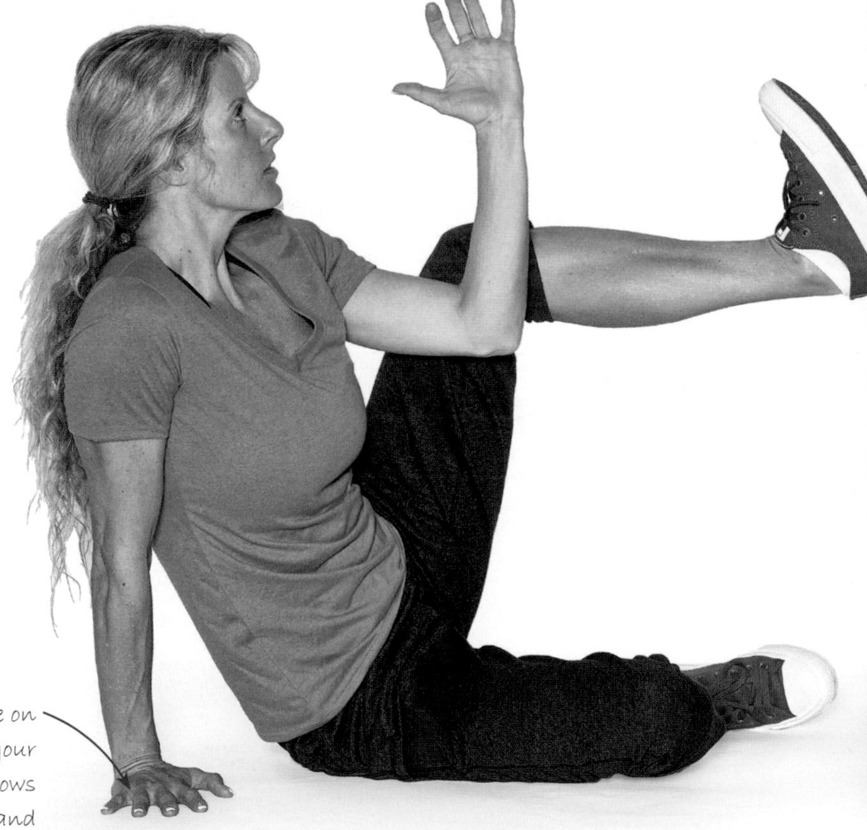

When you're on your side on the ground, shifting your weight to your hand allows you to turn faster and begins your upward movement.

1. From the Side Position, straighten your bottom arm and put your weight on the palm of your hand.

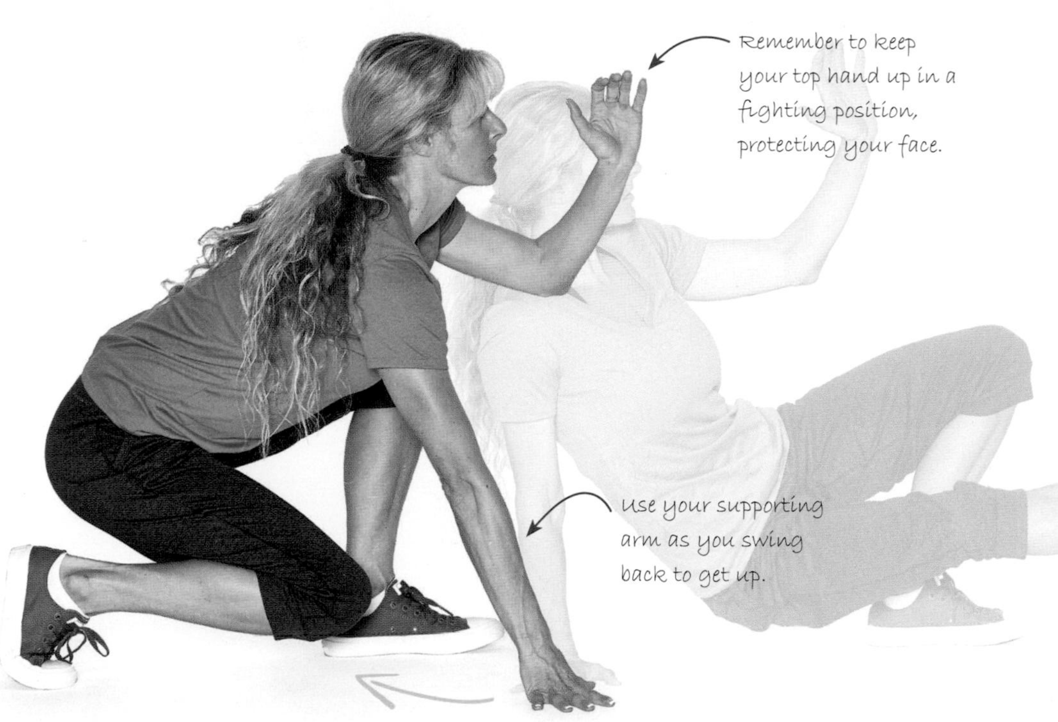

Remember to keep your top hand up in a fighting position, protecting your face.
Use your supporting arm as you swing back to get up.

2 Drop your top (chambered) leg to the floor, planting the sole of the foot close to your rear. Lift your hips from the ground by pressing off of your hand and base foot. Quickly recoil your leg and use the momentum to swing it back past your planted hand.

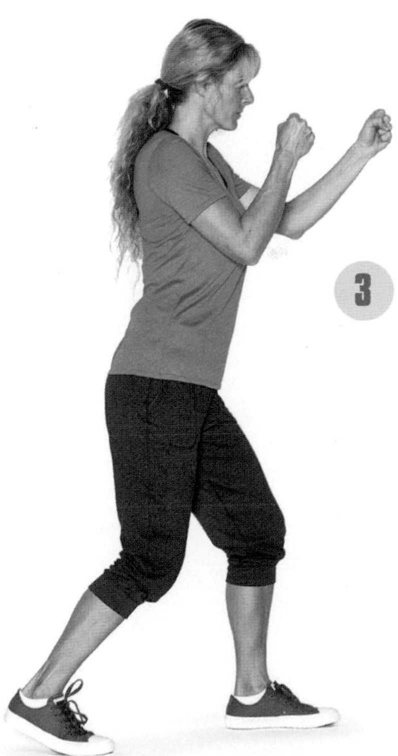

3 Push off with your other foot to drive your body backward and up to a standing position.

IF IT FAILS

The goal of getting up is to increase your mobility, create distance from your attacker, and escape. If you trip or fall, simply return to the Back Position. This will allow you to reassess the situation more safely.

FALL BREAKS

Fall breaks are an essential tool for minimizing injury when you're pushed, tripped, or thrown to the ground. They're even effective in daily life if you slip on a wet surface, for example.

Back Fall Break

This version of a fall break allows you to fall onto your back in a safe manner while also preparing you to attack as soon as you're there.

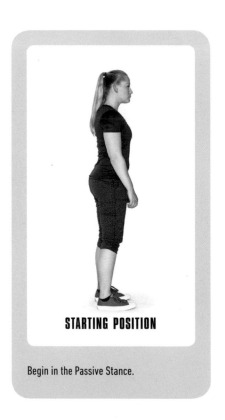

STARTING POSITION

Begin in the Passive Stance.

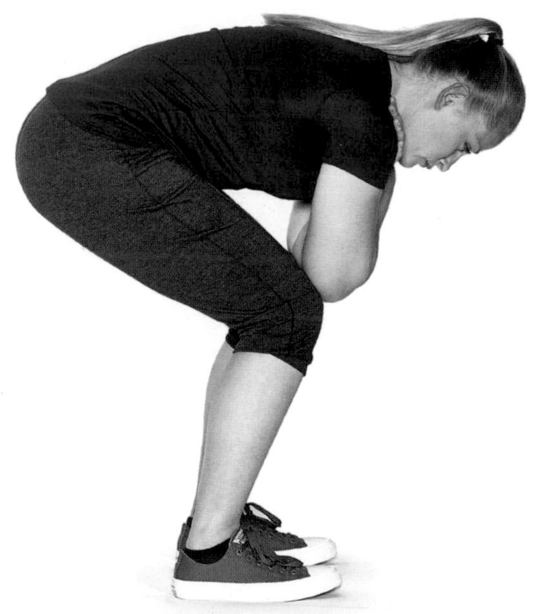

1 Squat low, bringing your chin and your arms into your chest for protection. (This is for training purposes only; you wouldn't do this in a real-world situation.)

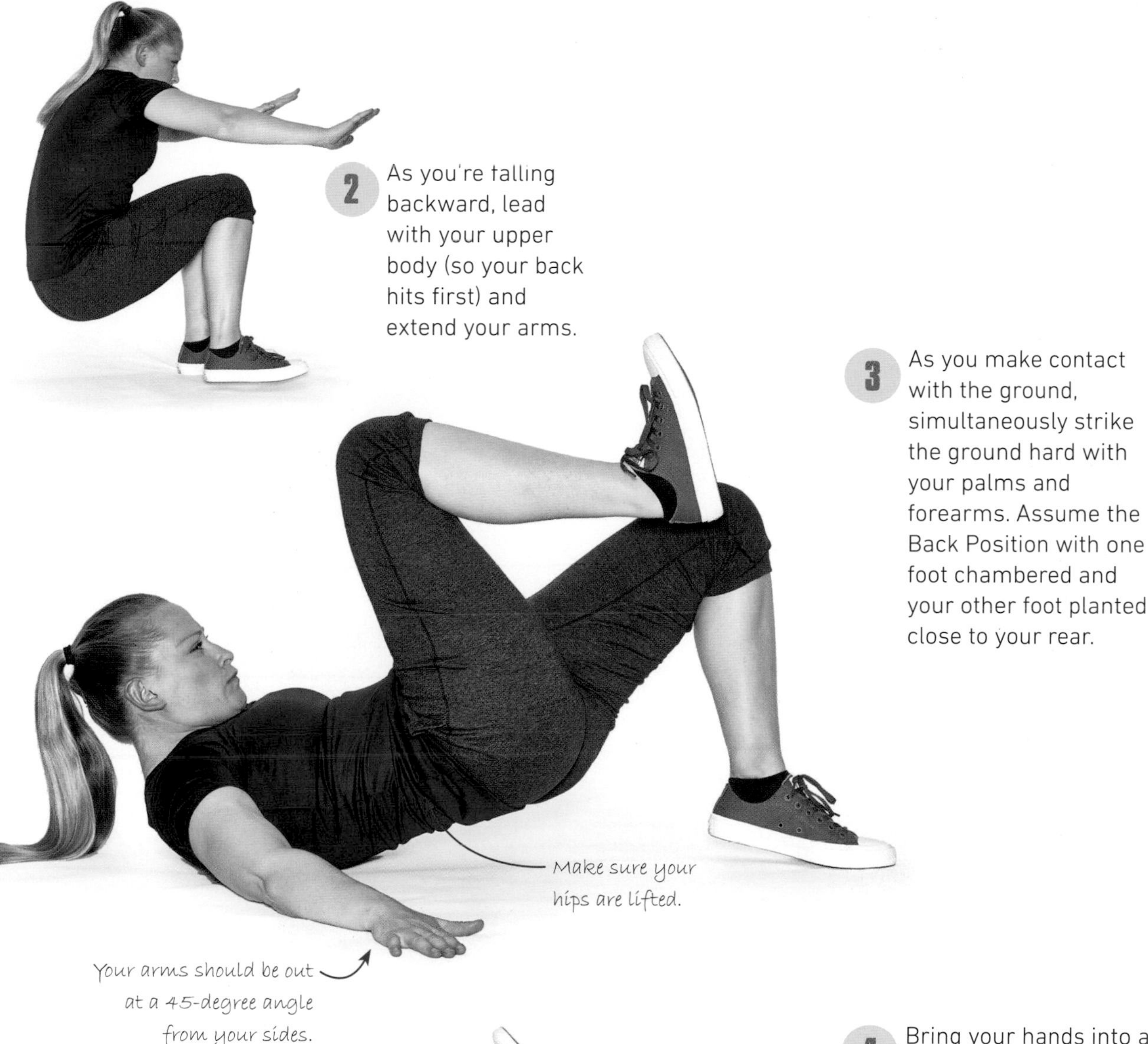

Make sure your hips are lifted.
Your arms should be out at a 45-degree angle from your sides.

2 As you're falling backward, lead with your upper body (so your back hits first) and extend your arms.

3 As you make contact with the ground, simultaneously strike the ground hard with your palms and forearms. Assume the Back Position with one foot chambered and your other foot planted close to your rear.

4 Bring your hands into a fighting position and prepare to strike.

Side Fall Break

This version of a fall break allows you to fall onto your side in a safe manner while also preparing you to attack as soon as you're there.

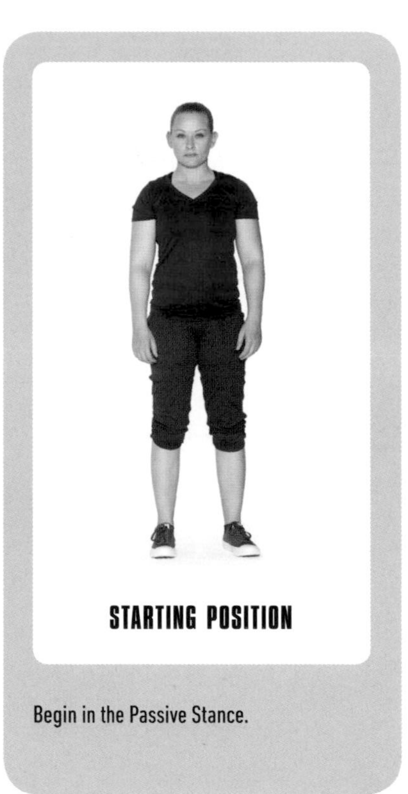

STARTING POSITION

Begin in the Passive Stance.

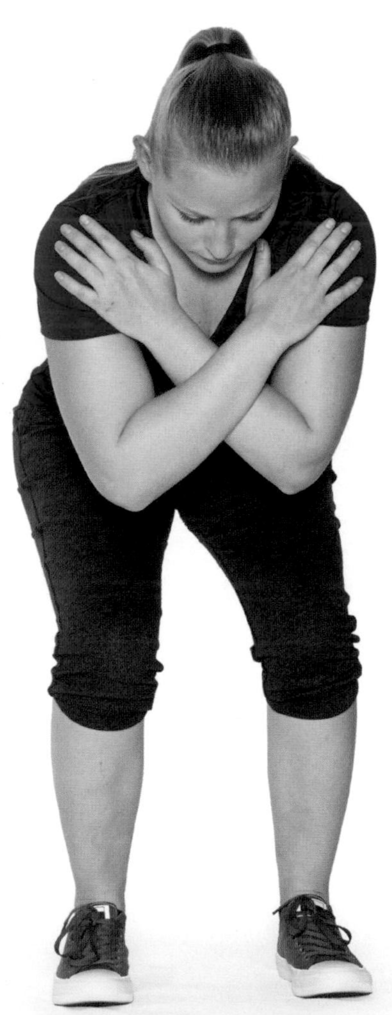

1 Squat low, bringing your chin and your arms into your chest for protection.

2 As you're falling to the side, lead with your upper body. Shoot the leg that will contact the ground forward and to the side.

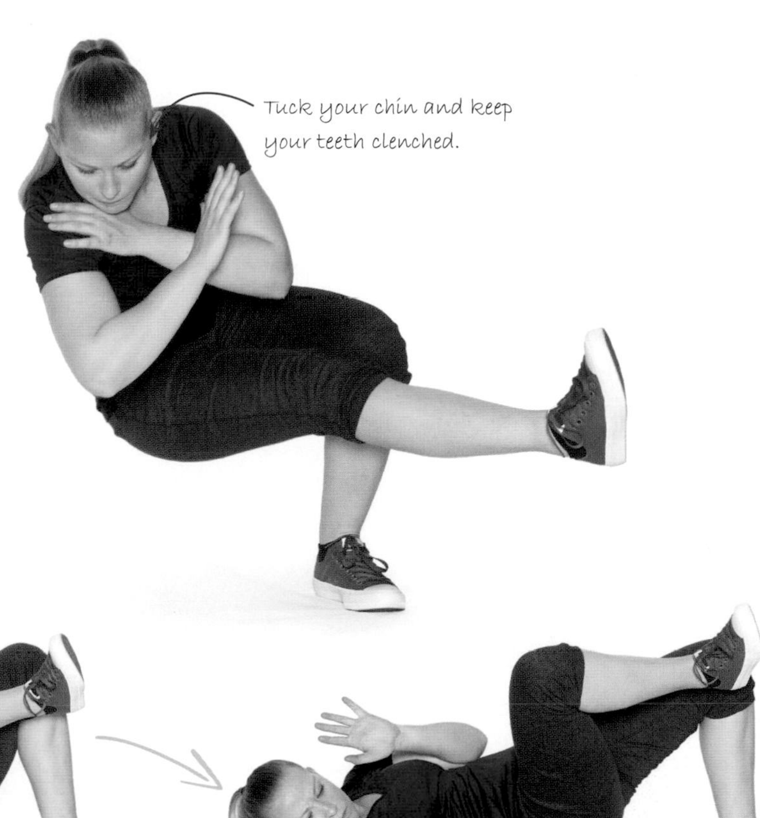

Tuck your chin and keep your teeth clenched.

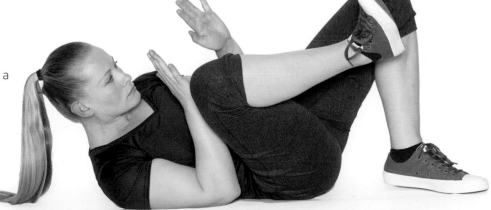

Your arm should be at a 45-degree angle from the side of your body.

3 As you make contact with the ground, simultaneously strike the ground hard with your palm and forearm. Assume the Back Position with one foot chambered and your other foot close to your rear.

4 Bring your hands into a fighting position and prepare to strike.

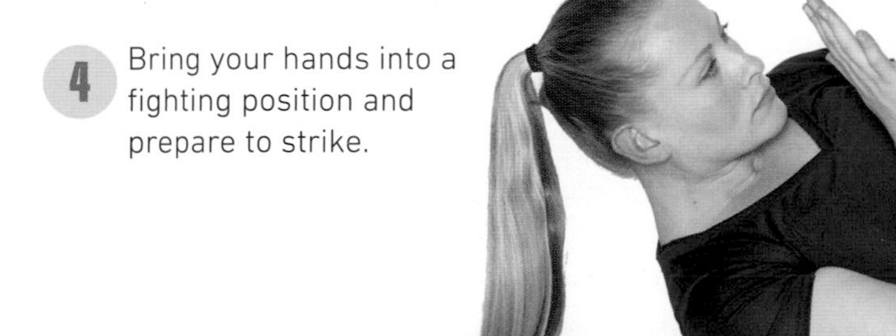

Sprawl

Out of desperation, your attacker may try to grab your legs from the front, lift you up, and slam you to the ground. You can use Sprawl to help you escape your attacker's hold on your lower body.

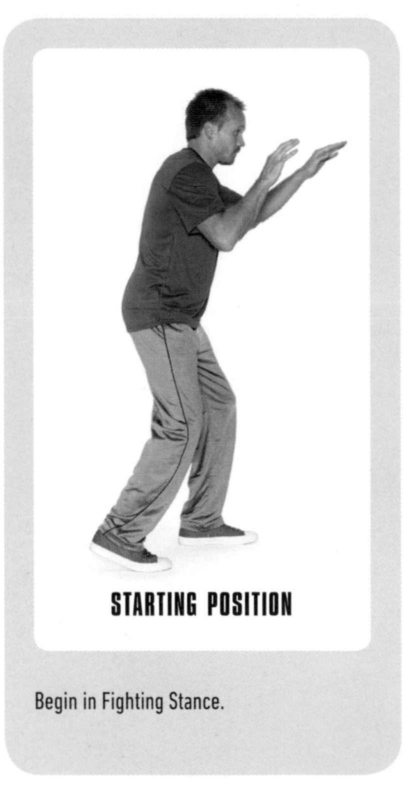

STARTING POSITION

Begin in Fighting Stance.

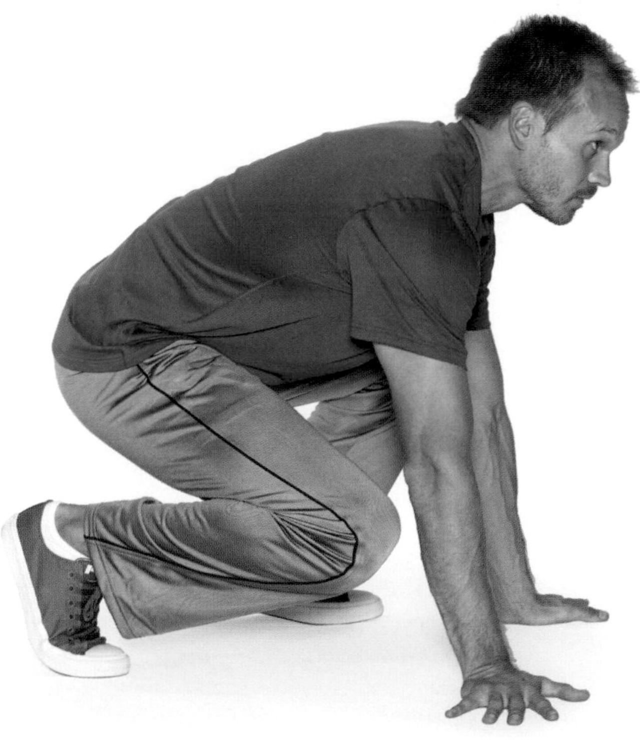

1 Shoot your hands down either side of your attacker and simultaneously shoot your hips back.

2 Throw your legs straight back. As your hands make contact with the ground, drop your hips and look to the sky.

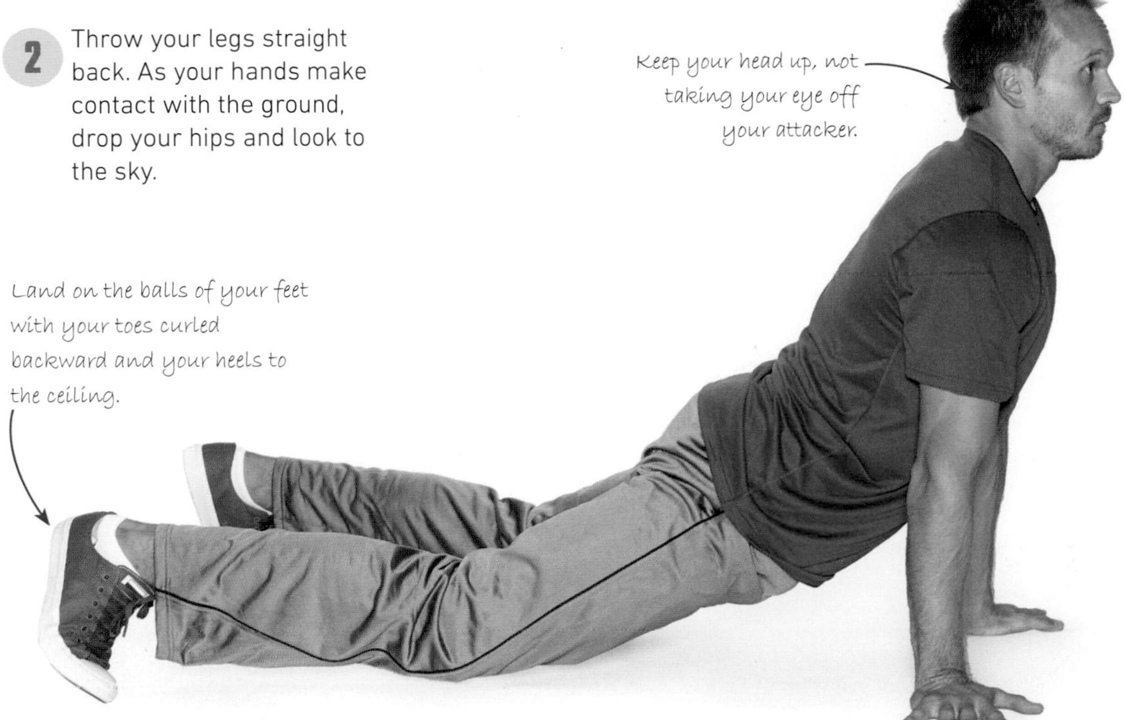

Keep your head up, not taking your eye off your attacker.
Land on the balls of your feet with your toes curled backward and your heels to the ceiling.

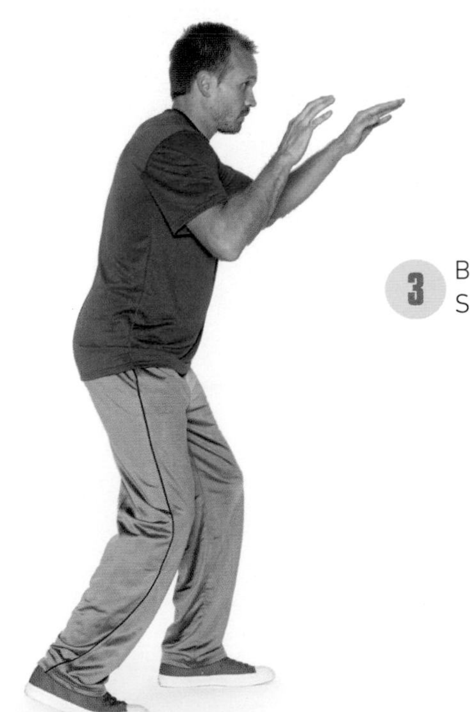

3 Burst upward into Fighting Stance.

DEFENSE TIP

Explosively shoot your legs back and send your hips to the ground simultaneously to prevent your attacker from getting a solid hold on you.

BASIC DEFENSES AND BLOCKING

Strikes toward your face or head are common in an attack. An attacker can strike in two ways—straight at you (inside) or from another angle (outside). You can defend against both in multiple ways.

Inside Defense

You can use the Inside Defense to block Straight Punches to the center of your body. While Outside Defenses stop an attack, Inside Defense redirects the attack offline. Defend with your hand and wrist to block your head and throat, and defend your midsection using your forearm.

DEFENSE TIP

Even if you're only able to move your head offline, you still lessen the impact.

STARTING POSITION

Begin in Fighting Stance.

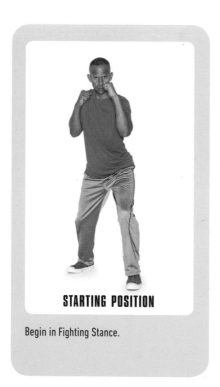

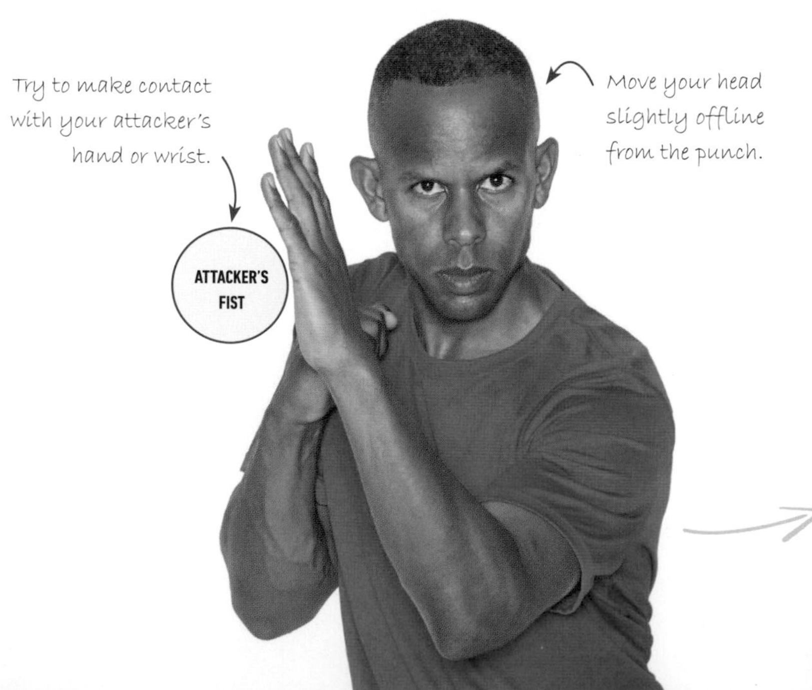

Try to make contact with your attacker's hand or wrist.
ATTACKER'S FIST
Move your head slightly offline from the punch.

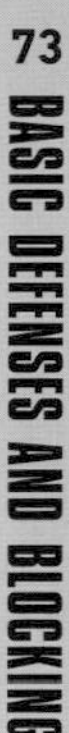

1 When your attacker throws the punch, move your hand forward and inward until it connects with the punch. Upon contact, hold your weight forward and keep tension in your arm.

2 Slightly move your head offline in the opposite direction of where you're defending. Recoil your arm and return to Fighting Stance.

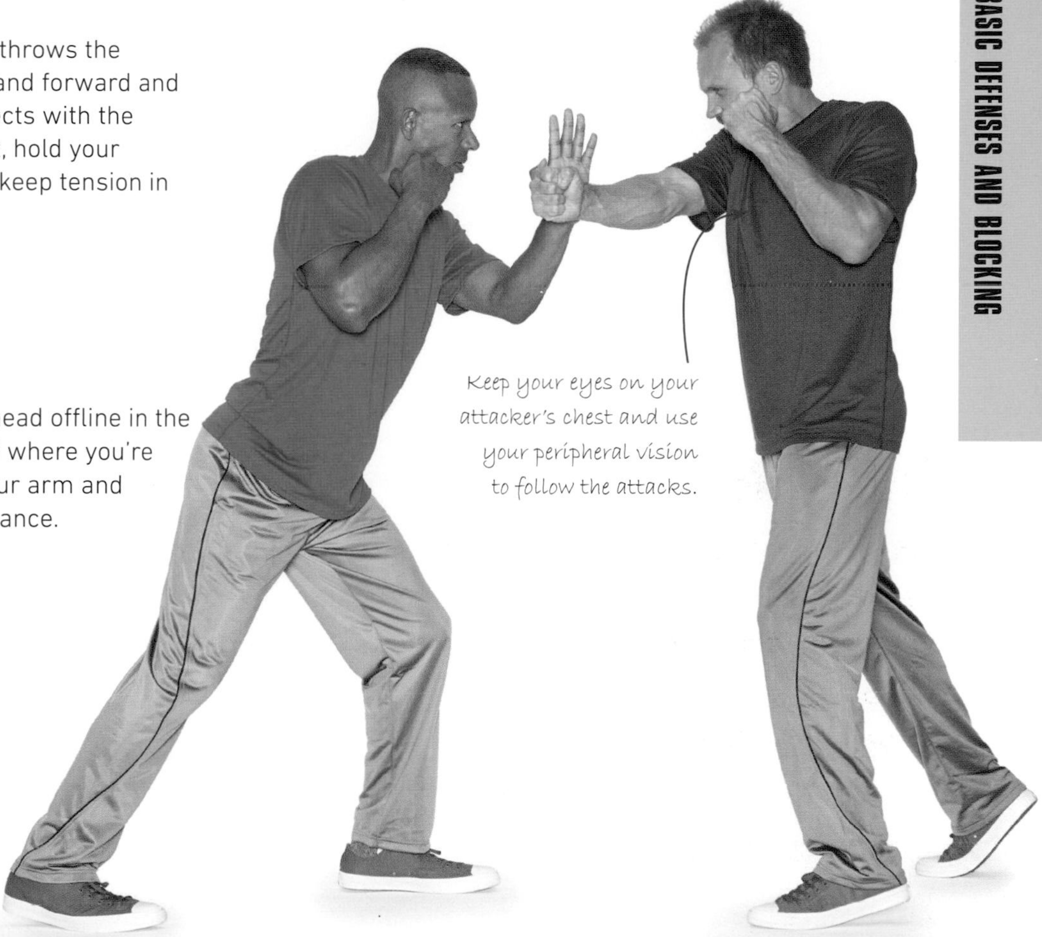

Keep your eyes on your attacker's chest and use your peripheral vision to follow the attacks.

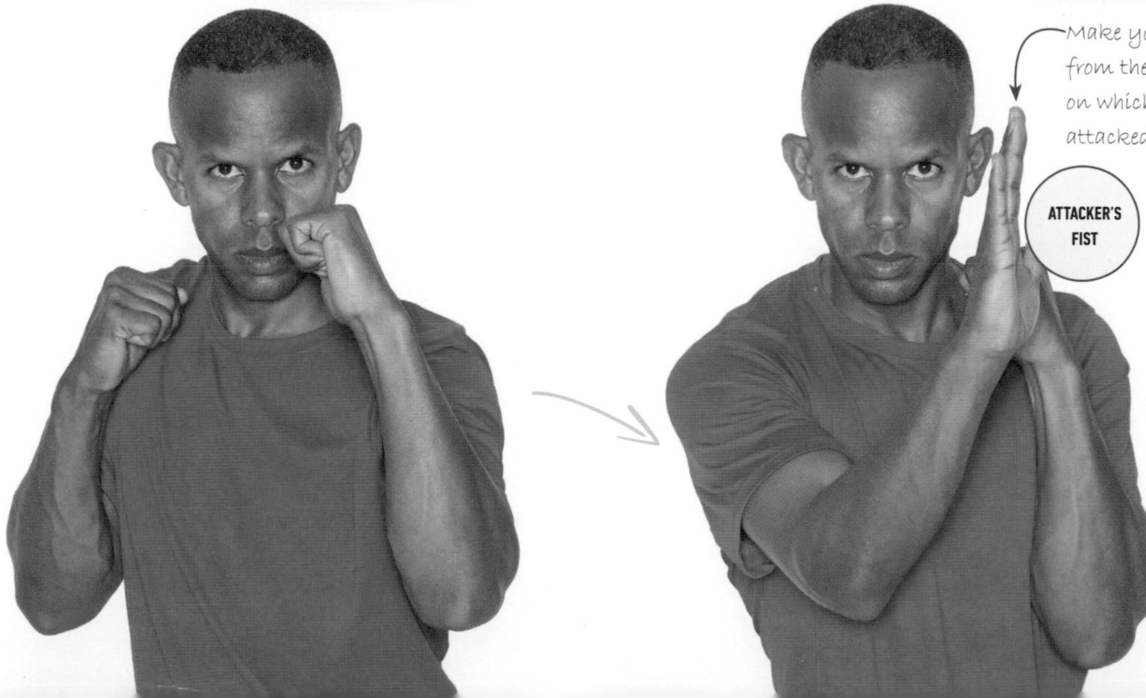

Make your defense from the same side on which you're attacked.

ATTACKER'S FIST

Outside Defenses

Outside Defenses satisfy your body's instinct to cover your head when attacked. While teachers often instruct the use of both hands to learn the positions, using one hand is usually more realistic. Although this book covers seven learning positions, you can use an Outside Defense at any angle by following the same principles.

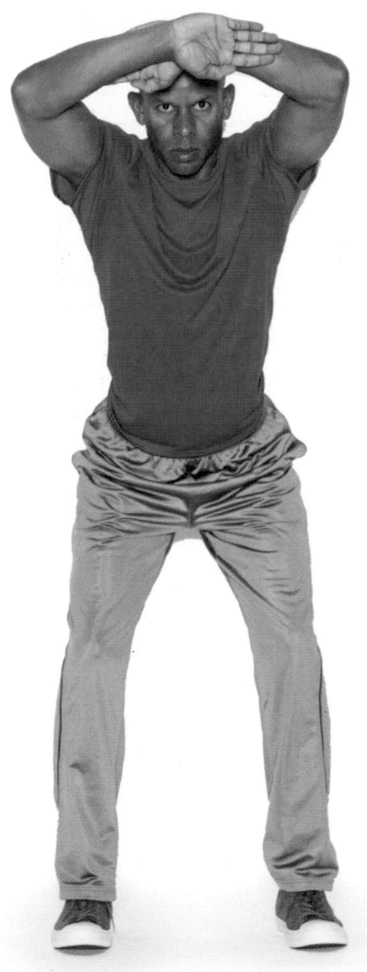

OUTSIDE DEFENSE 1

Use this to defend against an attack coming down at a 90-degree angle.

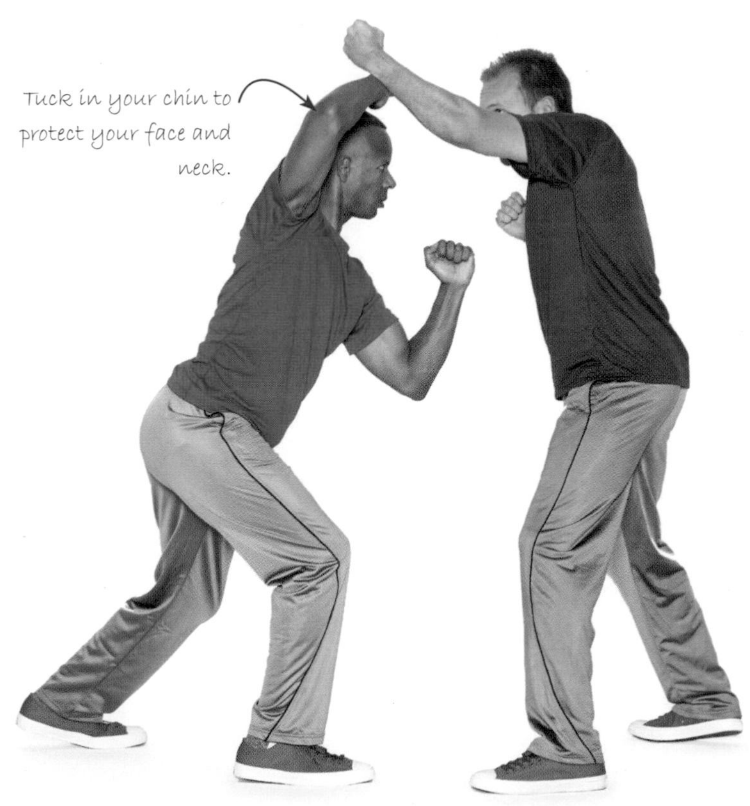

Tuck in your chin to protect your face and neck.

1 Bring both hands slightly in front of and above your head. Stack them so one is resting on the forearm of the arm in front, while the other is resting on the forearm of the arm in back.

2 Block with the wrist on the same side of the attack. Simultaneously move forward into the attack by slightly bending at your waist and bringing your head forward. Quickly recoil and return to Fighting Stance.

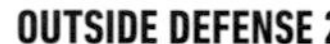

OUTSIDE DEFENSE 2

Use this to defend against an attack coming from a 45-degree angle.

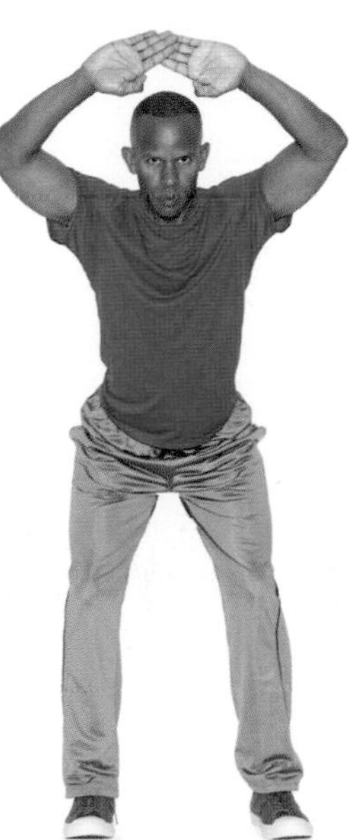

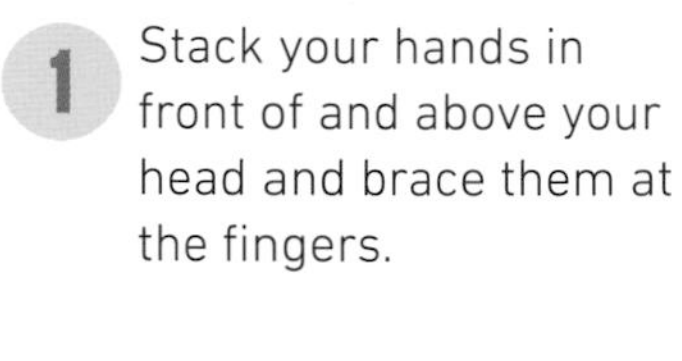

1. Stack your hands in front of and above your head and brace them at the fingers.

2. Block with the wrist on the same side of the attack. Simultaneously move forward into the attack by slightly bending at your waist and bringing your head forward. Quickly recoil and return to Fighting Stance.

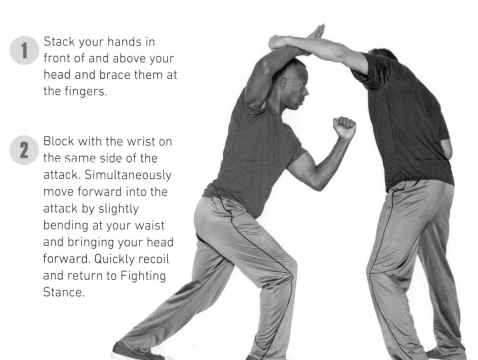

OUTSIDE DEFENSE 3

Use this to defend against an attack looping in from the outside.

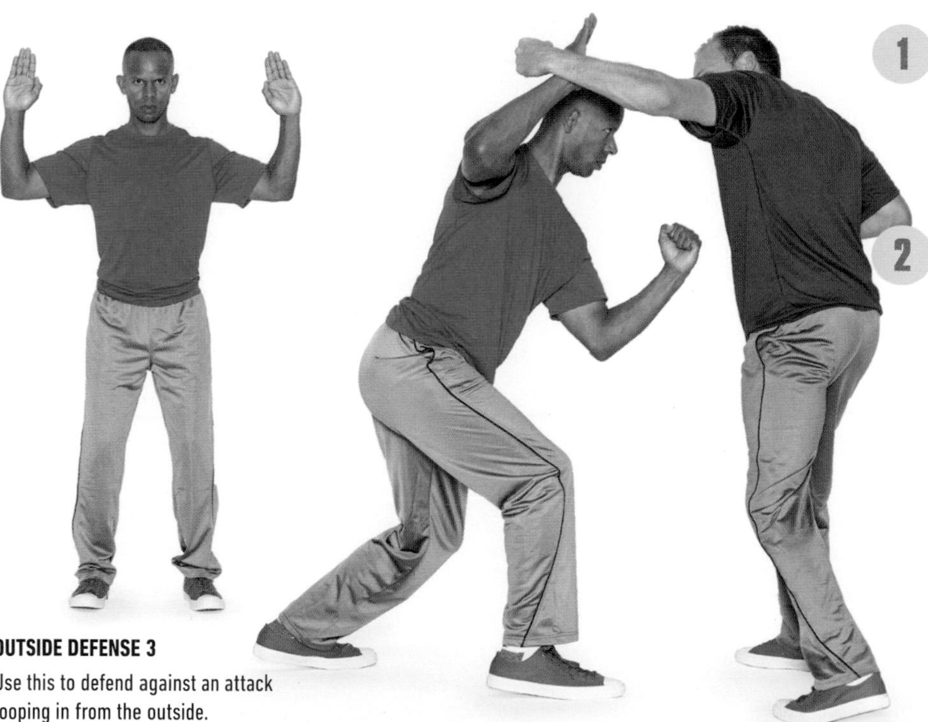

1. Bring your hands to face level with your arms bent at 90-degree angles.

2. Block with the wrist on the same side of the attack. Simultaneously move forward into the attack by slightly bending at your waist and bringing your head forward. Quickly recoil and return to Fighting Stance.

1 Position your hands slightly below face level with your arms bent at 45-degree angles.

2 Block with the wrist on the same side of the attack. Simultaneously move forward into the attack by slightly bending at your waist and bringing your head forward. Quickly recoil and return to Fighting Stance.

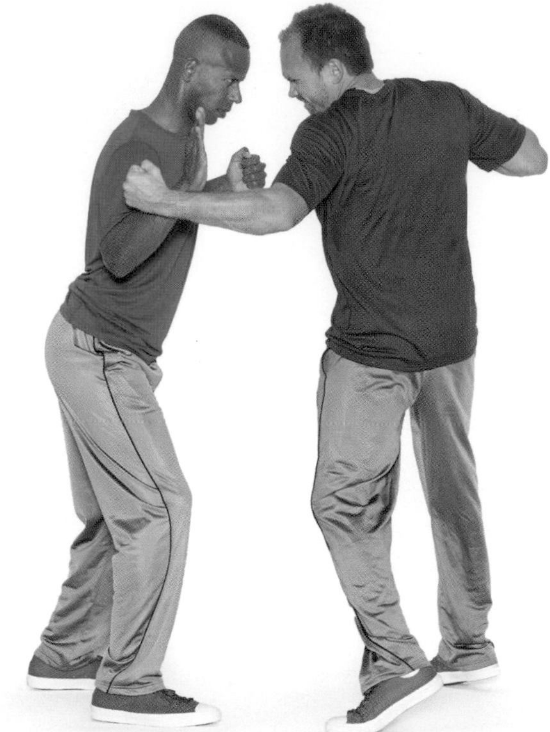

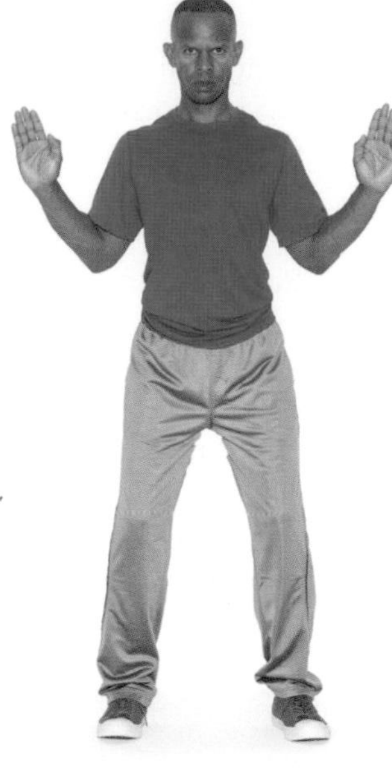

OUTSIDE DEFENSE 4

Use this to help you defend against a side attack to your ribs.

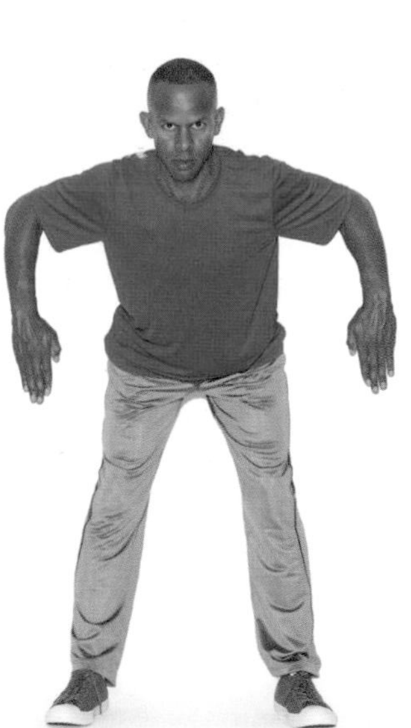

OUTSIDE DEFENSE 5

Use this to defend against a side attack to your ribs.

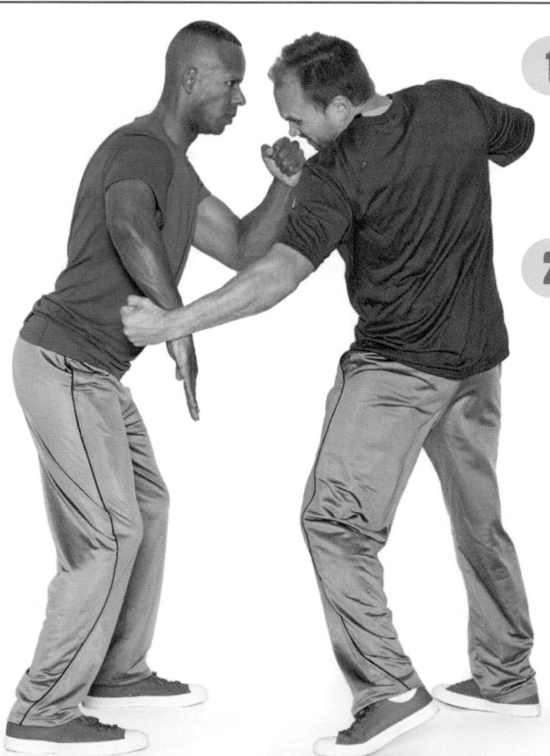

1 Bend over slightly and bring your arms to 90-degree angles, palms facing out.

2 Block with the wrist on the same side of the attack. Simultaneously move forward into the attack by slightly bending at your waist and bringing your head forward. Quickly recoil and return to Fighting Stance.

1 Bend at the waist and bring your arms to 45-degree angles, palms facing in.

2 Block with the wrist on the same side of the attack. Simultaneously move forward into the attack by slightly bending at your waist and bringing your head forward. Quickly recoil and return to Fighting Stance.

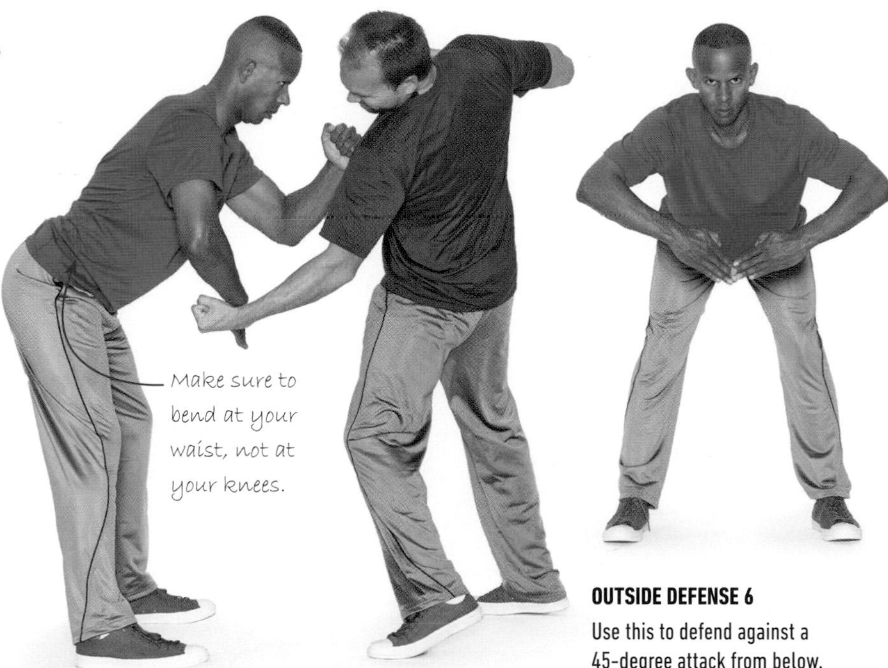

Make sure to bend at your waist, not at your knees.

OUTSIDE DEFENSE 6

Use this to defend against a 45-degree attack from below.

---

1 Bend at the waist and fold your arms together so they're parallel to the ground.

2 Block with the wrist on the same side of the attack. Simultaneously move forward into the attack by slightly bending at your waist and bringing your head forward. Quickly recoil and return to Fighting Stance.

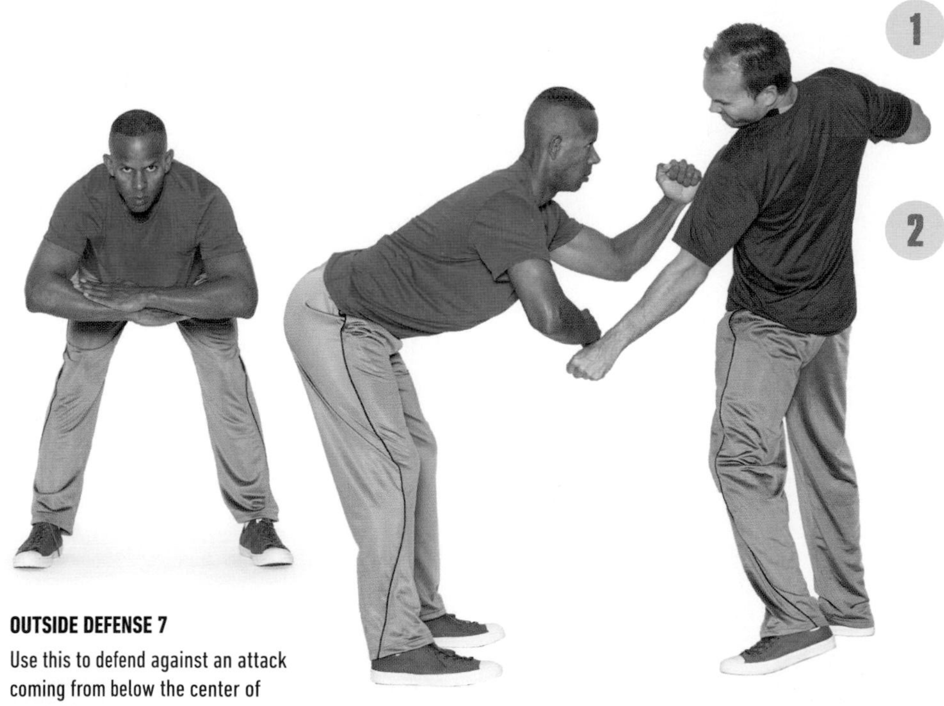

OUTSIDE DEFENSE 7

Use this to defend against an attack coming from below the center of your body.

Covering Defense

If you're assaulted from multiple directions or an attacker rapidly sends hook punches to the side of your head, the Covering Defense will protect your head from injury. By bursting toward the attack with your head covered, you avoid the full force of the strikes.

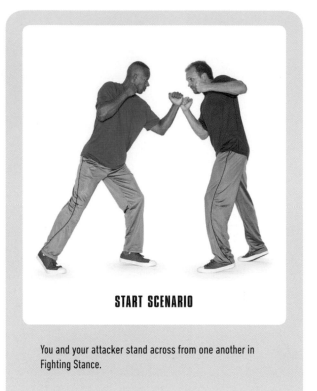

START SCENARIO

You and your attacker stand across from one another in Fighting Stance.

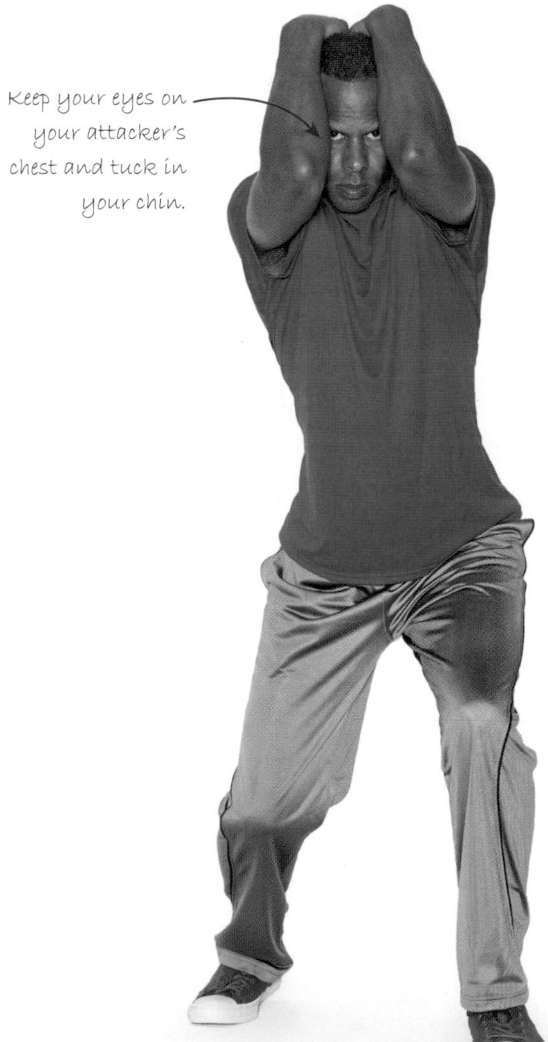

Keep your eyes on your attacker's chest and tuck in your chin.

1. As your attacker throws a punch at you, move your hands to the back of your head and tighten your forearms and biceps to the sides of your head.

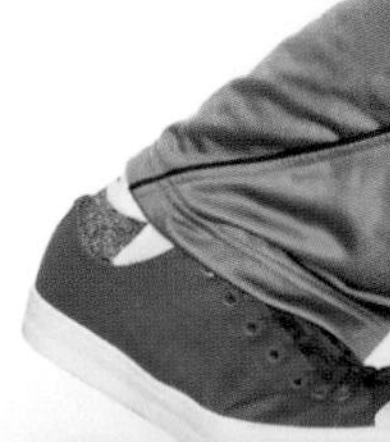

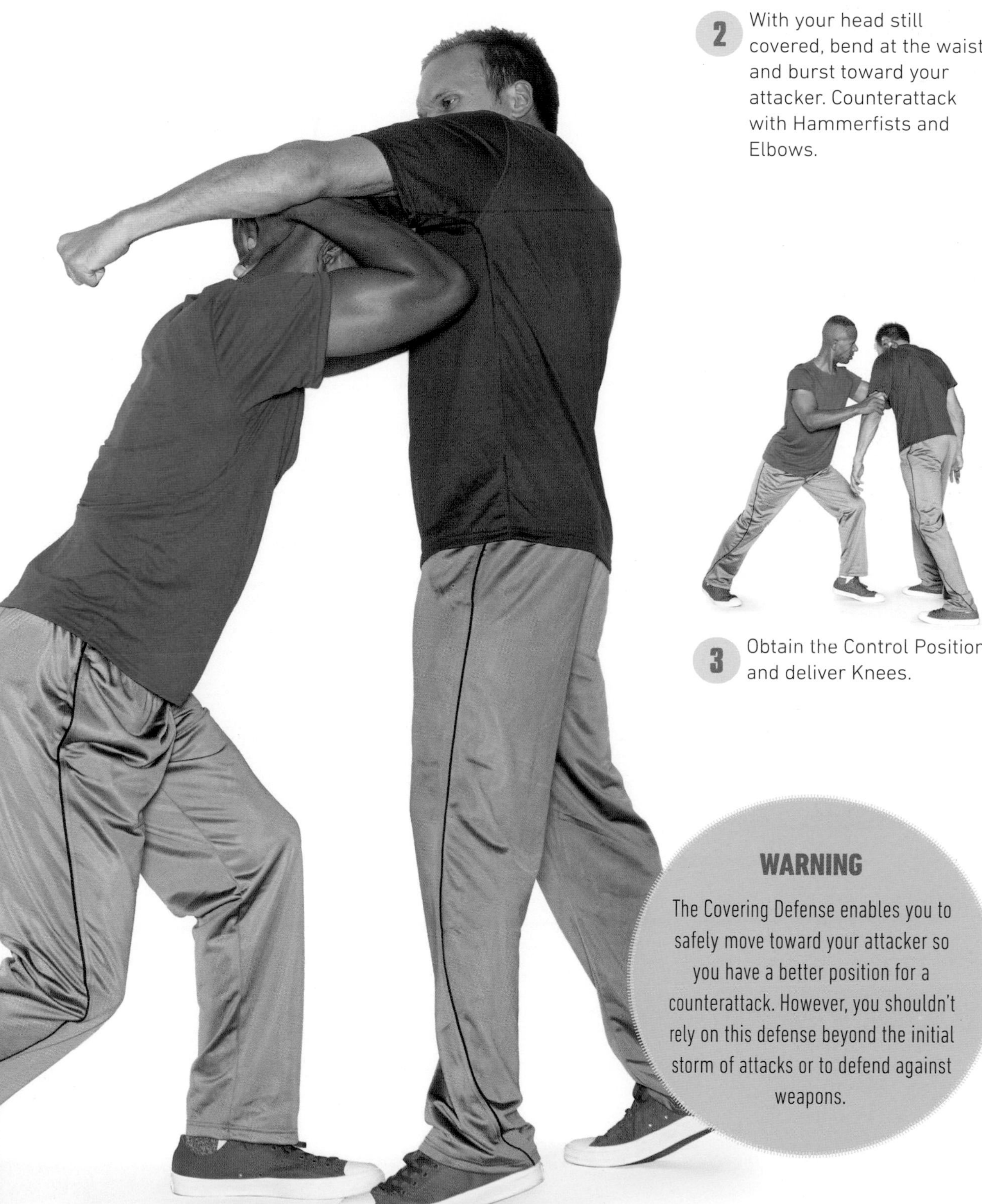

2 With your head still covered, bend at the waist and burst toward your attacker. Counterattack with Hammerfists and Elbows.

3 Obtain the Control Position and deliver Knees.

WARNING

The Covering Defense enables you to safely move toward your attacker so you have a better position for a counterattack. However, you shouldn't rely on this defense beyond the initial storm of attacks or to defend against weapons.

Inside Defense Against Punches on the Ground

Use this when your attacker is punching directly at you while you're on the ground beneath him or her. This keeps you from being vulnerable to choking, headlocks, and severe strikes.

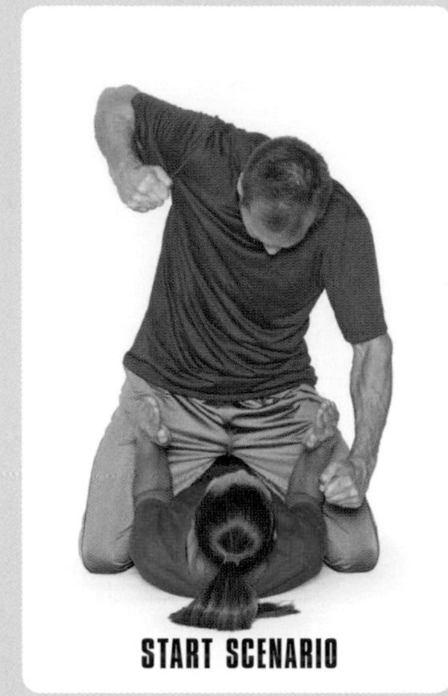
START SCENARIO

Begin on the ground with your attacker mounted on top of you, winding up to punch directly.

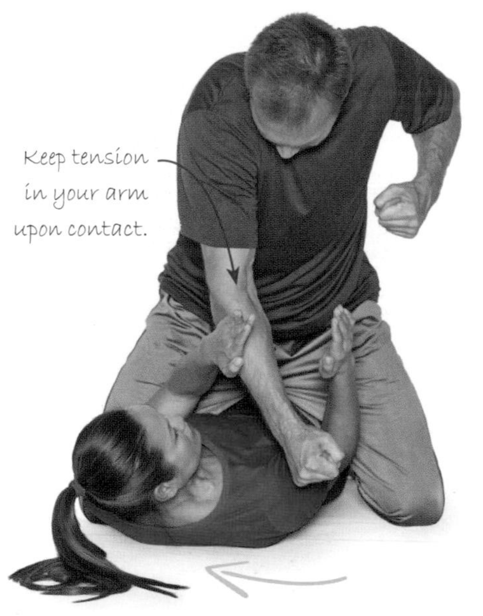
Keep tension in your arm upon contact.

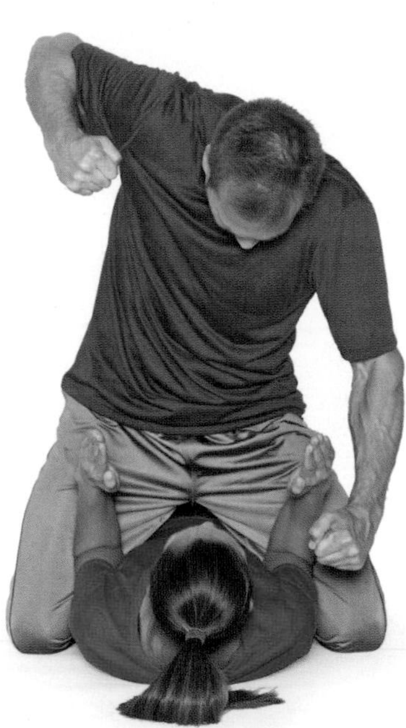

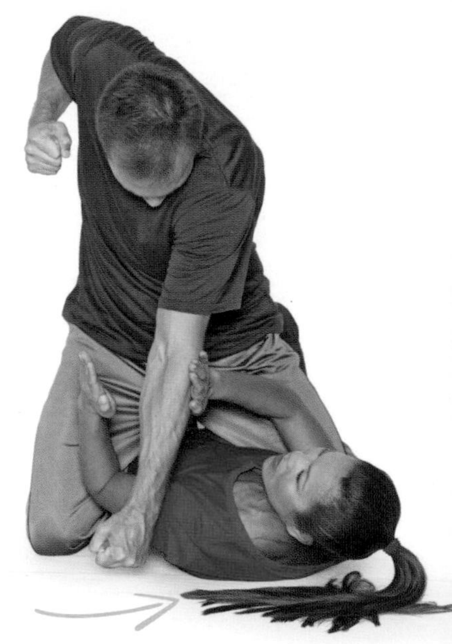

1 When your attacker throws the punch, move your hand forward and inward until it connects with the punch. As you make contact with your attacker, slightly move your head in the opposite direction of where you're defending.

2 Buck your hips explosively, like in the Buck, Trap, and Roll. When you buck, your attacker will likely fall forward onto his or her hands; trap your attacker's arms and legs and roll on top of him or her.

Outside Defense Against Punches on the Ground

Use this when your attacker is punching from outside while you're on the ground beneath him or her. This high-level threat requires you to make an immediate combination of defenses to escape.

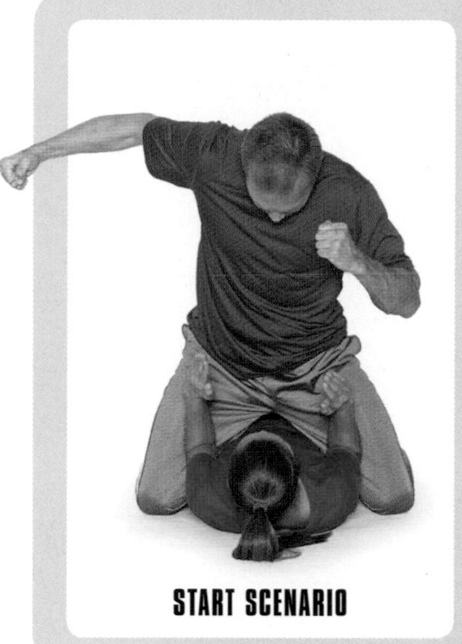
START SCENARIO

Begin on the ground with your attacker mounted on top of you, winding up to punch from outside.

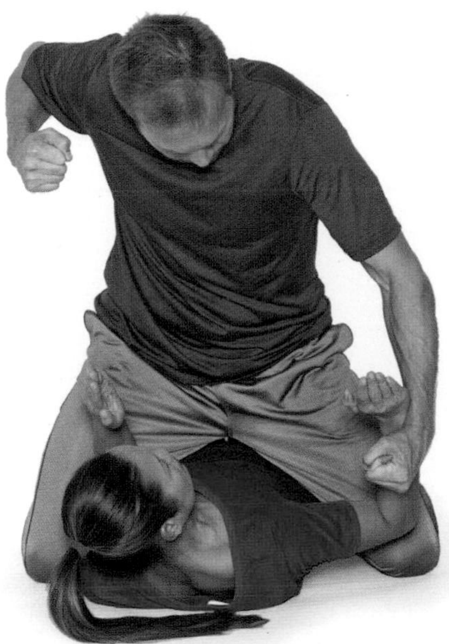

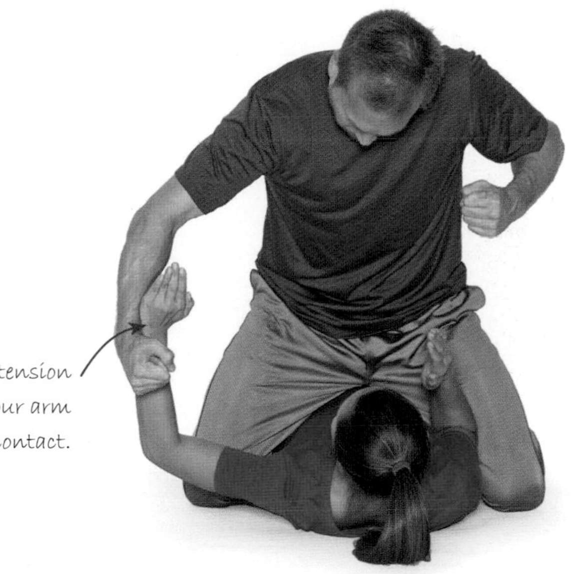
Keep tension in your arm upon contact.

1. When your attacker throws the punch, block with the wrist on the same side as the punch using any Outside Defense. As you make contact with your attacker, slightly move your head in the opposite direction of where you're defending.

2. When you buck, the attacker will likely fall forward onto his or her hands; trap your attacker's arms and legs and roll on top of him or her.

STRIKING

Strikes are closely associated with defense. From penetrating hits with the fingers, to closed-fist punches, to Knees, these techniques can damage your attacker and set you up to gain the upper hand.

Straight Punch

The Straight Punch is a primary weapon in your arsenal—a foundational technique to quickly devastate your attacker. From this core punch, you can set up countless combinations of counterstrikes to achieve your primary goal: escaping safely.

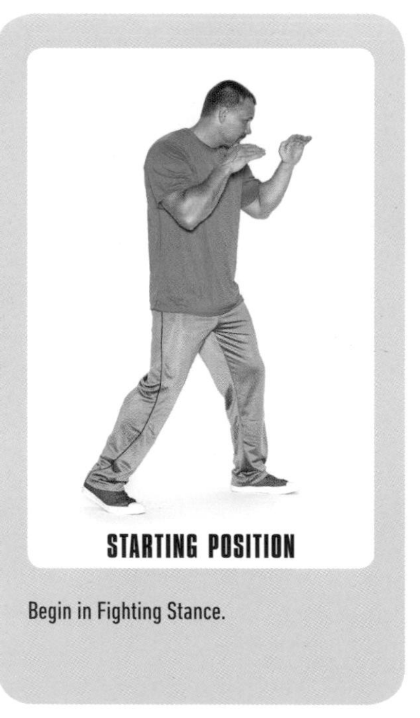

STARTING POSITION

Begin in Fighting Stance.

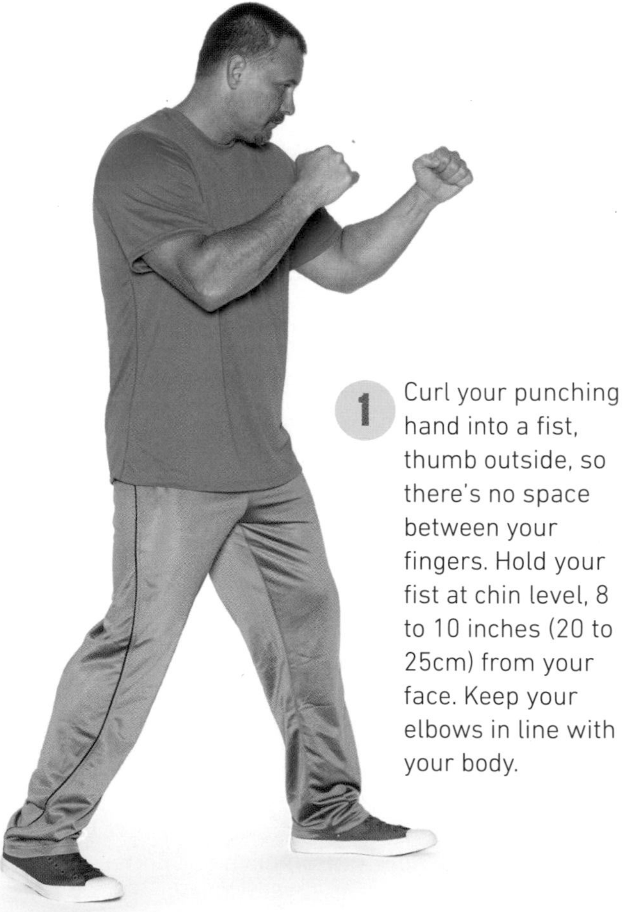

1 Curl your punching hand into a fist, thumb outside, so there's no space between your fingers. Hold your fist at chin level, 8 to 10 inches (20 to 25cm) from your face. Keep your elbows in line with your body.

2 Drive your hips and shoulders forward and explosively extend your fist toward the target. Keeping your wrist straight, slightly rotate your fist inward so you hit the target with your first two knuckles. To maximize force, exhale completely as you deliver the punch.

IF IT FAILS

If the Straight Punch fails, don't give up. By recoiling quickly, you'll always be prepared to defend yourself or aggressively counterattack with Palm Strikes, Elbows, or any of the other strikes. If your attacker is protecting his or her face, you can try a Front Kick to the Groin on the exposed lower body.

Keep your other hand up to defend or to quickly deliver another strike.

Explosively punch *through* the target, not just to the target.

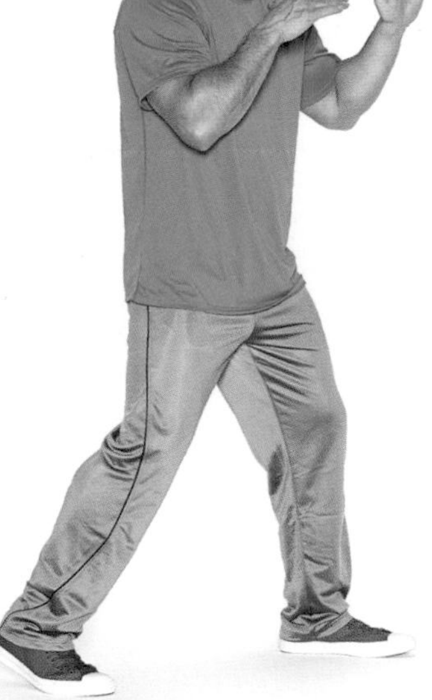

3 Recoil your fist and arm as quickly as you sent out the punch and return to Fighting Stance.

Hammerfist Forward

The Hammerfist Forward is an unorthodox strike to the face, generally to the bridge of the nose. This can cause your attacker to become disoriented (an OODA loop interruption) and can bring tears to his or her eyes.

DEFENSE TIP

Strike with the meaty part of your fist, on the opposite side of your thumb. Although the thumb and knuckles can do more damage, this protects you from hand injuries.

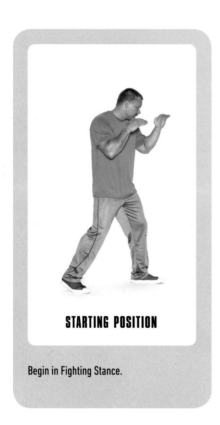

STARTING POSITION

Begin in Fighting Stance.

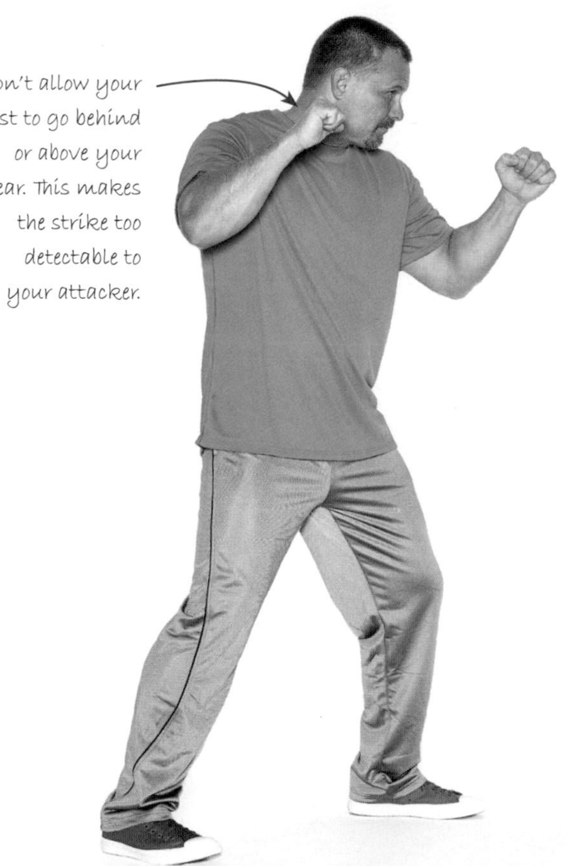

Don't allow your fist to go behind or above your ear. This makes the strike too detectable to your attacker.

1 Raise your fist in a small wind-up, with your knuckles facing your attacker.

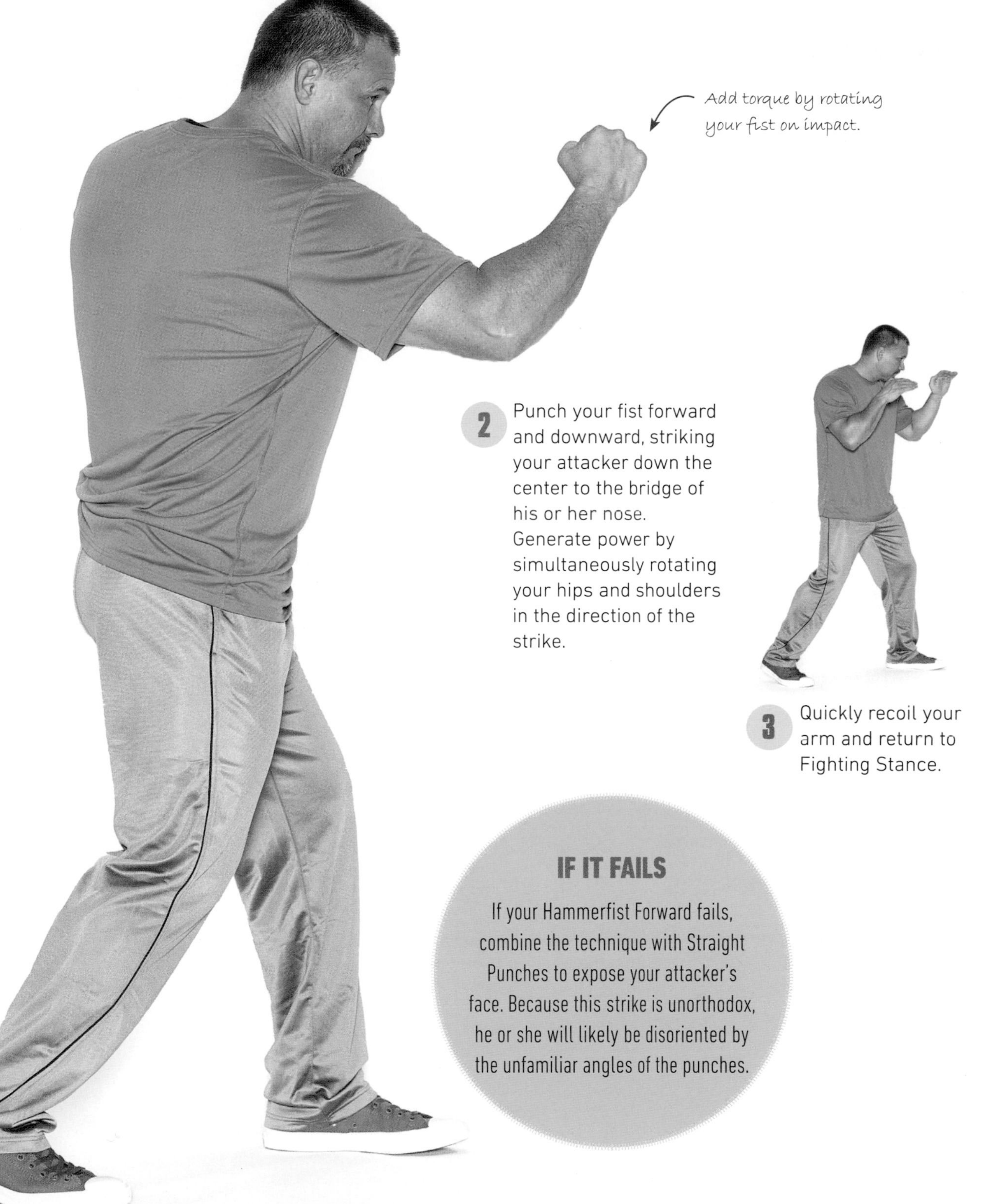

Add torque by rotating your fist on impact.

2 Punch your fist forward and downward, striking your attacker down the center to the bridge of his or her nose. Generate power by simultaneously rotating your hips and shoulders in the direction of the strike.

3 Quickly recoil your arm and return to Fighting Stance.

IF IT FAILS

If your Hammerfist Forward fails, combine the technique with Straight Punches to expose your attacker's face. Because this strike is unorthodox, he or she will likely be disoriented by the unfamiliar angles of the punches.

Hammerfist to the Side

You can perform the Hammerfist to the Side from Fighting Stance or Passive Stance, which allows you to use this technique in reaction to surprise attacks or changing directions in a fight.

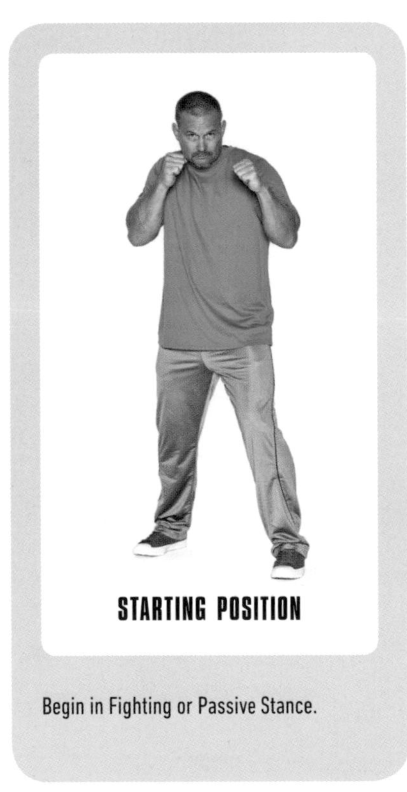

Begin in Fighting or Passive Stance.

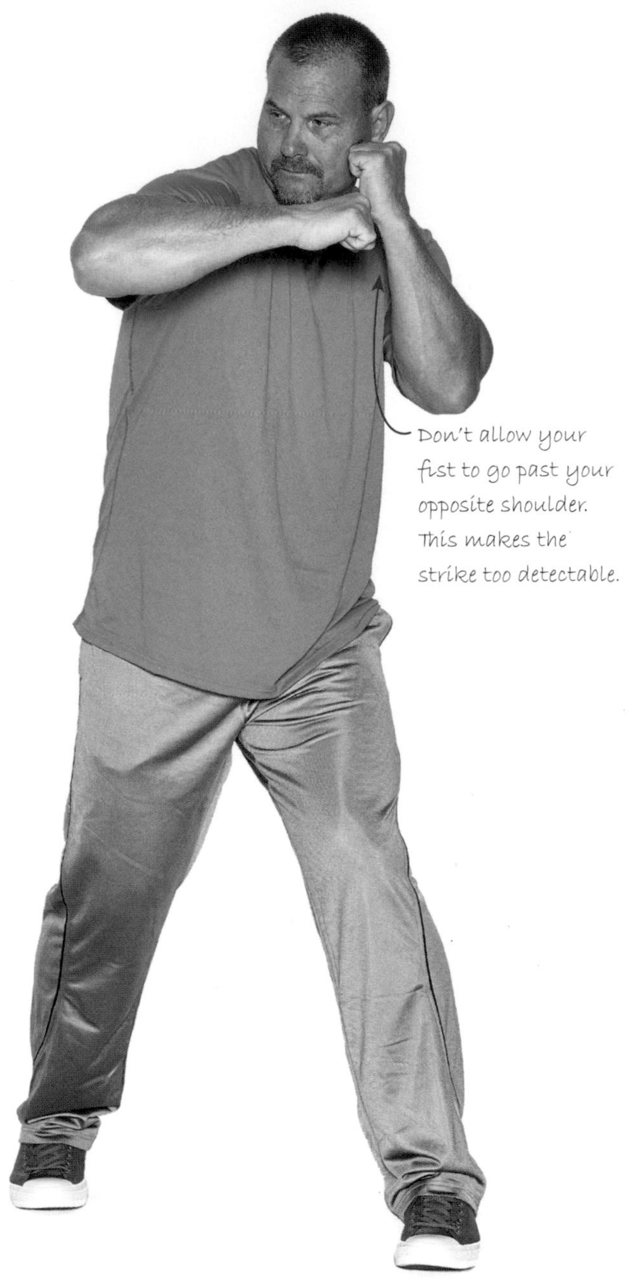

Don't allow your fist to go past your opposite shoulder. This makes the strike too detectable.

1 Raise your elbow and fist to shoulder height, horizontal to the ground. Bring your fist in front of your face.

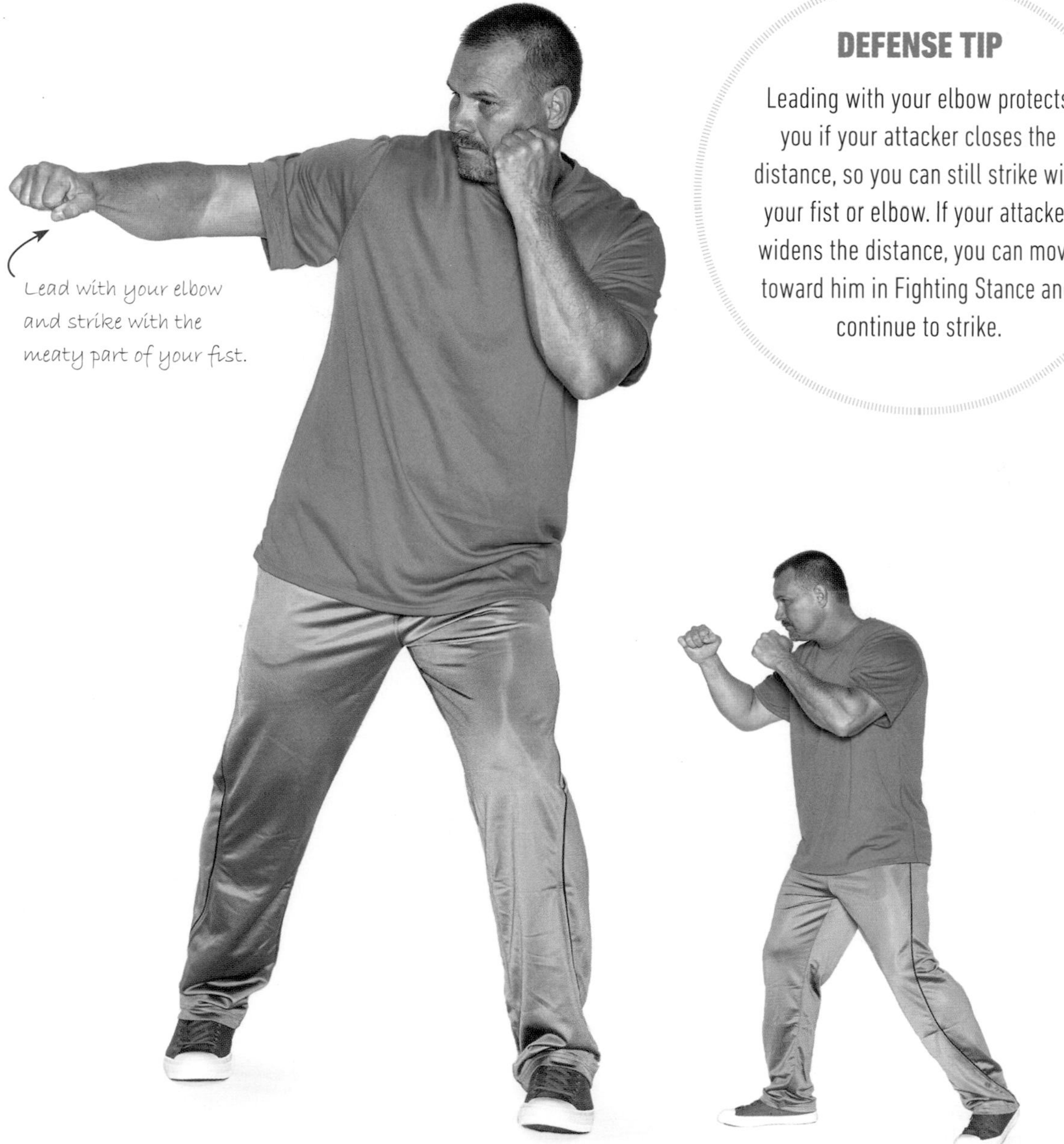

Lead with your elbow
and strike with the
meaty part of your fist.

DEFENSE TIP

Leading with your elbow protects you if your attacker closes the distance, so you can still strike with your fist or elbow. If your attacker widens the distance, you can move toward him in Fighting Stance and continue to strike.

2 Send your fist out, generating power by rotating your hips and shoulders in the direction of the strike.

3 After your strike, complete your rotation toward your attacker and return to Fighting Stance.

Palm Strike

You may often have to strike a hard surface when counterattacking. The Palm Strike technique will prevent you from damaging your knuckles and allow you to stay in the fight.

STARTING POSITION

Begin in Fighting Stance.

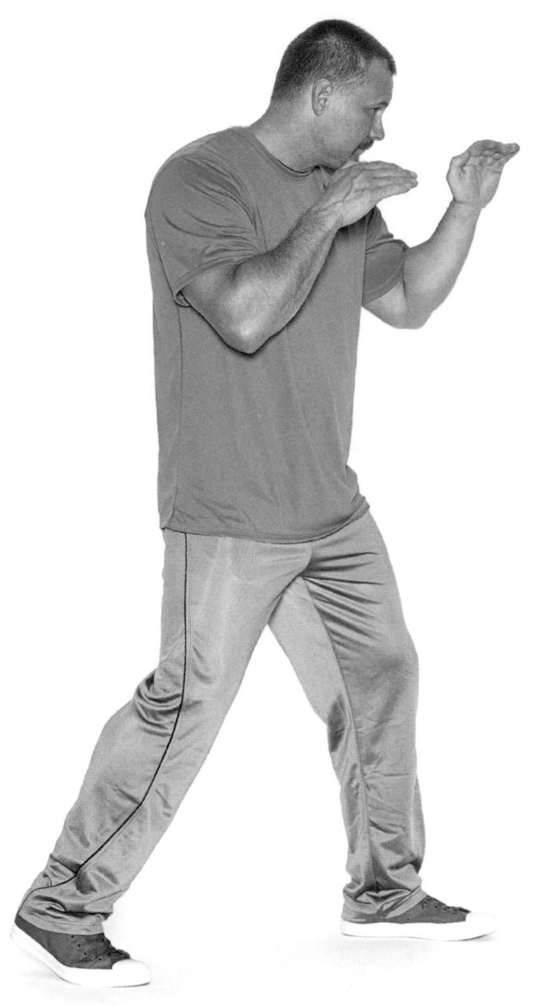

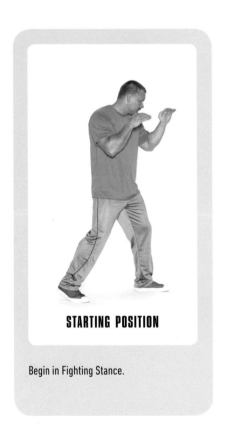

1 From Fighting Stance, drive forward with your hips and shoulders.

2 Explosively extend your hand toward the target. Just before impact, flex your wrist back and slightly rotate your hand inward so you make contact with the heel of your palm.

IF IT FAILS

If your Palm Strike isn't effective, continue it with other combinations, such as Knees. Because this strike can distribute its force, causing extra damage, try using it in different areas. For example, striking the chin can also send the head up and back.

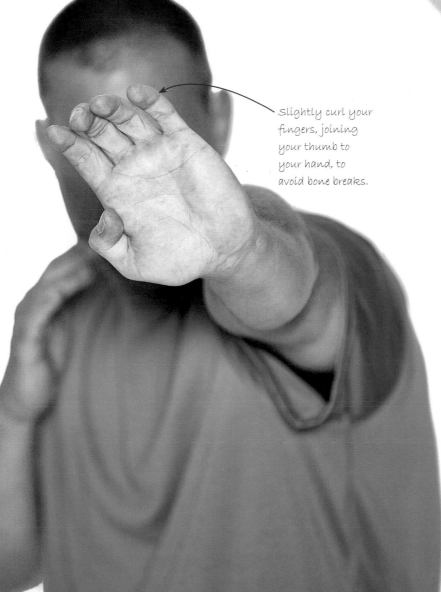

Slightly curl your fingers, joining your thumb to your hand, to avoid bone breaks.

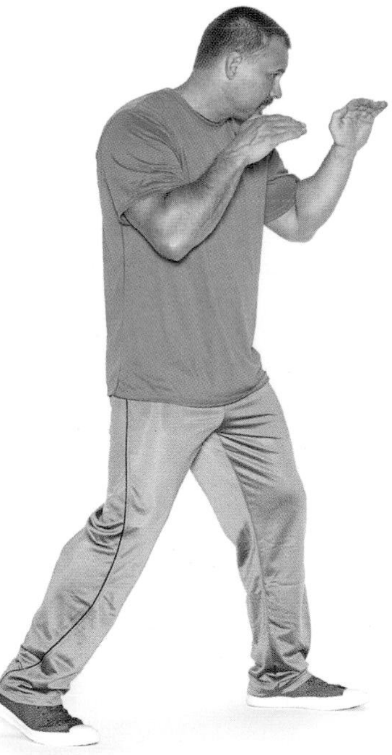

3 Quickly recoil your arm and return to Fighting Stance.

Eye Strike

Use this technique to strike your attacker in the eyes with your fingertips. You can perform Eye Strikes in combination with Straight Punches to further disorient your attacker.

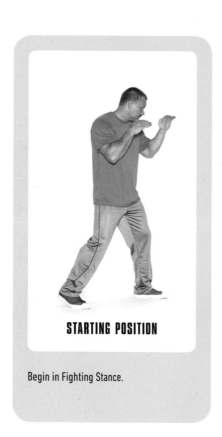

STARTING POSITION

Begin in Fighting Stance.

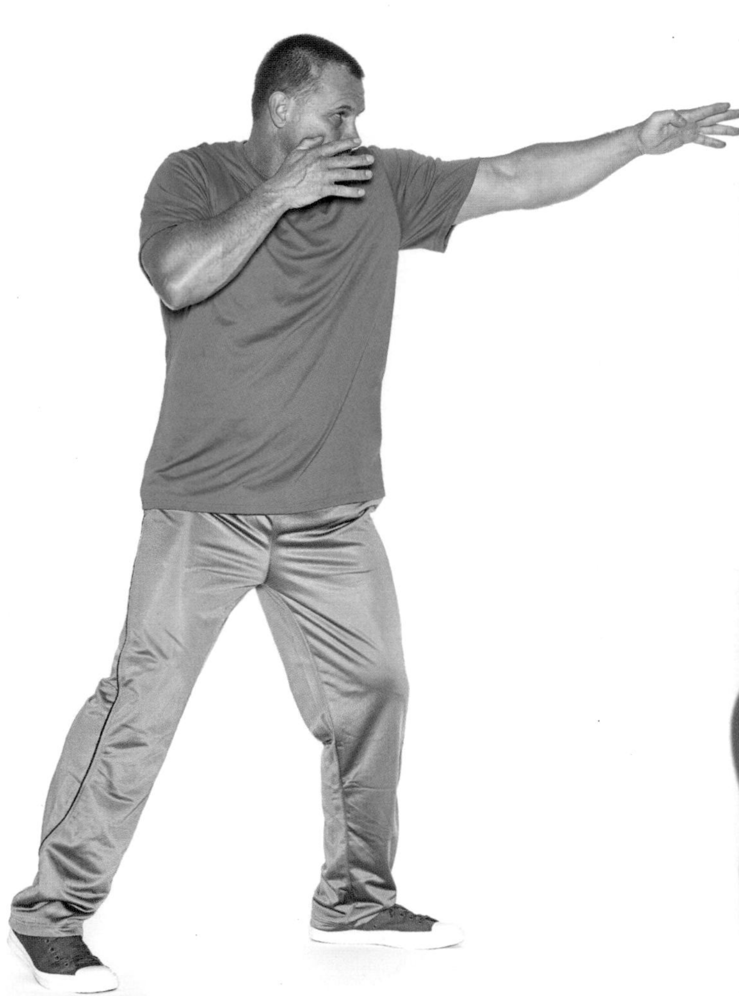

1. From Fighting Stance, explosively launch forward with your legs. With your fingers tensed and your knuckles slightly bent, extend your hand toward your attacker's eyes.

DEFENSE TIP

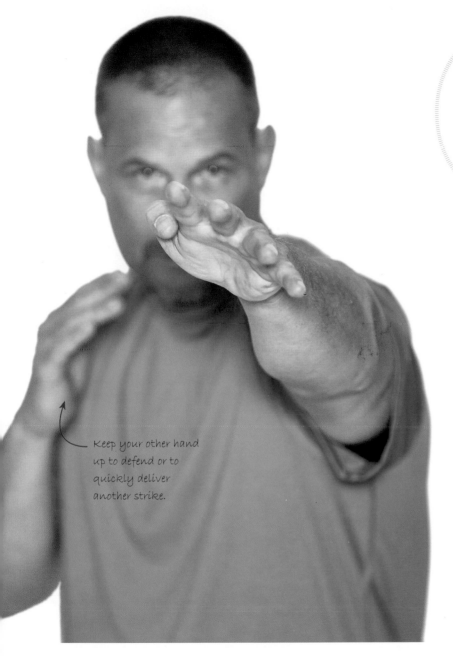

By rotating your hand 45 degrees while delivering the Eye Strike, you increase your chance of getting at least one finger into your attacker's eyes.

Keep your other hand up to defend or to quickly deliver another strike.

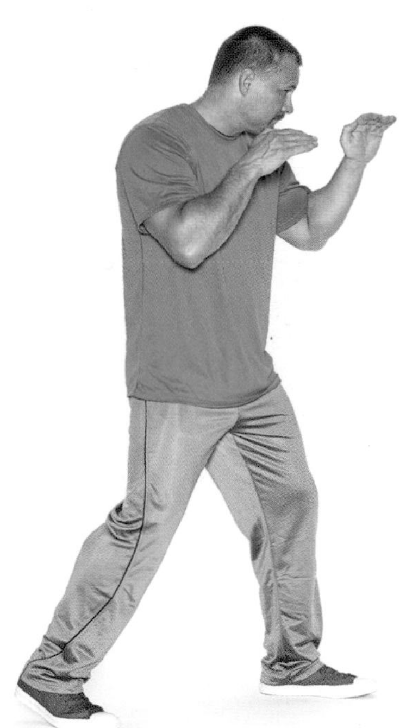

2 Just before impact, rotate your hand 45 degrees to angle your fingers toward your attacker's face.

3 Quickly recoil your arm and return to Fighting Stance.

Throat Strike

This strike helps you disorient your attacker by going after one of his or her vital processes—breathing. The Throat Strike can favorably change the momentum of your fight.

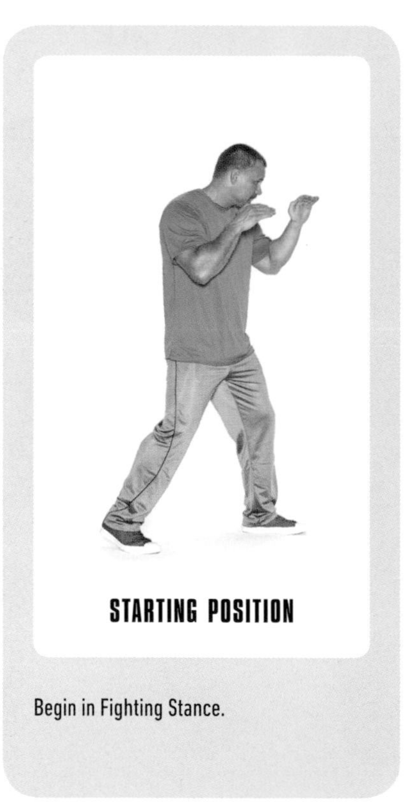

STARTING POSITION

Begin in Fighting Stance.

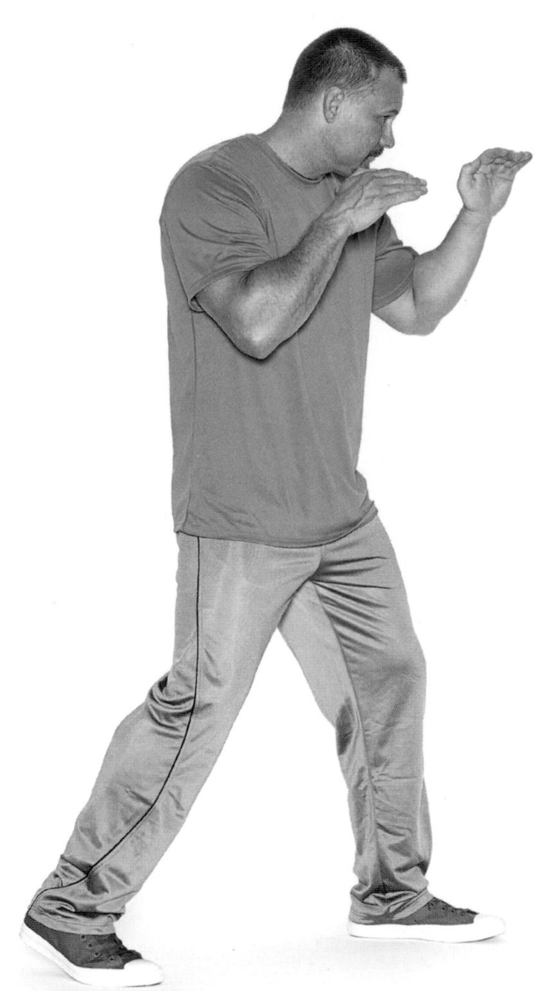

1 From your Fighting Stance, explosively launch forward with your legs.

2 Keeping your fingers together, separate your thumb to make a Y shape and extend your hand toward your attacker's throat. Strike your attacker with the inside of the Y, or the webbing of your hand.

DEFENSE TIP

Don't limit yourself to one type of Throat Strike. Even if your opponent is heavier, taller, or stronger, all attackers are vulnerable at the throat. You can vary the movement by targeting the throat with a Hammerfist to the Side.

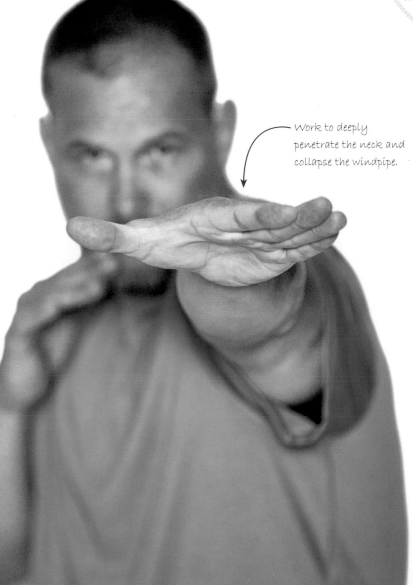

Work to deeply penetrate the neck and collapse the windpipe.

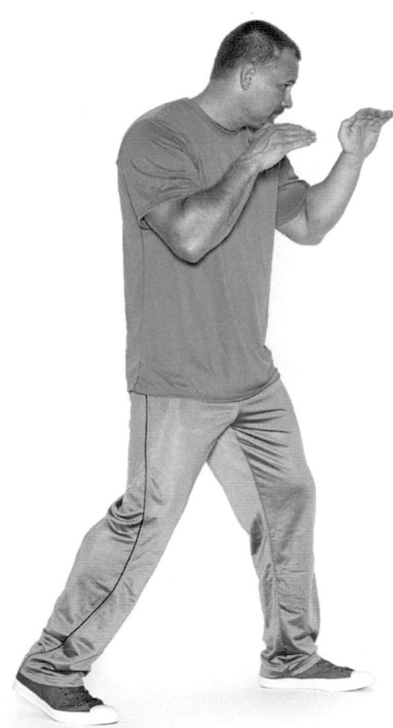

3 Quickly recoil your arm and return to Fighting Stance.

Elbows

Elbow strikes allow you to respond to an attack and then reposition yourself to deliver counterattacks. Because of their devastating power, they are often your best friends in a fight. You can deliver elbows in front of or behind you, as well as to the side, at many different angles.

Elbow 1: Forward (Horizontal)

You can use a forward horizontal motion to blindside your attacker from the front with a powerful strike to his or her face or throat.

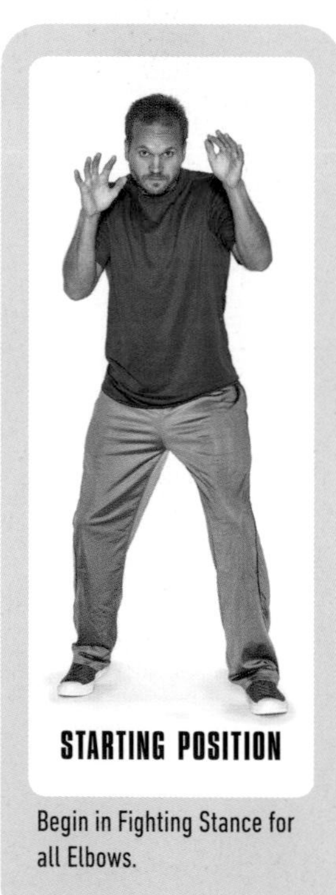

STARTING POSITION

Begin in Fighting Stance for all Elbows.

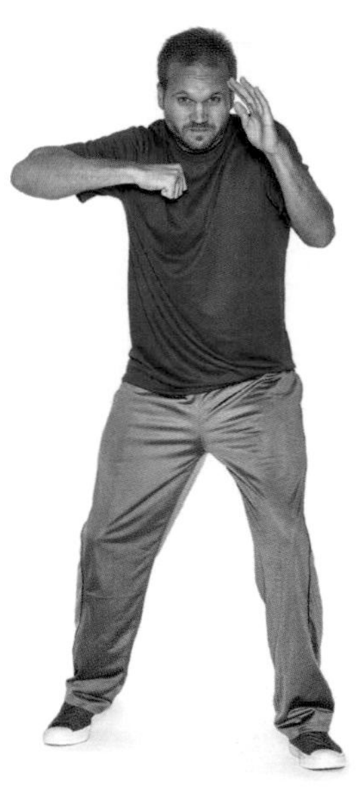

1 Hold one arm parallel to the ground at chest level.

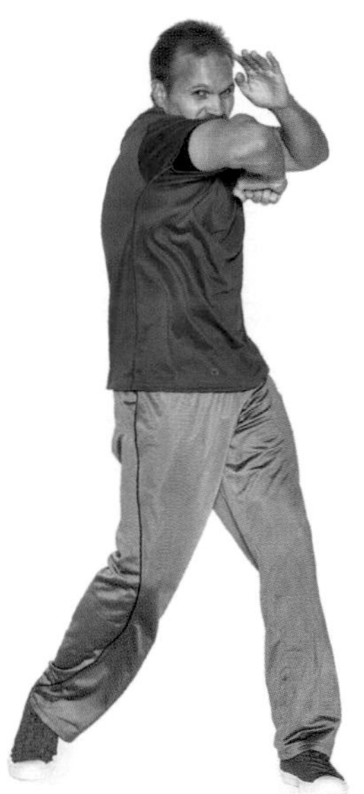

2 Bring your hand toward your other shoulder to expose your elbow. Rotate your body and drive it into your attacker.

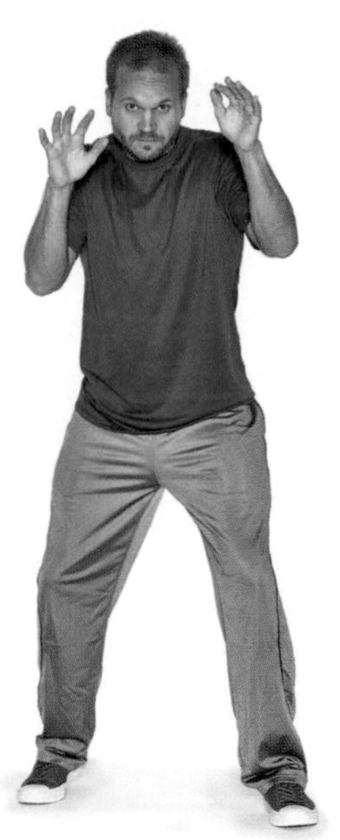

3 Quickly recoil your elbow and continue with counterattacks.

Elbow 2: Forward (Vertical)
You can use a vertical forward motion to strike your attacker's throat, jaw, or chin at a close range. It's also useful for splitting your attacker's hands when they're being used as shield in front of his or her face.

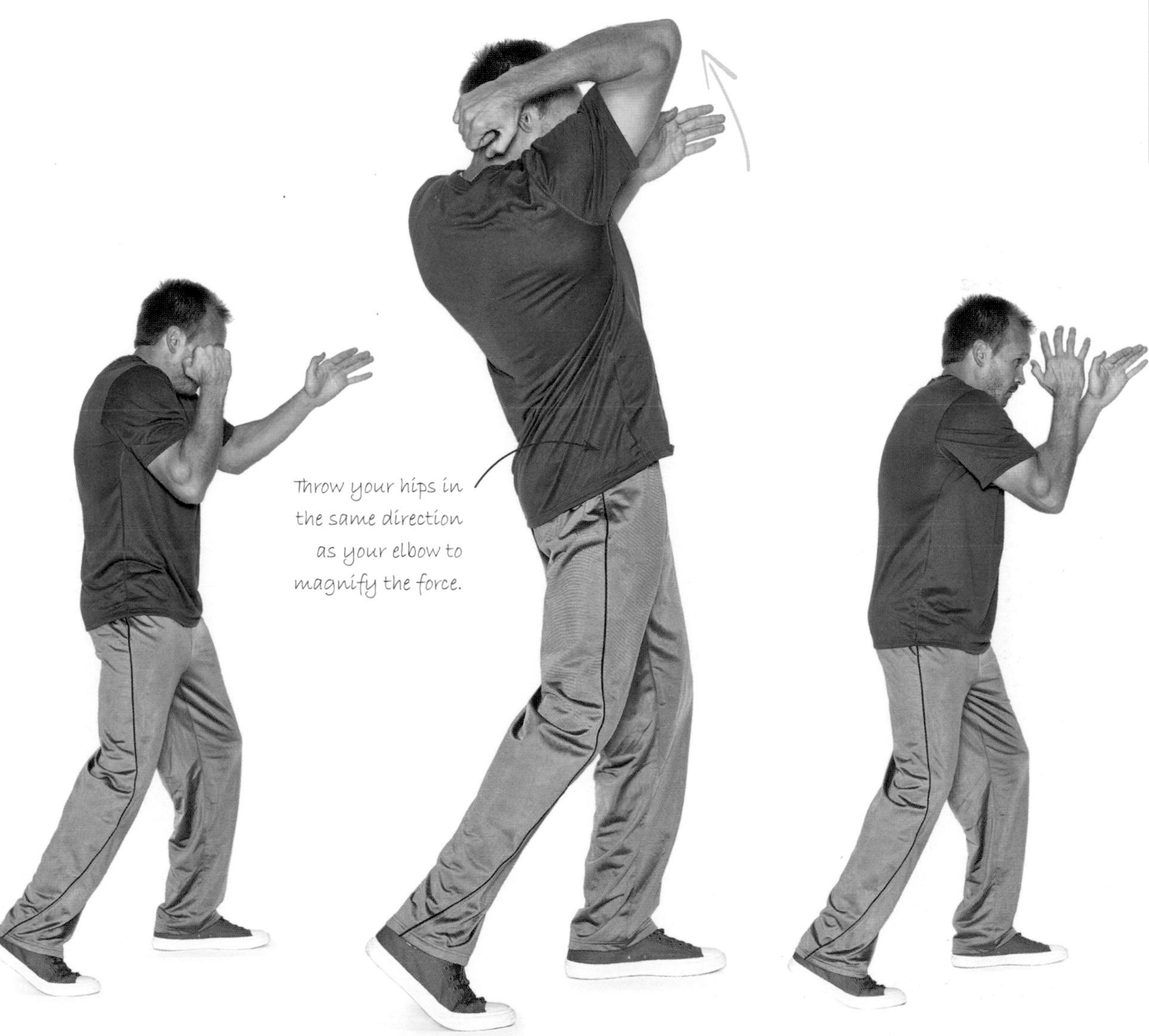

Throw your hips in the same direction as your elbow to magnify the force.

1. Hold one arm vertically near your face.
2. Bring your hand toward the same shoulder to expose your elbow. Thrust your elbow forward and upward into the target.
3. Quickly recoil your elbow and continue with counterattacks.

Elbow 3: To the Side (Horizontal)

Rather than turning immediately toward your attacker if he or she is next to you at close range, you can instead use a horizontal side elbow. This can be directed toward your attacker's face, throat, or midsection.

DEFENSE TIP

If you counterattack with your dominant elbow, your Fighting Stance may be reversed once you finish your attack and turn. When you're able, step forward into your familiar Fighting Stance and continue to fight.

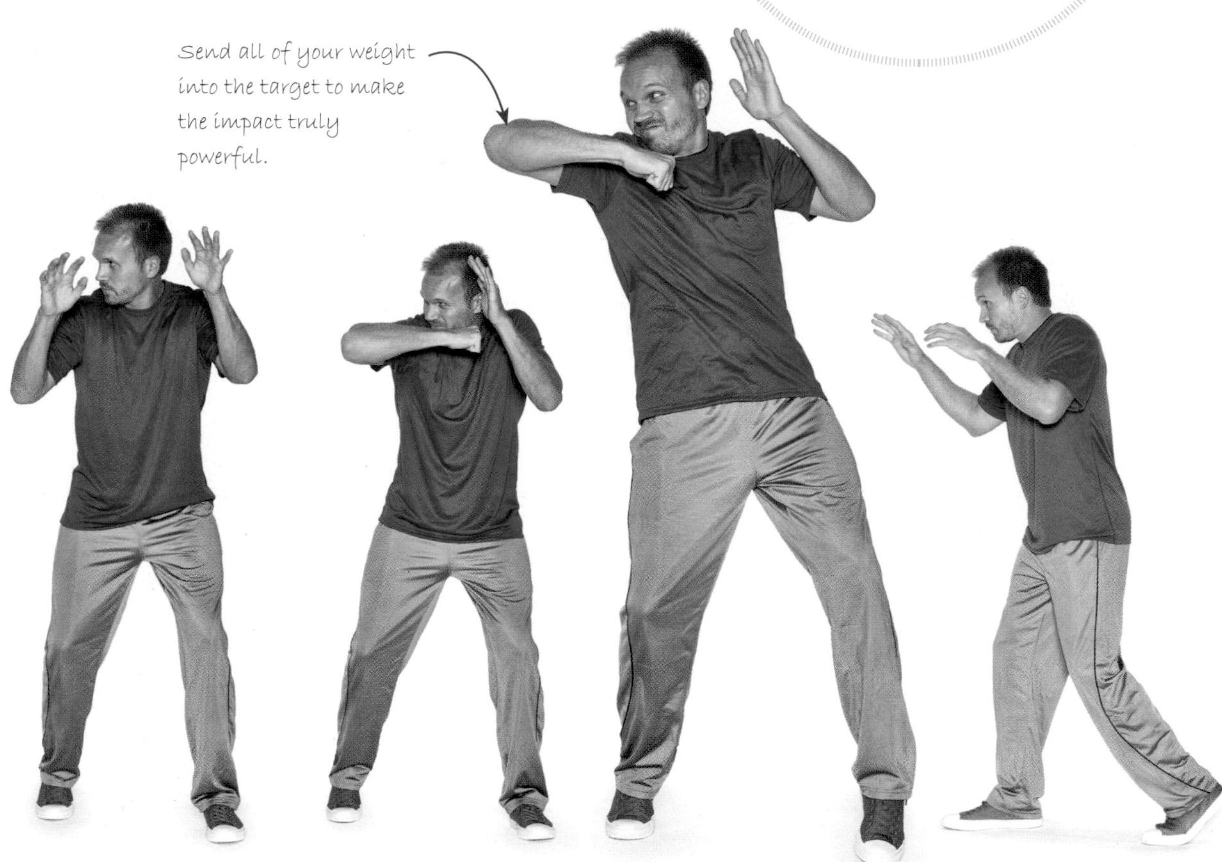
Send all of your weight into the target to make the impact truly powerful.

1. Turn your head to the side to look toward your attacker.
2. Hold one arm horizontal. Bring your hand toward your opposite shoulder to expose your elbow.
3. Explosively thrust your elbow sideways at the target.
4. Quickly recoil your elbow, turn toward your attacker, and continue with counterattacks.

Elbow 4: Down (Vertical)

If your attacker is bent over (maybe because you kicked him or her in the groin), you can use a downward vertical elbow to strike the brain stem or spine.

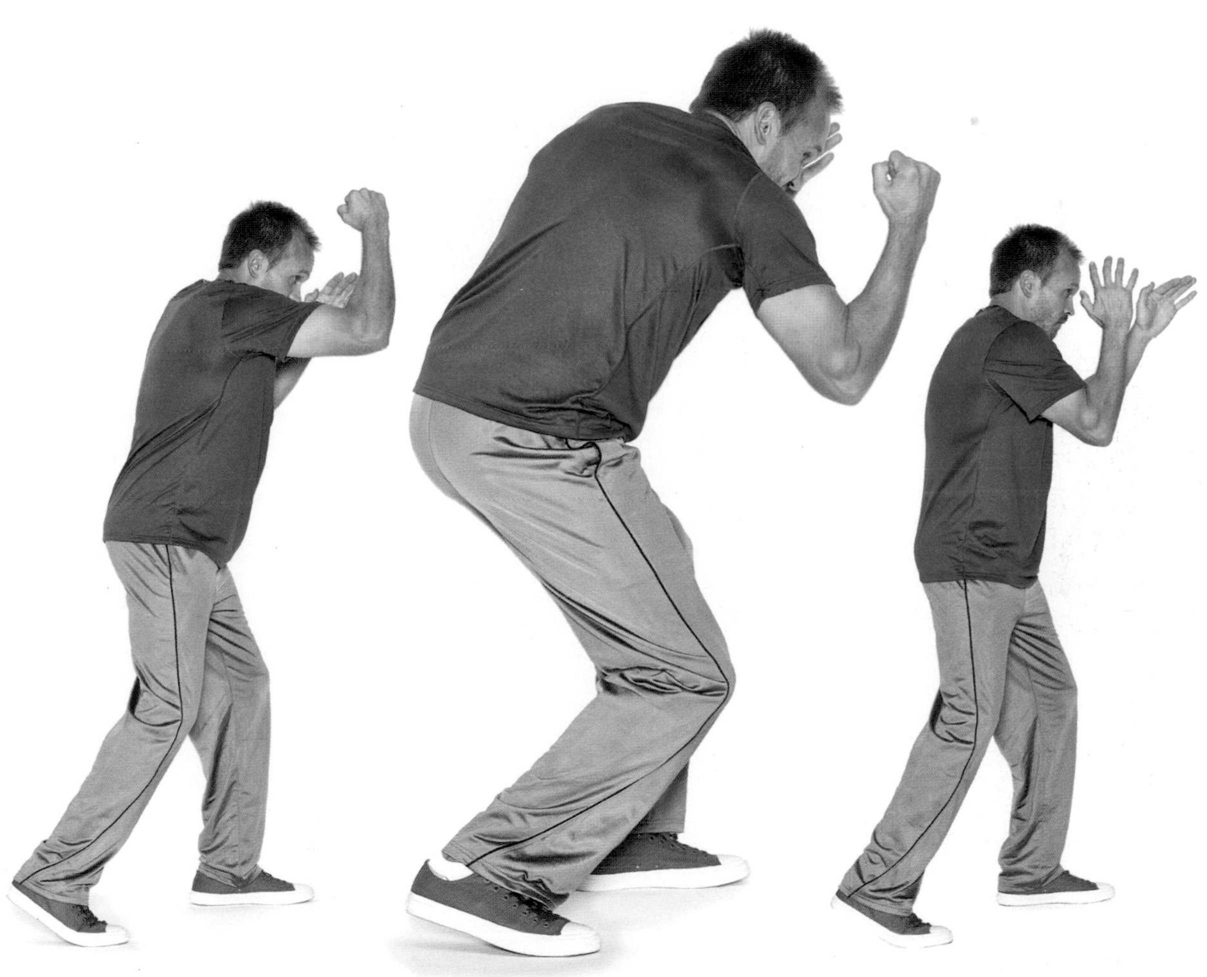

1. Hold your arm vertically near your face. Bring your hand toward the same shoulder to expose your elbow.
2. Explosively send your elbow downward, dropping all of your weight onto the target.
3. Quickly recoil your elbow and continue with counterattacks.

Elbow 5: Behind (Horizontal)
If your attacker is behind you at a close range, a horizontal strike back is a quick, immediate counterattack that can allow you to then turn around to fight.

DEFENSE TIP

Immediately follow up Elbow Behind (Horizontal) with a second Elbow or with Hammerfists, depending on the distance from your attacker. Further counterstrikes might include punches, kicks, Knees, or more Elbows.

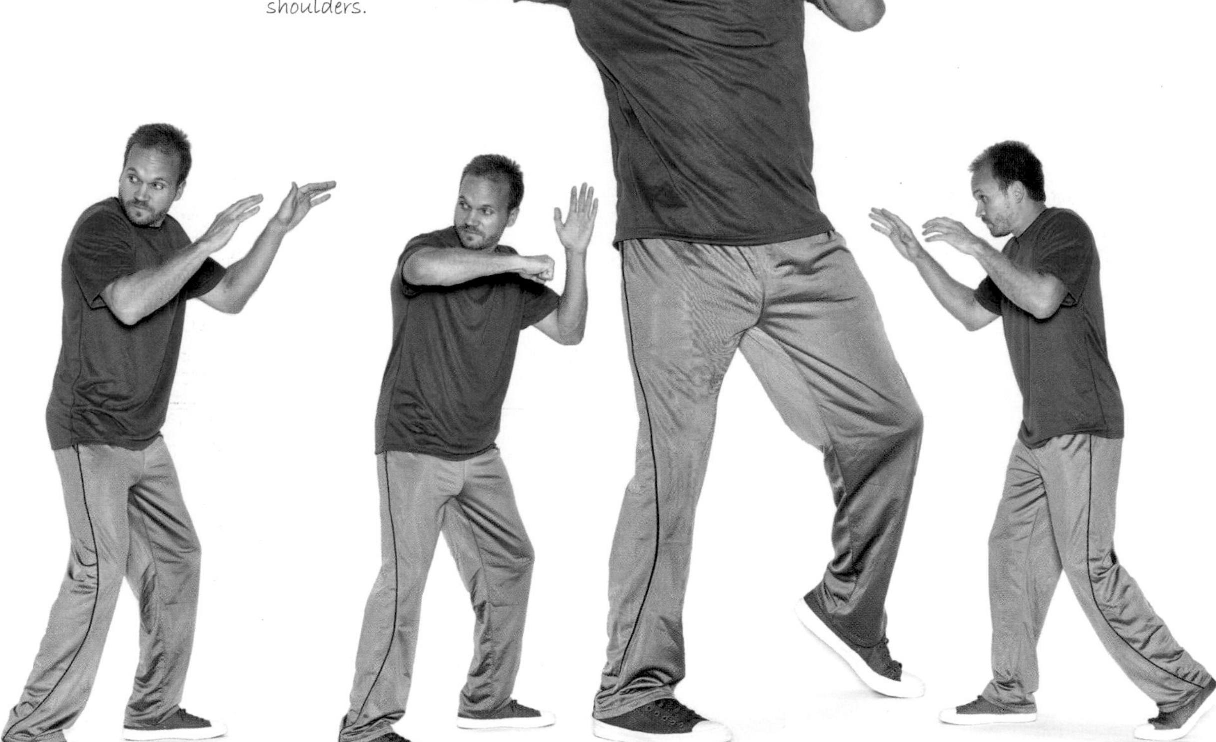

Generate force by pushing off with your opposite foot and rotating your hips and shoulders.

1. Turn your head to the side to look toward your attacker, in order to sight your target.
2. Hold one arm horizontal. Bring your hand toward your opposite shoulder to expose your elbow.
3. Explosively rotate your hips in the direction of your attack and drive your elbow into the target behind.
4. Quickly recoil your elbow, complete your turn toward your attacker, and continue with counterattacks.

Elbow 6: Behind (Vertical)
A vertical elbow back is an effective counterattack if your attacker is behind you. Use this movement to strike his or her groin, midsection, or face.

DEFENSE TIP

You can use this movement on higher targets, like an attacker's jaw. To do this, simultaneously bend at the waist and send your elbow up to the higher target.

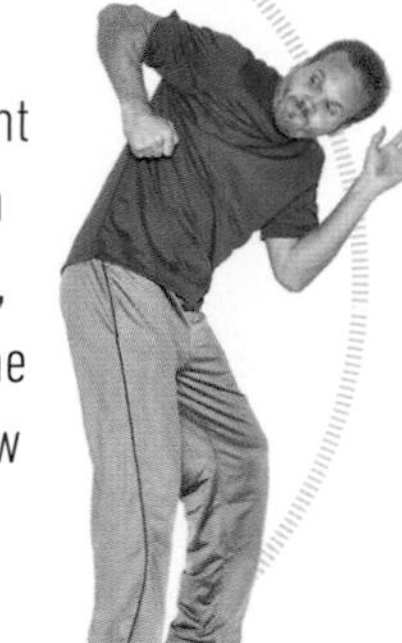

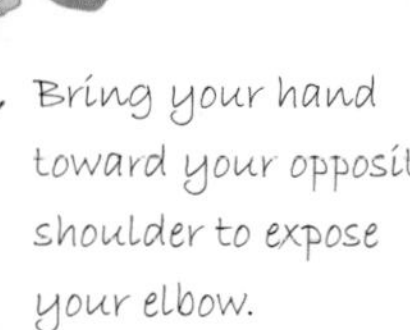

Bring your hand toward your opposite shoulder to expose your elbow.

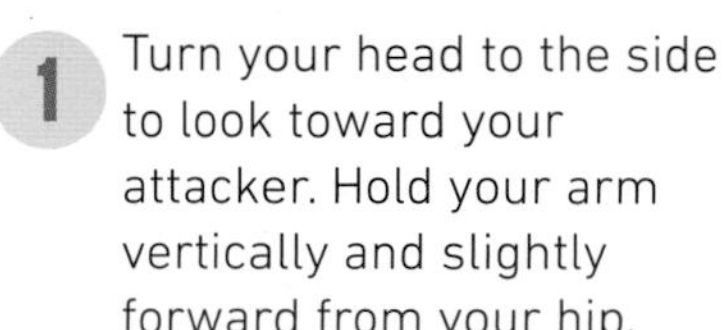

1. Turn your head to the side to look toward your attacker. Hold your arm vertically and slightly forward from your hip.
2. Explosively rotate your hips in the direction of your attacker and drive your elbow backward into the target.
3. Quickly recoil your elbow, complete your turn toward your attacker, and continue with counterattacks.

Knees

Similar to Elbows, you'll use Knees when your attacker is at a close distance. It can be an effective and devastating strike to your attacker's groin, midsection, or head.

DEFENSE TIP

As you pull your attacker in, keep a 90-degree angle in your arm with your elbow down while pressing your forearm into his or her chest. Your forearm tells you where your attacker's weight is and how much fight he or she has left, as well as blocking the attacker from closing the distance.

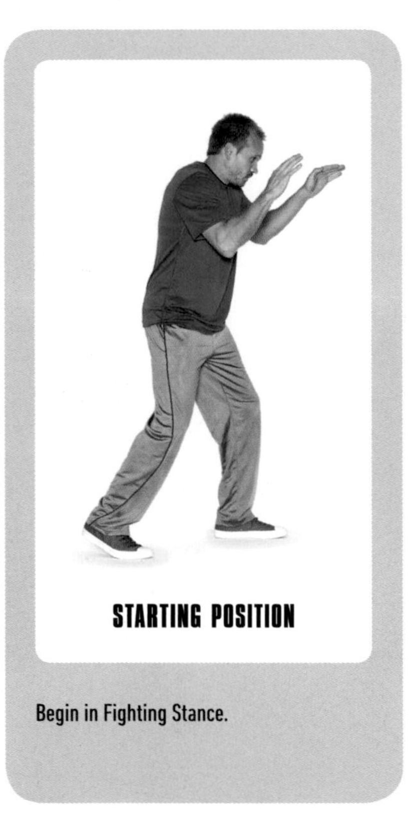

STARTING POSITION

Begin in Fighting Stance.

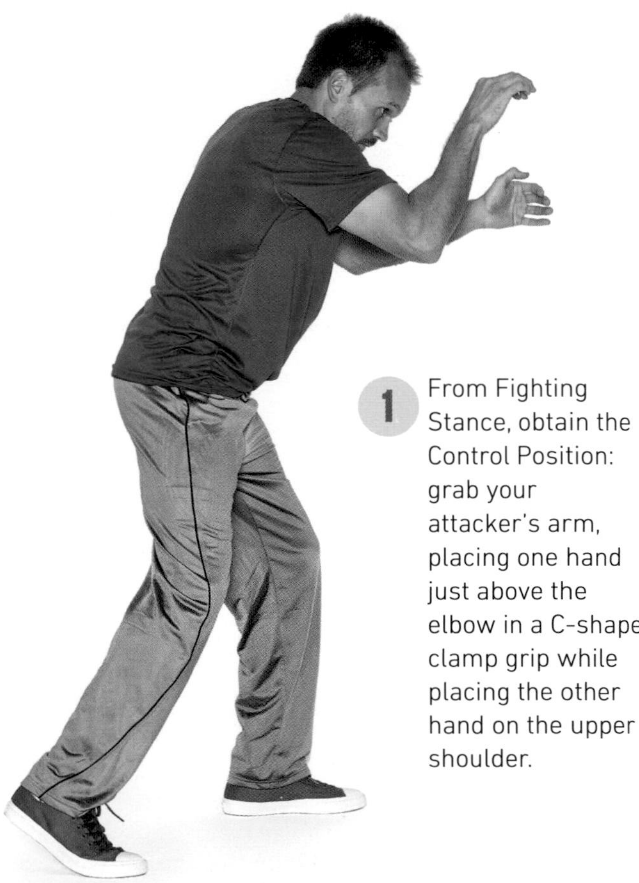

1 From Fighting Stance, obtain the Control Position: grab your attacker's arm, placing one hand just above the elbow in a C-shape clamp grip while placing the other hand on the upper shoulder.

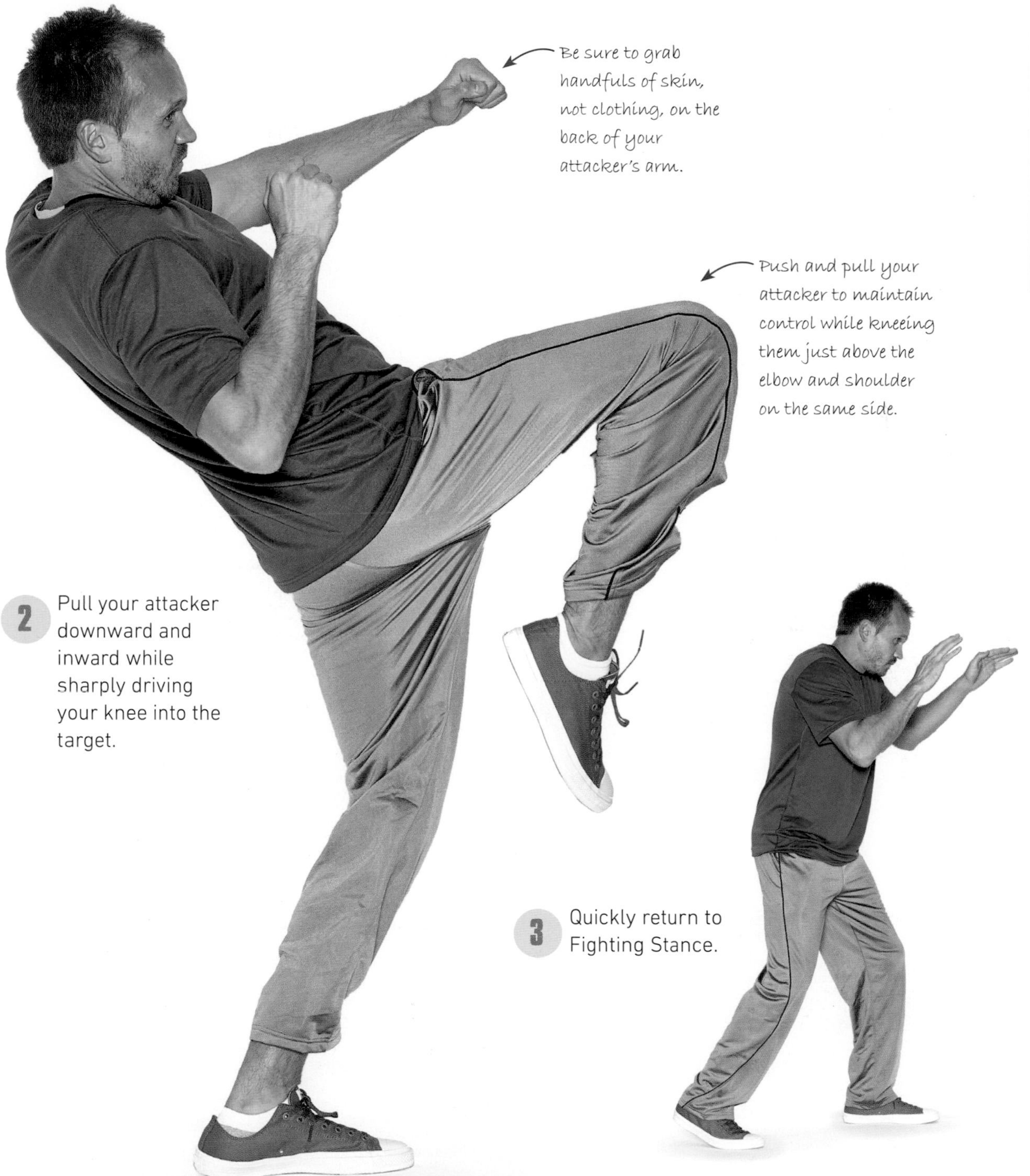
Be sure to grab handfuls of skin, not clothing, on the back of your attacker's arm.
Push and pull your attacker to maintain control while kneeing them just above the elbow and shoulder on the same side.

2 Pull your attacker downward and inward while sharply driving your knee into the target.

3 Quickly return to Fighting Stance.

KICKING

Kicks keep you beyond the reach of closer-range attacks. You can use them offensively and defensively by changing the strike location and striking surface (ball versus full bottom of your foot).

Front Kick to the Groin

With Front Kick to the Groin, you can strike this vulnerable area to cause enough pain to devastate your attacker and help you achieve control.

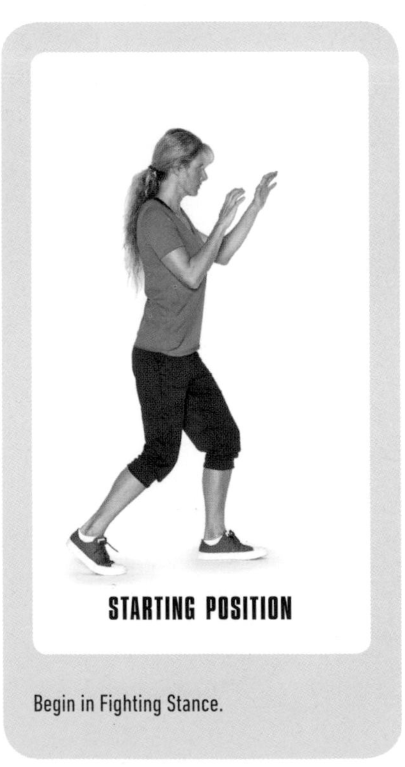

STARTING POSITION

Begin in Fighting Stance.

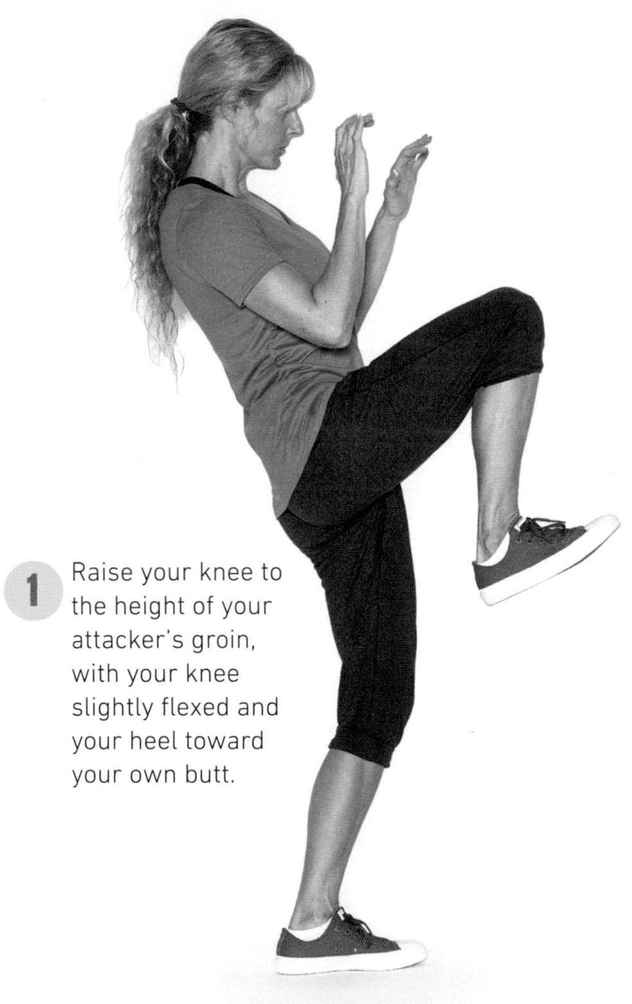

1 Raise your knee to the height of your attacker's groin, with your knee slightly flexed and your heel toward your own butt.

DEFENSE TIP

Use a combination of kicks and upper-body movements to disorient your attacker. If he or she is bent over after the Front Kick, follow up with Hammerfists and Knees. If upright, follow with Straight Punches, Hammerfists, and Eye Strikes.

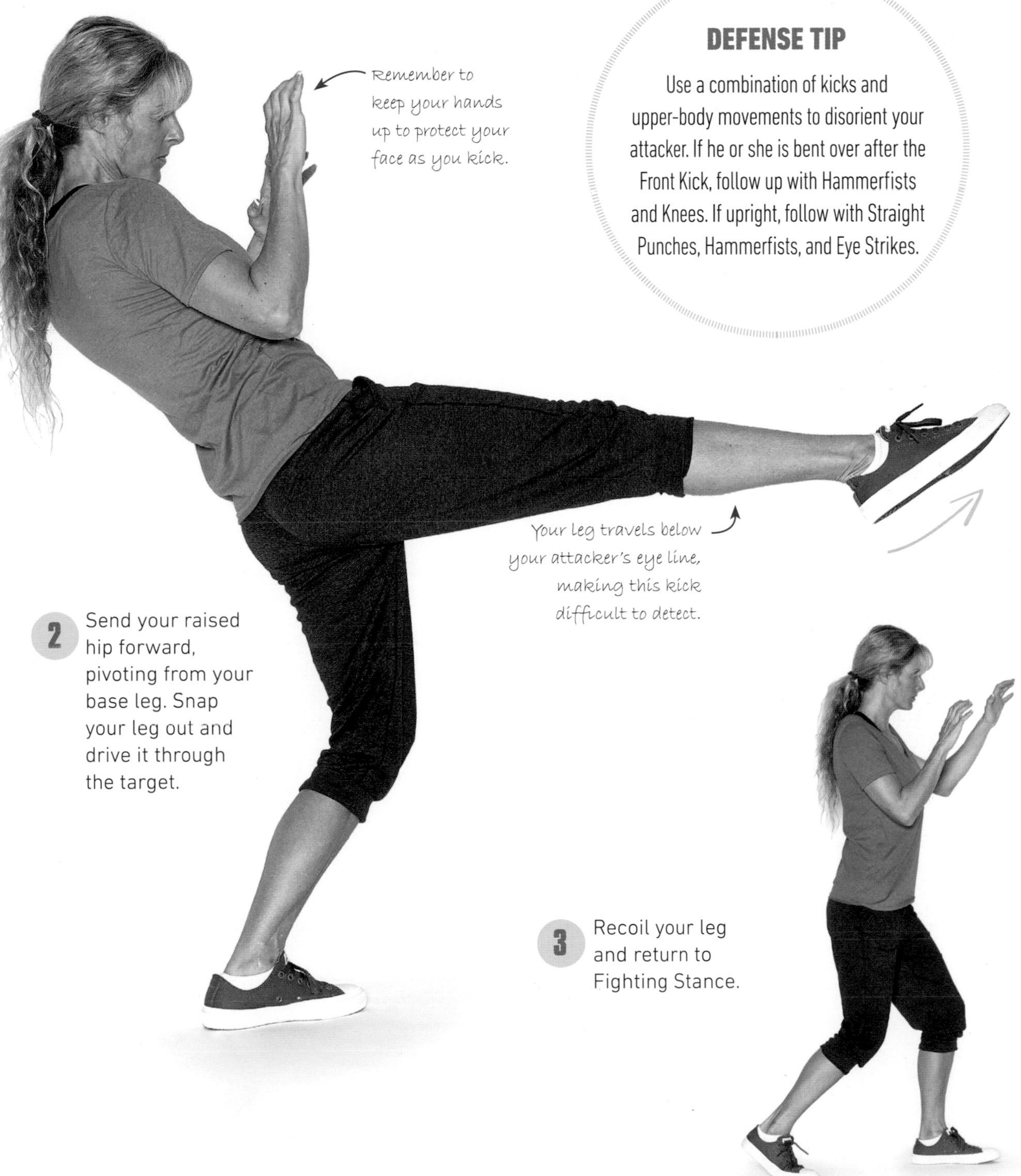

Remember to keep your hands up to protect your face as you kick.

Your leg travels below your attacker's eye line, making this kick difficult to detect.

2 Send your raised hip forward, pivoting from your base leg. Snap your leg out and drive it through the target.

3 Recoil your leg and return to Fighting Stance.

Front Kick to a Vertical Target (Defensive)

Use this kick to stop your attacker if he or she is trying to close the distance between the two of you. Front Kick to a Vertical Target (Defensive) can halt your attacker and give you a chance to break contact or counterattack.

IF IT FAILS

If your kick was off target or if your attacker is larger, continue with other counterattacks such as punches, Knees, and Elbows to try to create distance. Always return to Fighting Stance in anticipation of further attack.

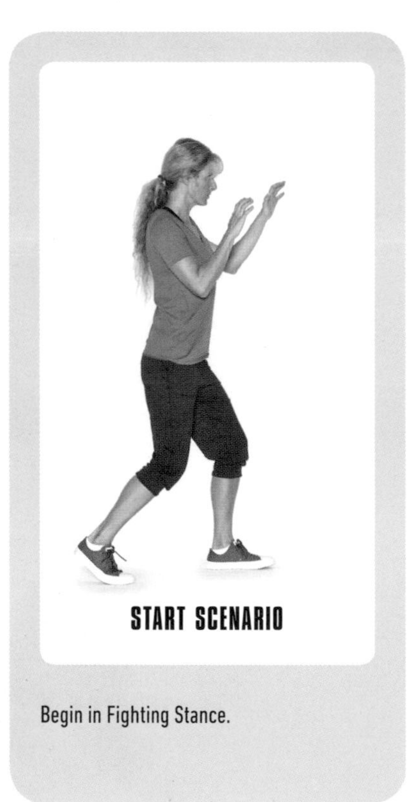

START SCENARIO

Begin in Fighting Stance.

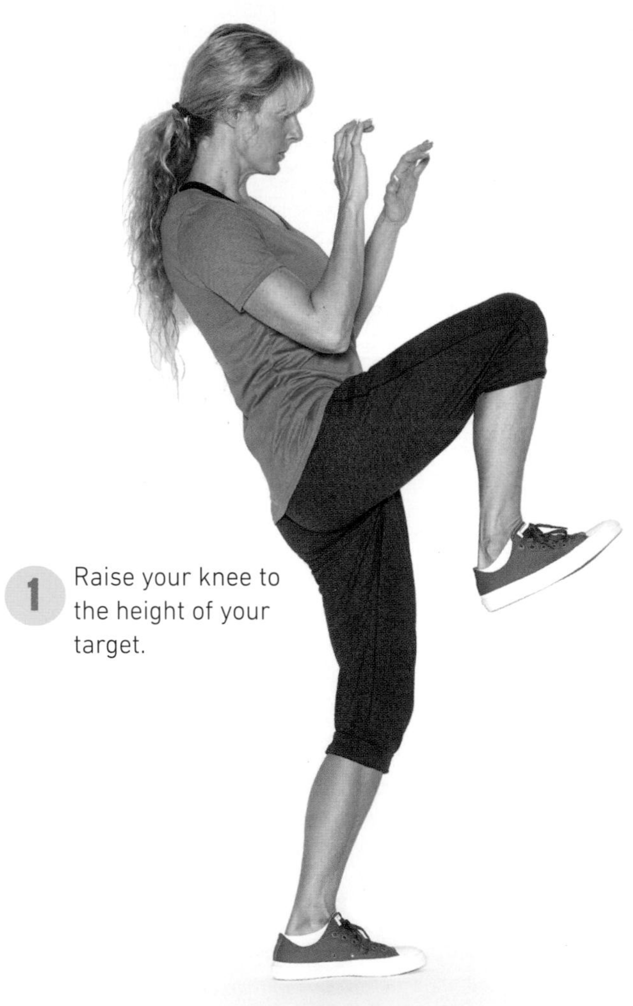

1 Raise your knee to the height of your target.

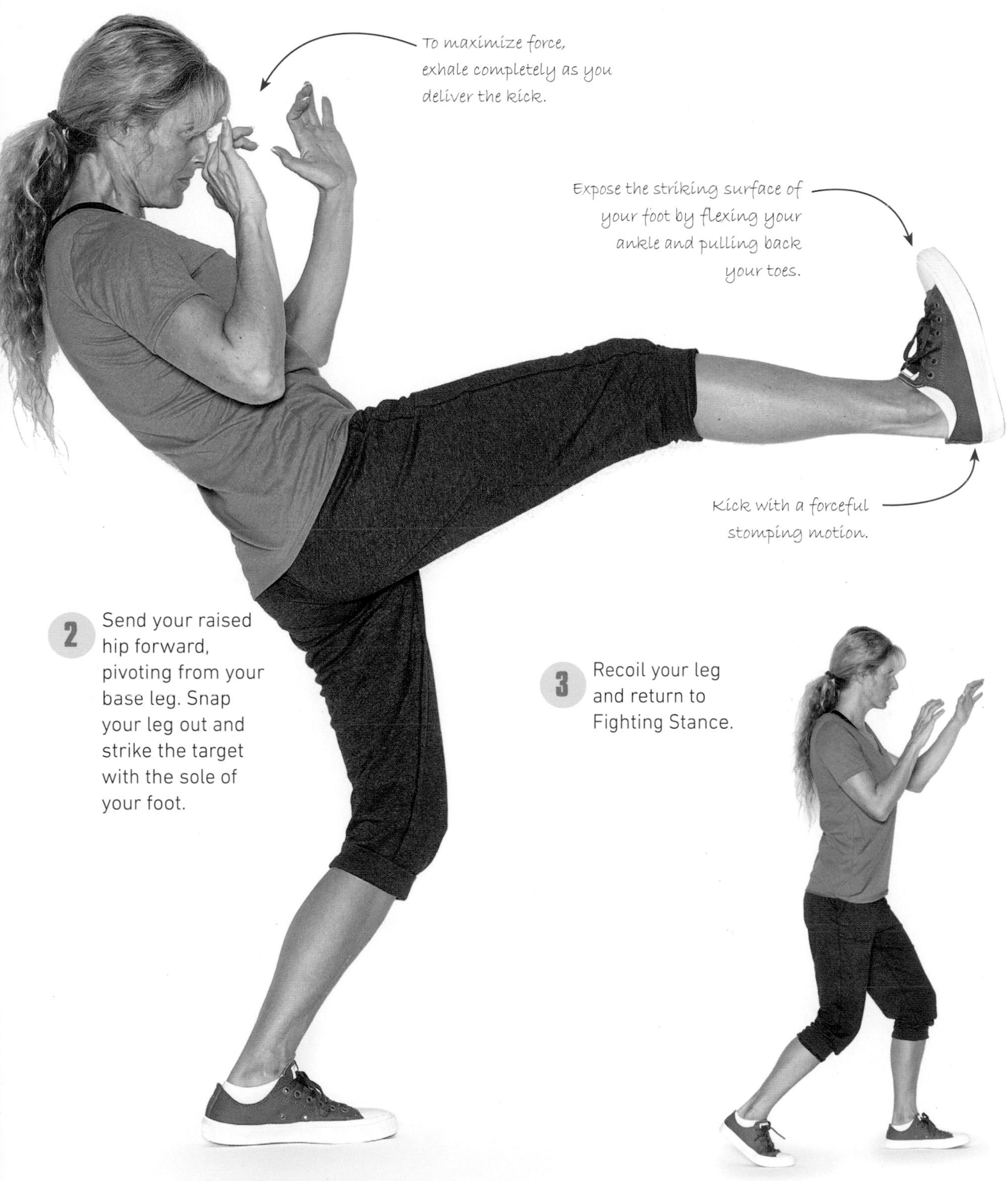

To maximize force, exhale completely as you deliver the kick.
Expose the striking surface of your foot by flexing your ankle and pulling back your toes.
Kick with a forceful stomping motion.

2 Send your raised hip forward, pivoting from your base leg. Snap your leg out and strike the target with the sole of your foot.

3 Recoil your leg and return to Fighting Stance.

Stomp Kick

With the Stomp Kick, you can stop forward progress of an attacker. You can also loosen him or her up by making a distraction strike just prior to performing a self-defense technique (such as stomping on a foot while in a bear hug).

WARNING

While the Stomp Kick can disorient your attacker, it shouldn't be treated as a finishing move. Instead, it's a technique that should be followed up with more aggressive attacks or defenses.

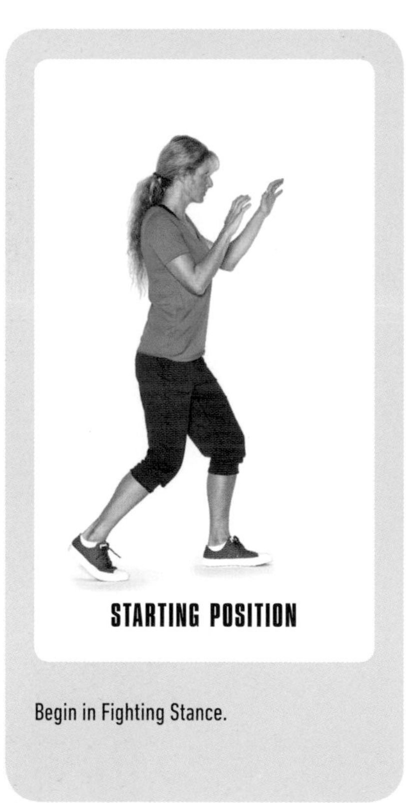

STARTING POSITION

Begin in Fighting Stance.

1. Lift your knee to waist height and pull back your foot to expose your heel.

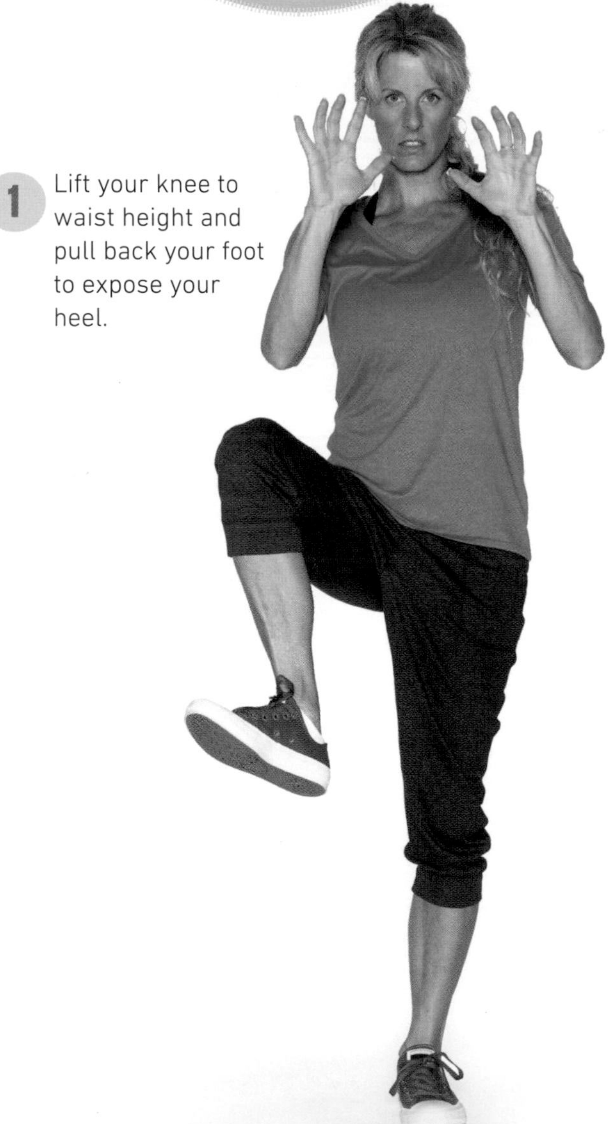

2 Stomp your heel downward onto the target.

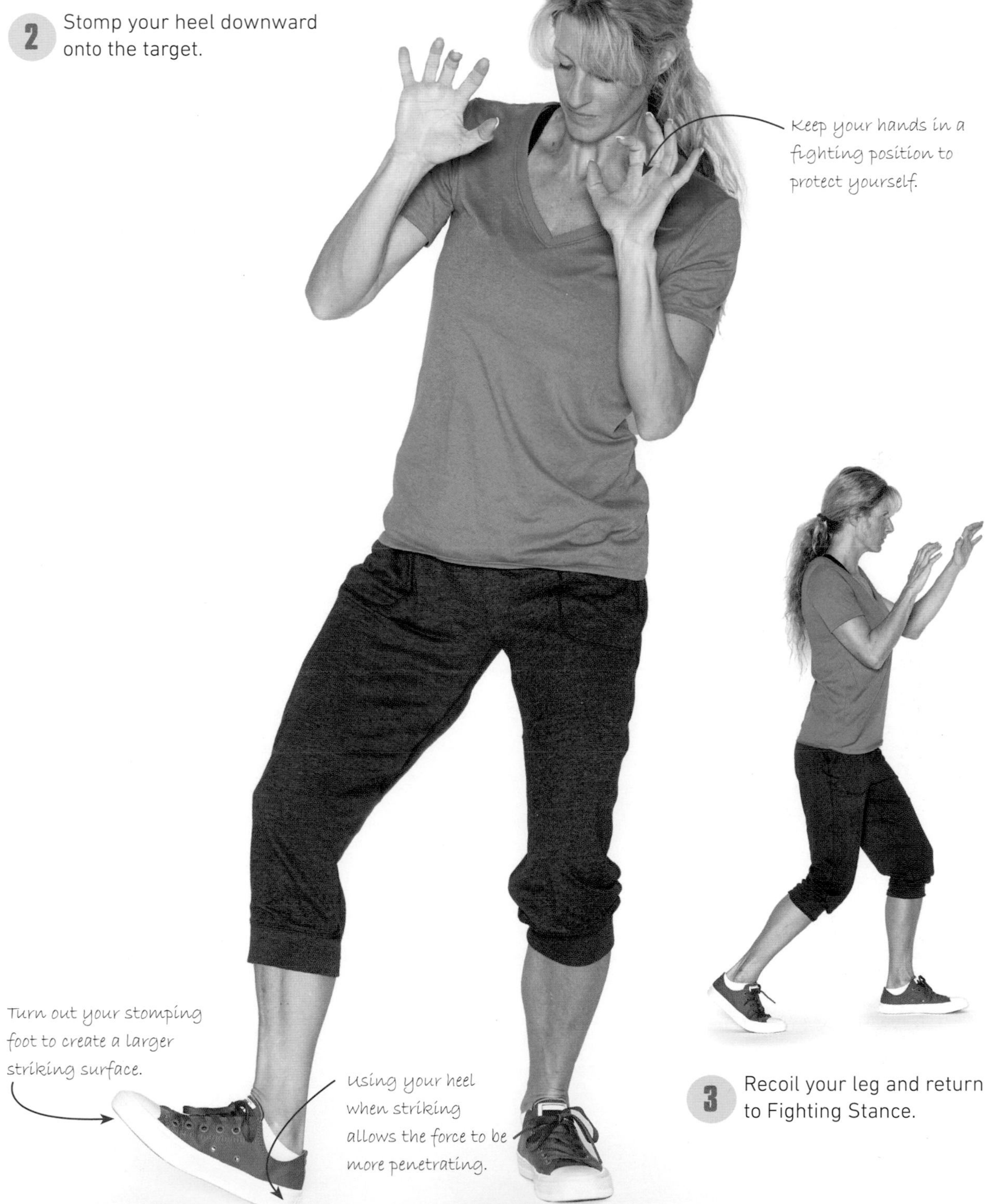

Keep your hands in a fighting position to protect yourself.
Turn out your stomping foot to create a larger striking surface.
Using your heel when striking allows the force to be more penetrating.

3 Recoil your leg and return to Fighting Stance.

Back Kick Standing

If an attacker is approaching from behind, you can use the Back Kick Standing to put some distance between the two of you and inflict damage on your attacker.

IF IT FAILS

If your kick was off target or if your attacker is larger, continue with other counterattacks such as punches, Knees, and Elbows to try to create distance. Always return to Fighting Stance in anticipation of further attack.

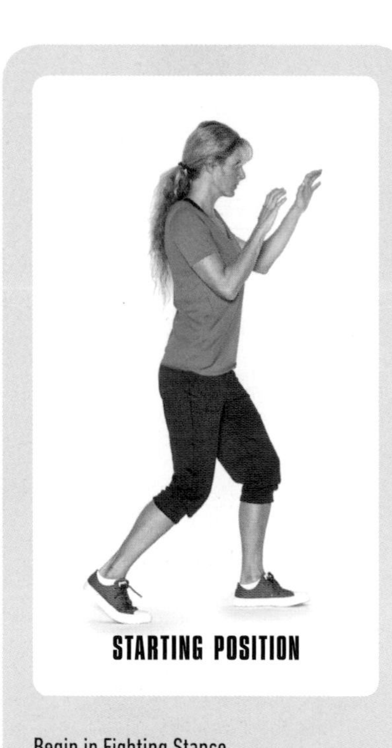

STARTING POSITION

Begin in Fighting Stance.

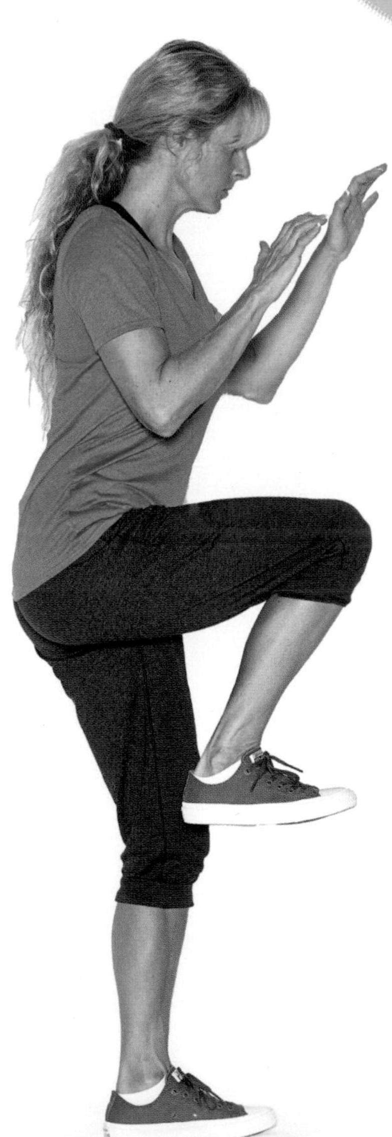

1. Lift your knee to waist height in front of you. Pull back your toes to expose your heel.

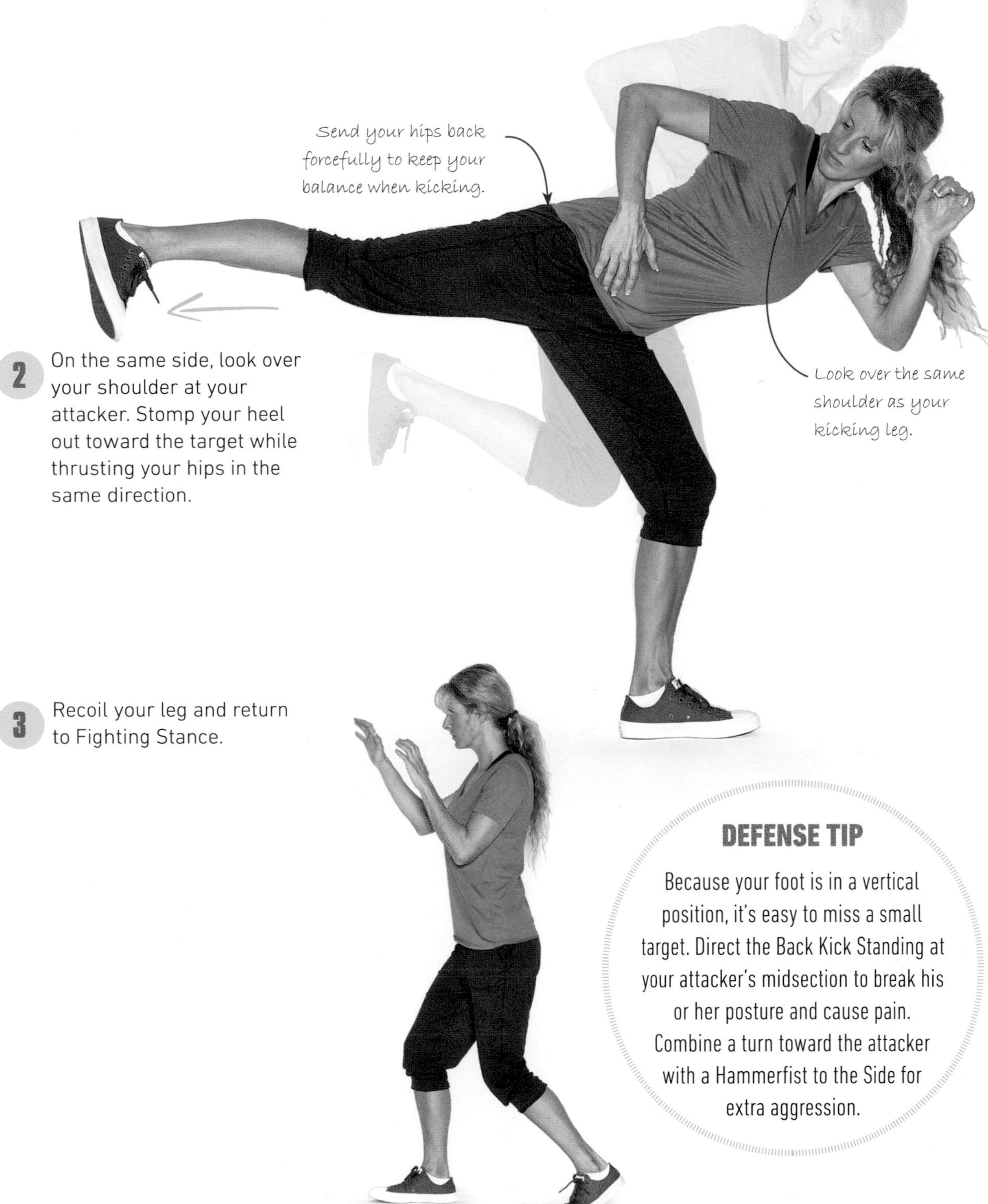

Send your hips back
forcefully to keep your
balance when kicking.
Look over the same
shoulder as your
kicking leg.

2 On the same side, look over your shoulder at your attacker. Stomp your heel out toward the target while thrusting your hips in the same direction.

3 Recoil your leg and return to Fighting Stance.

DEFENSE TIP

Because your foot is in a vertical position, it's easy to miss a small target. Direct the Back Kick Standing at your attacker's midsection to break his or her posture and cause pain. Combine a turn toward the attacker with a Hammerfist to the Side for extra aggression.

Ground Side Kick

If you find yourself lying sideways on the ground, you can deliver Ground Side Kicks up to your attacker's knees, midsection, or face.

WARNING

Particularly when you're in an extra-vulnerable position like lying on the ground sideways, you must always try to combine your defense with offensive counterattacks. One kick may not be enough. If your attacker persists, you may need to drop to the Back Position to better protect your head.

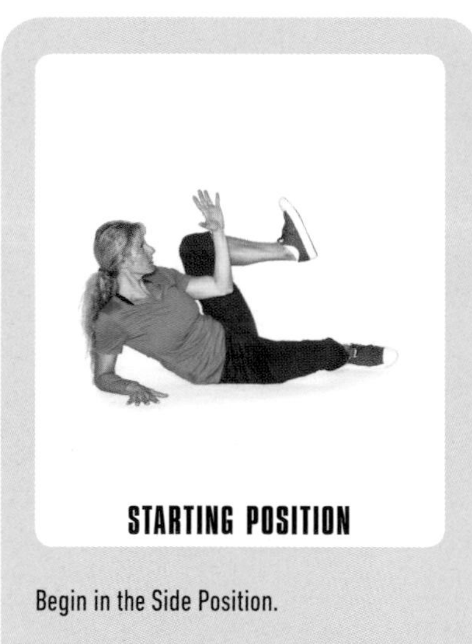

STARTING POSITION

Begin in the Side Position.

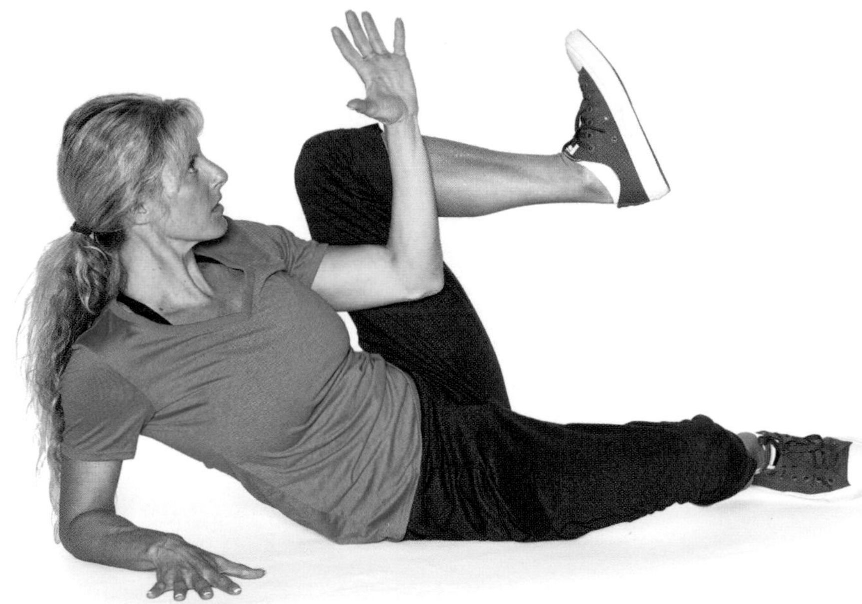

1. Lift your hips off the ground and draw your knee into your chest with your foot flexed and your toes pulled back to your shin (chambered).

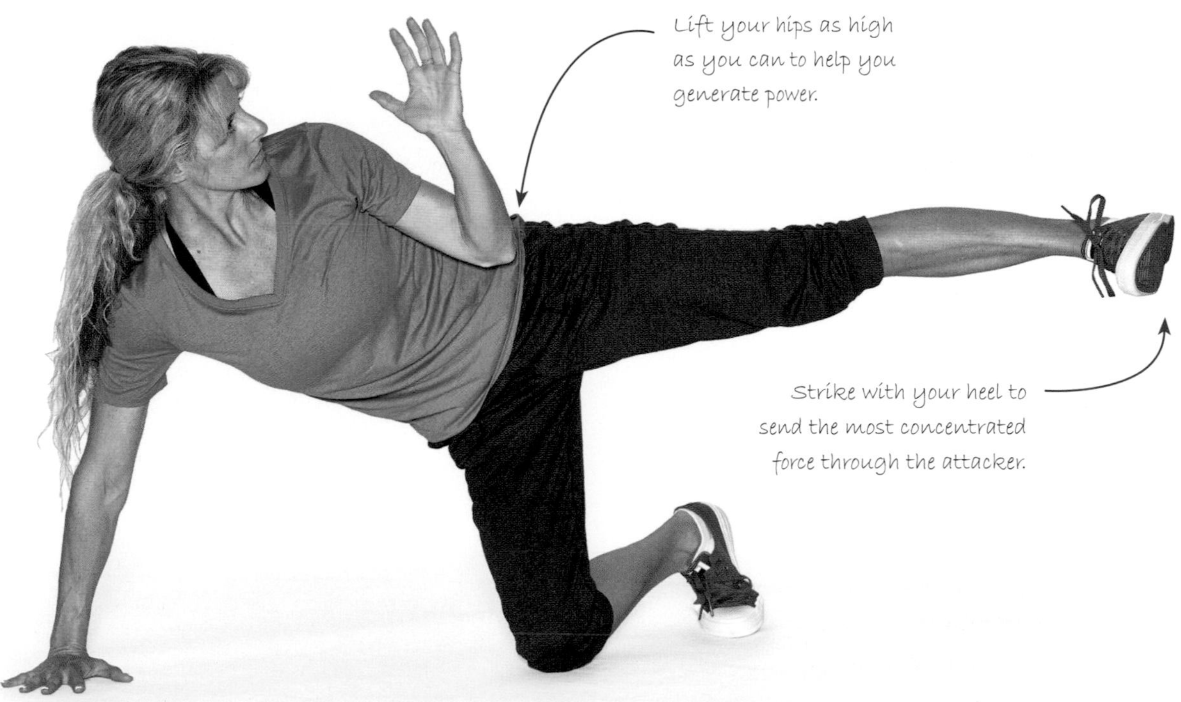

Lift your hips as high as you can to help you generate power.
Strike with your heel to send the most concentrated force through the attacker.

2 With your kicking foot horizontal to the floor, strike your heel into your attacker's knee, face, or midsection.

3 Immediately recoil your leg to the Side Position and prepare to deliver more kicks.

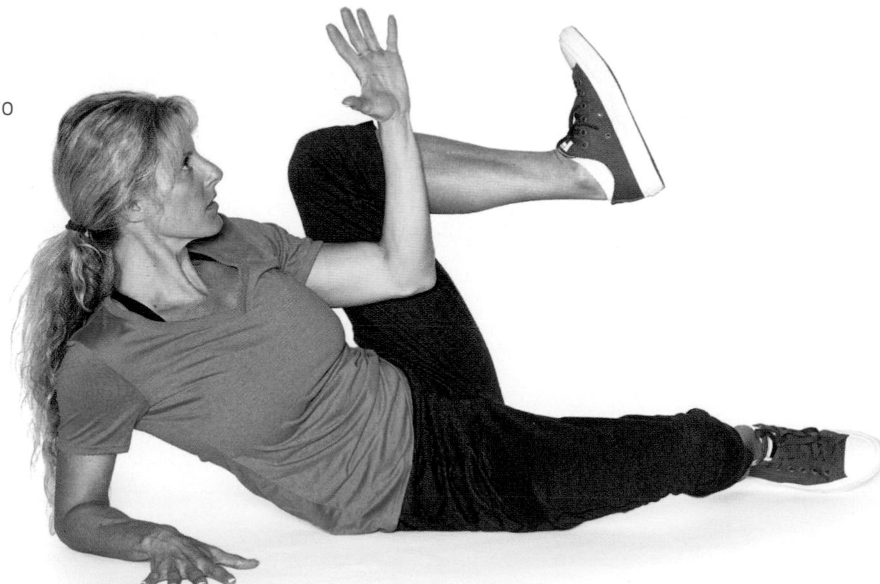

Ground Stomp Forward

When on your back in a fighting position, you can use a Ground Stomp Forward to keep your attacker at a distance and to inflict damage until you have space to get to your feet.

WARNING

Particularly when you're in a vulnerable position like lying on the ground, you must try to combine your defense with offensive counterattacks. After all, one kick may not be enough. Use movement or multiple strikes to protect your head or to get him or her to back off.

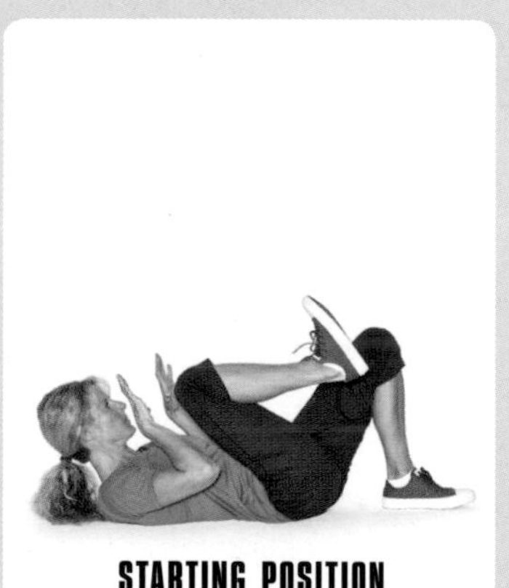

STARTING POSITION

Begin on your back with your kicking leg pulled toward your chest (chambered) and your hands in fighting position.

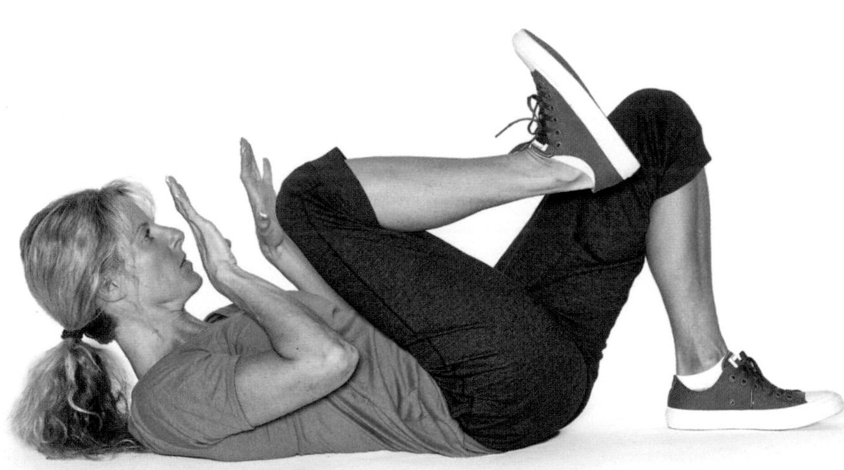

1. Tuck your chin against your chest and round your shoulders off the ground while keeping your hands in fighting position.

2 Drive your hips up using your base foot and stomp your attacker's midsection or face.

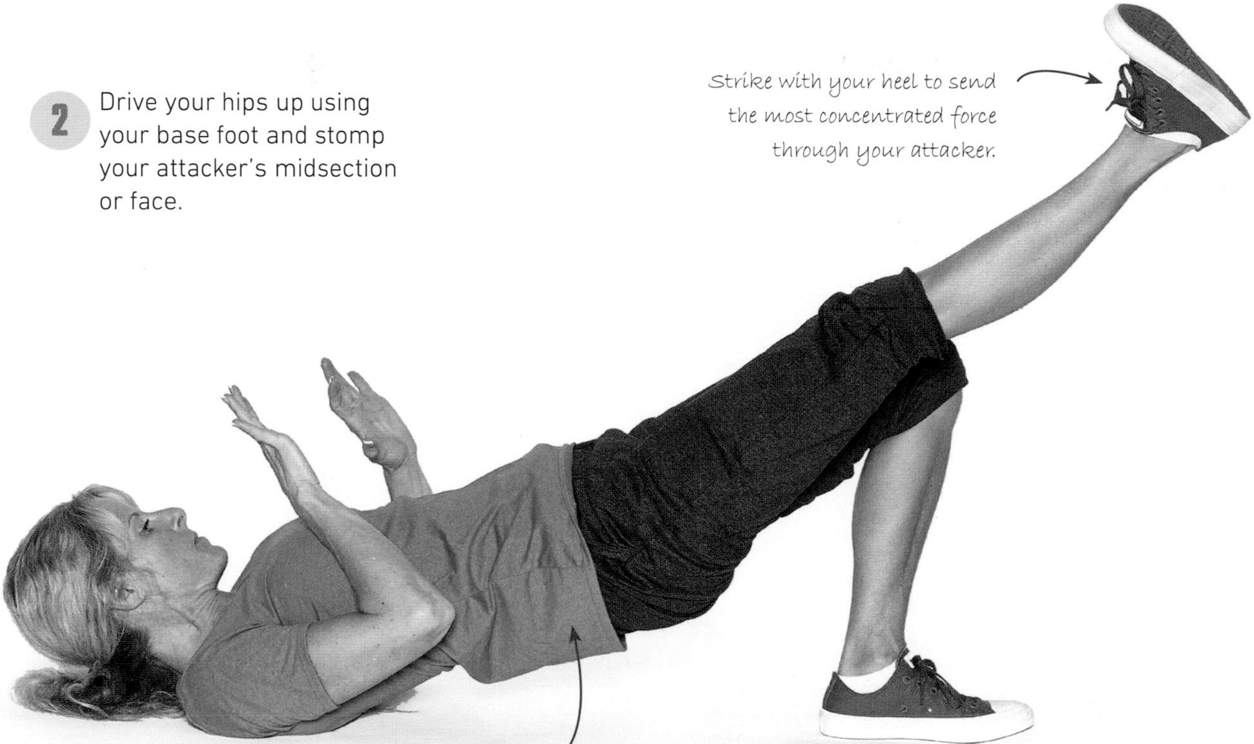

Strike with your heel to send the most concentrated force through your attacker.

Lift your hips as high as you can to help you generate power.

3 Recoil to the back fighting position and be ready to send another kick.

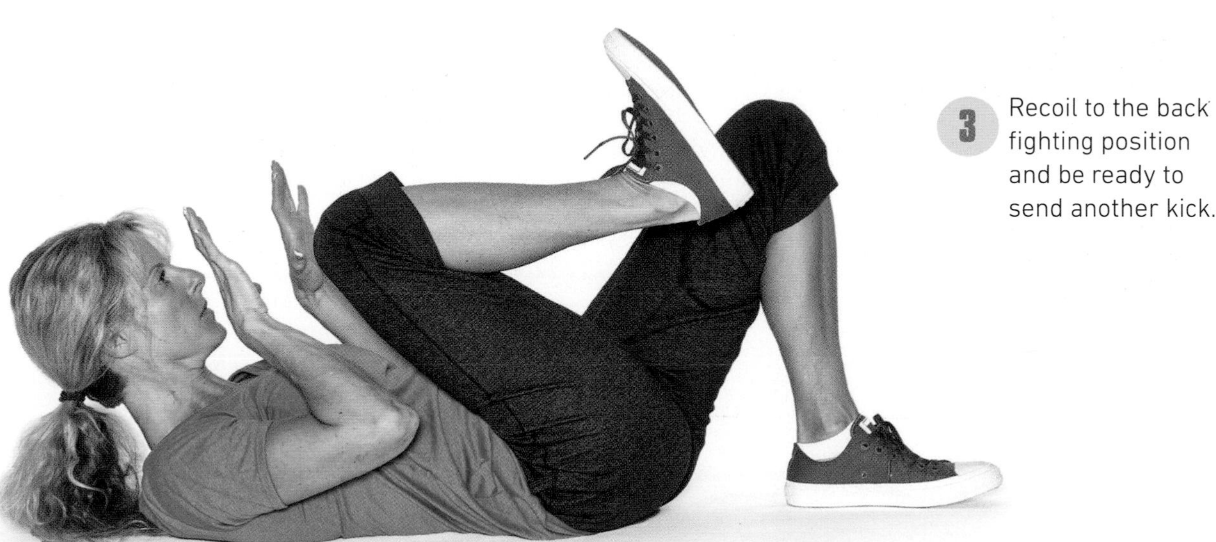

DEFENSE STRATEGIES

In certain attack situations, you may be choked or physically restrained, have your purse or backpack snatched, or confront an attack on the ground. In this section, you take the basic moves and strike fundamentals learned previously and combine them to throw off your attacker and defend yourself.

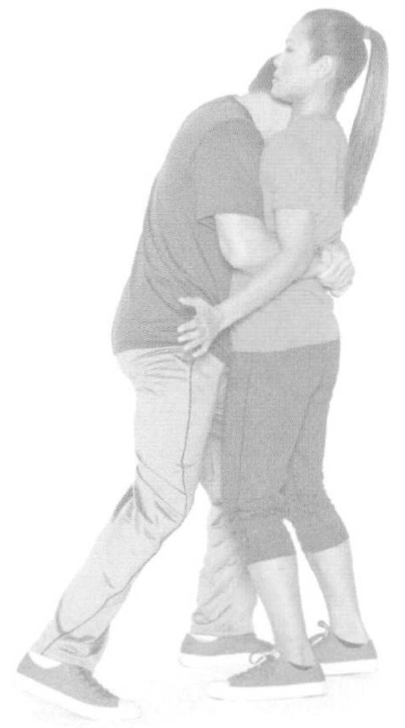

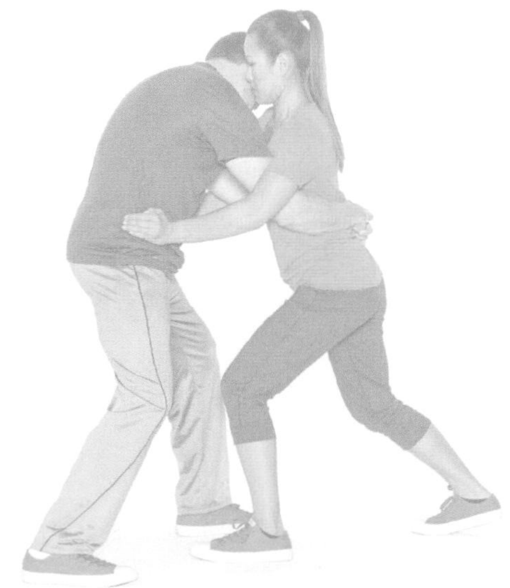

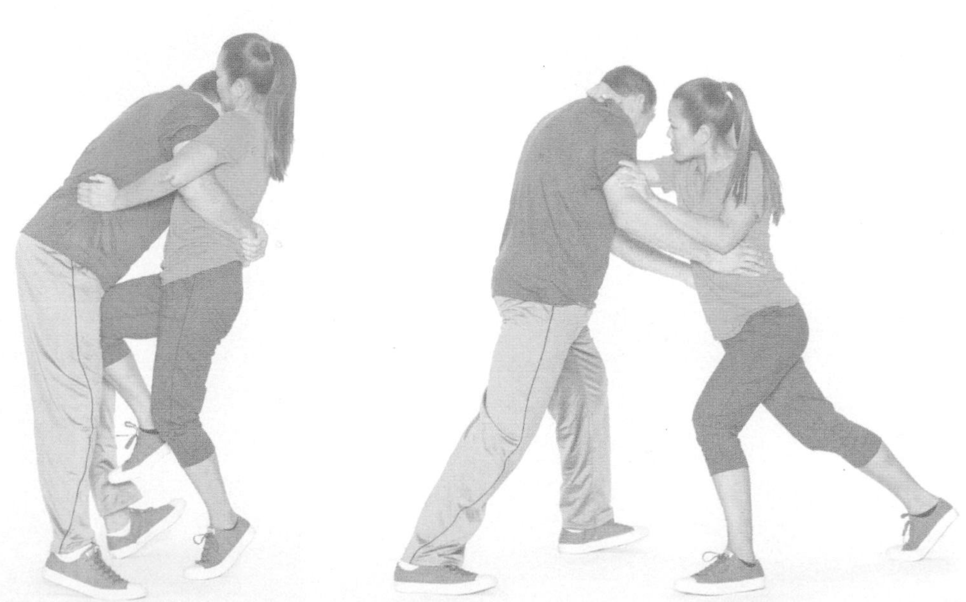

MASTERING ESCAPES

In training, you put yourself in the position of being caught to prepare for real-life scenarios. After a simulated attack from your partner, such as a choke or a bear hug, you perform a defense to escape.

Choke from the Front

This technique uses a two-handed pluck with both hands to relieve the pressure (while a one-handed pluck is equally effective, it's less instinctual than with two hands). By combining this defense with a counterattack, you reset your attacker's thought process and make it easier to further attack or to escape.

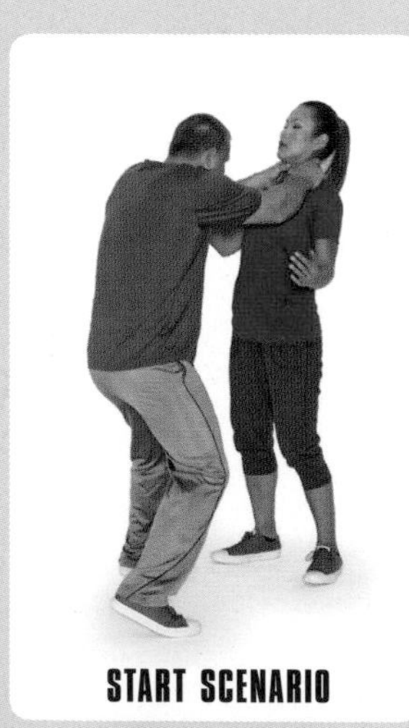

START SCENARIO

The attacker stands with feet shoulder width apart. Both hands are around your throat, thumbs crossed, making a wringing motion.

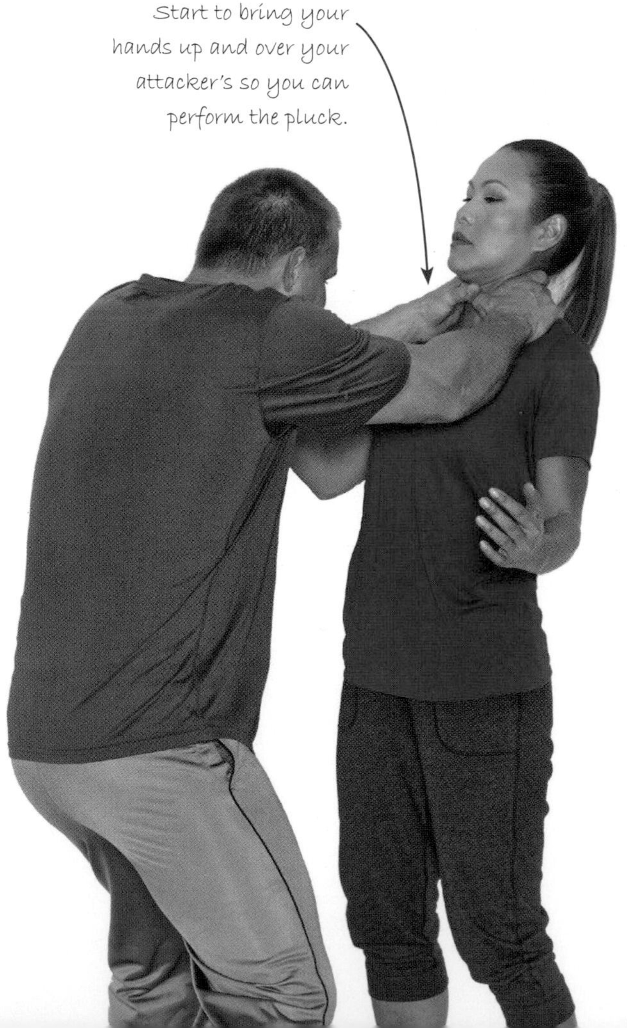

Start to bring your hands up and over your attacker's so you can perform the pluck.

1 Relying on speed (rather than strength), use both hands to explosively pluck at your attacker's thumbs by reaching deep inside where the attacker's wrists and thumbs meet and pulling up and out. Simultaneously perform a Front Kick to the Groin.

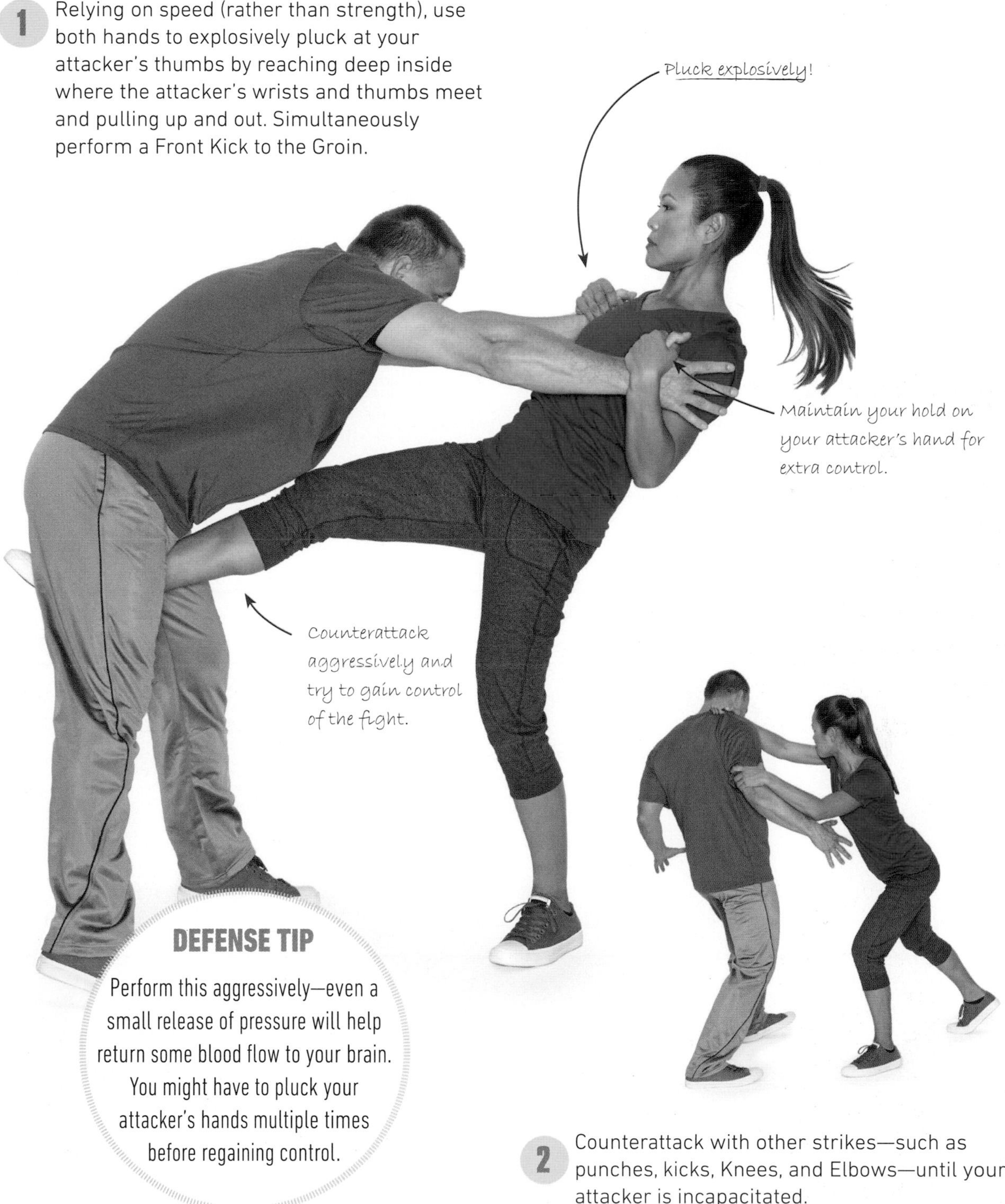

Pluck explosively!
Maintain your hold on your attacker's hand for extra control.
Counterattack aggressively and try to gain control of the fight.

DEFENSE TIP

Perform this aggressively—even a small release of pressure will help return some blood flow to your brain. You might have to pluck your attacker's hands multiple times before regaining control.

2 Counterattack with other strikes—such as punches, kicks, Knees, and Elbows—until your attacker is incapacitated.

Choke from the Side

You may find yourself next to an attacker and being choked from the side (which can happen when you turn away from an initial attack). Your attacker's arm would then partially block your instinctive reaction to bring both hands to the choke. For this escape technique, you'll use one hand to defend and your other hand to counterattack.

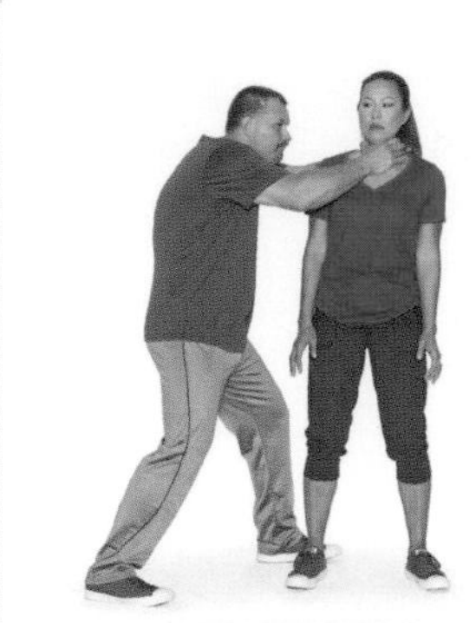

START SCENARIO

The attacker stands with feet shoulder width apart. Both hands are around your throat, with one hand in front of your neck and the other behind your neck, thumbs crossed.

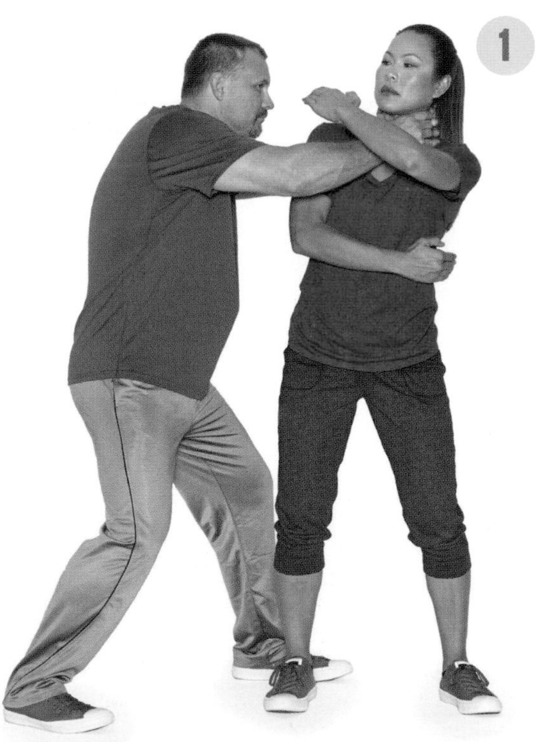

1 With your outside hand, reach past your attacker's hand and explosively pluck your attacker's thumb. With your closest hand, simultaneously deliver a Palm Strike to the groin.

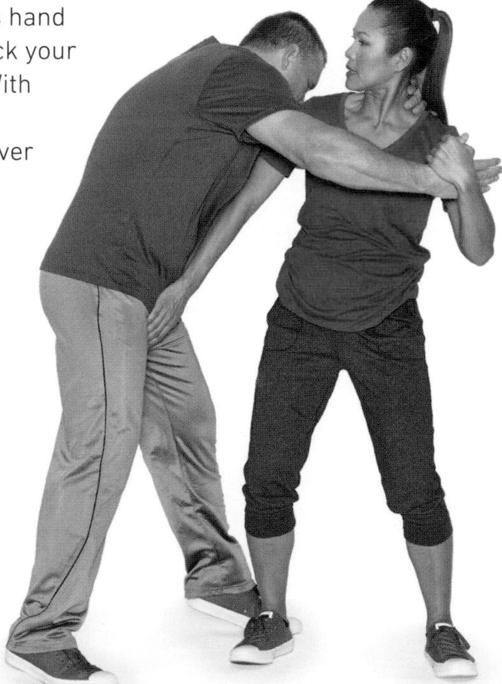

2 Turn toward your attacker and counterattack with other strikes—such as punches, kicks, Knees, and Elbows—until he or she is incapacitated.

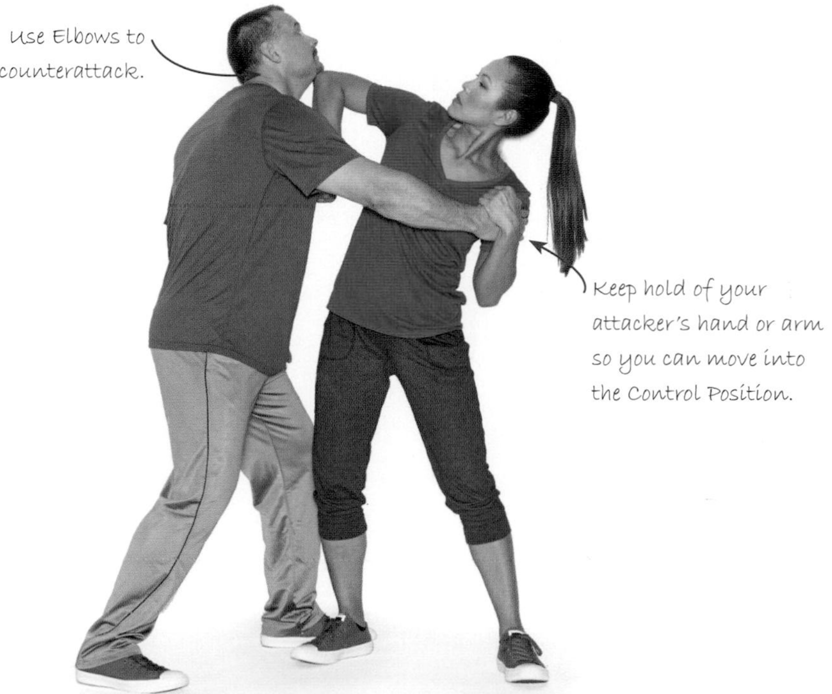
Use Elbows to counterattack.
Keep hold of your attacker's hand or arm so you can move into the Control Position.

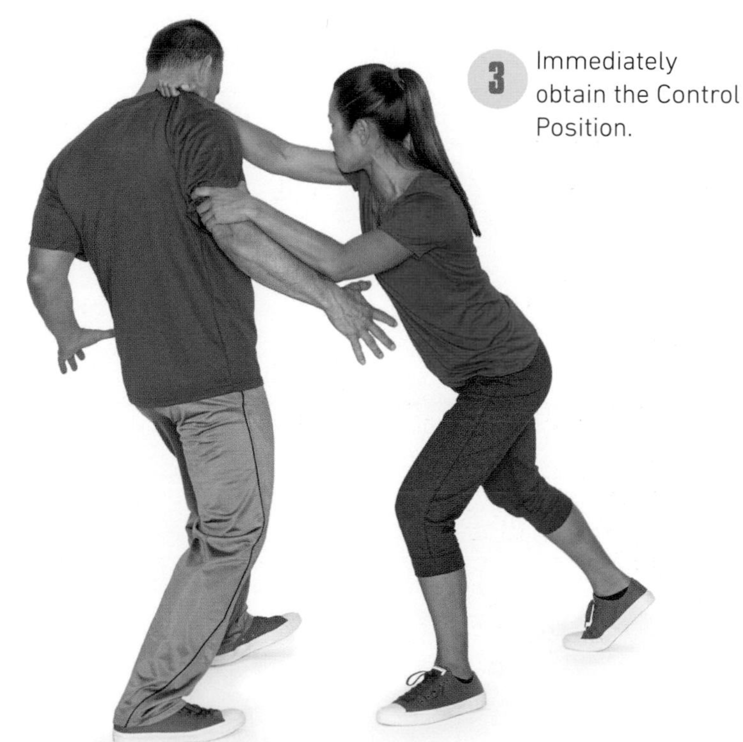

3 Immediately obtain the Control Position.

DEFENSE TIP

By using this technique to escape a choke from the side, turning toward your attacker may place you very close to him or her. This is the perfect opportunity to perform close-range strikes, like Elbows and Knees.

Choke from Behind

When you're choked from behind, you might instinctively round your shoulders and tuck in your chin. We build on this by increasing the shrug of the shoulders and tucking of the chin. This will expose your attacker's thumbs on the back of your neck and enable you to effectively pluck his or her thumbs to release the choke.

START SCENARIO

The attacker stands behind you in a strong stance and chokes you with two hands around your neck to cut off blood supply to your brain.

Reach as deeply as you can to pluck effectively.

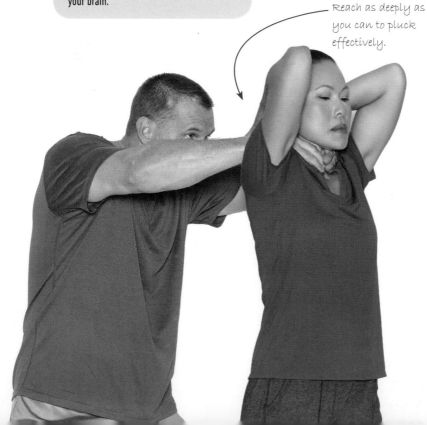

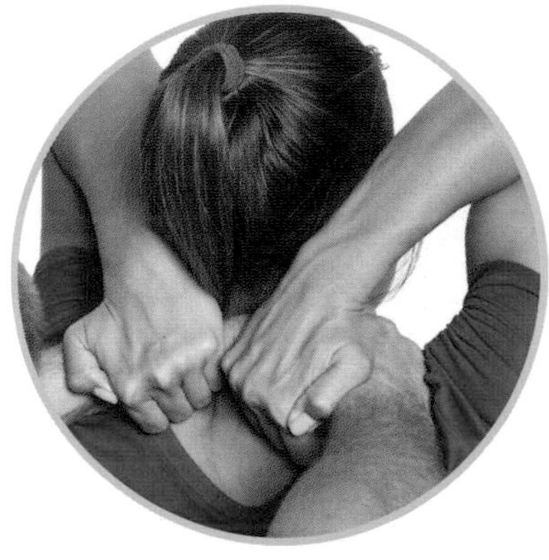

1 Tuck in your chin, round your shoulders forward, and pluck out at your attacker's thumbs with both hands.

2 Step diagonally forward and to the left while maintaining a hold on one of your attacker's hands with your left hand. Use your right hand to perform a Palm Strike to the groin.

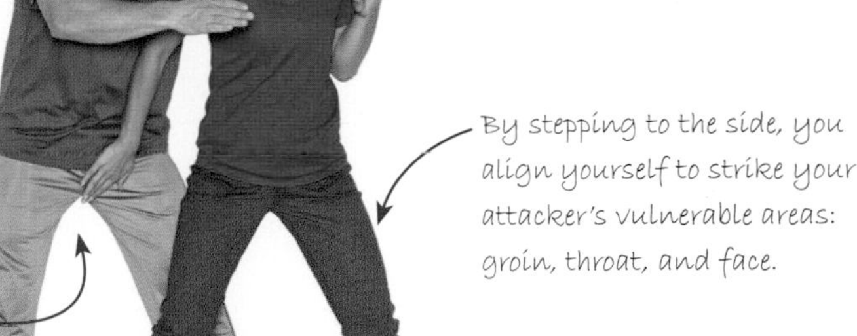

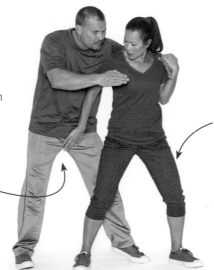

By stepping to the side, you align yourself to strike your attacker's vulnerable areas: groin, throat, and face.

Strike with an open palm to maximize the surface area.

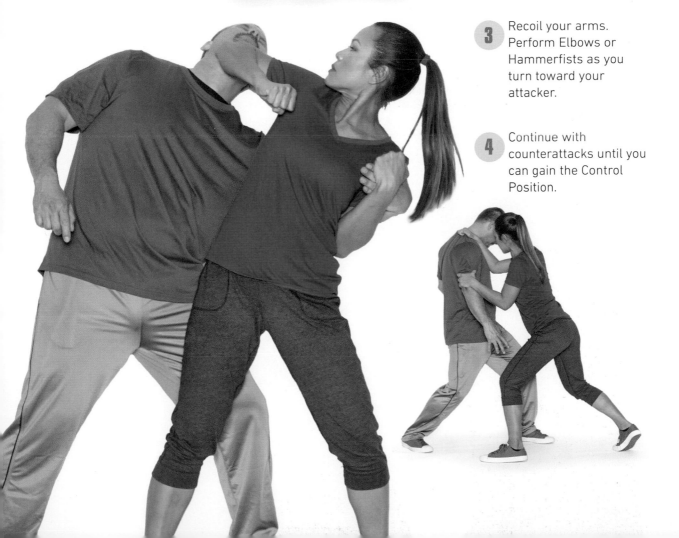

3 Recoil your arms. Perform Elbows or Hammerfists as you turn toward your attacker.

4 Continue with counterattacks until you can gain the Control Position.

Choke Against the Wall (From the Front)

If an attacker throws your back to a wall and chokes you, your arms won't be free to use a pluck to escape. This escape uses a turning technique instead to clear an attacker's hands from your throat.

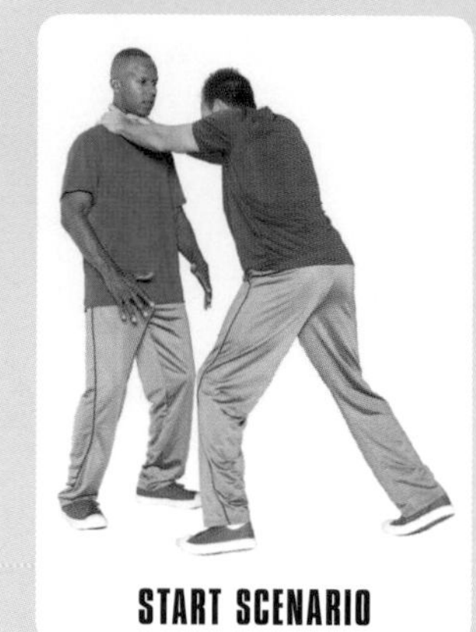

START SCENARIO

The attacker pushes you back by driving you toward a wall with his or her hands around your neck.

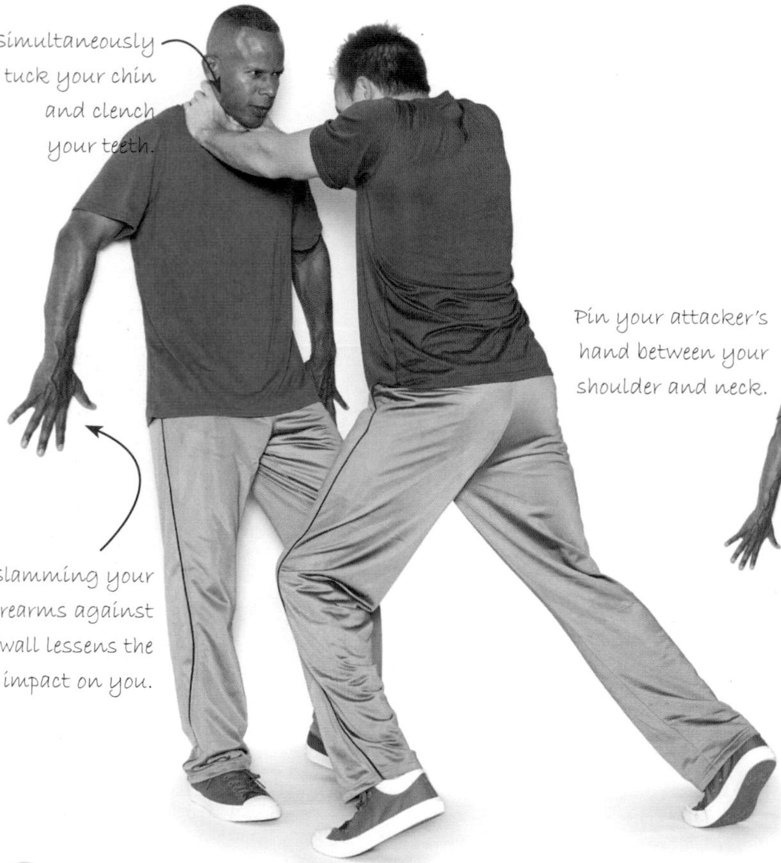

Simultaneously tuck your chin and clench your teeth.

Slamming your forearms against the wall lessens the impact on you.

Pin your attacker's hand between your shoulder and neck.

1. On impact, slam your forearms and hands into the wall to minimize the force to your body.

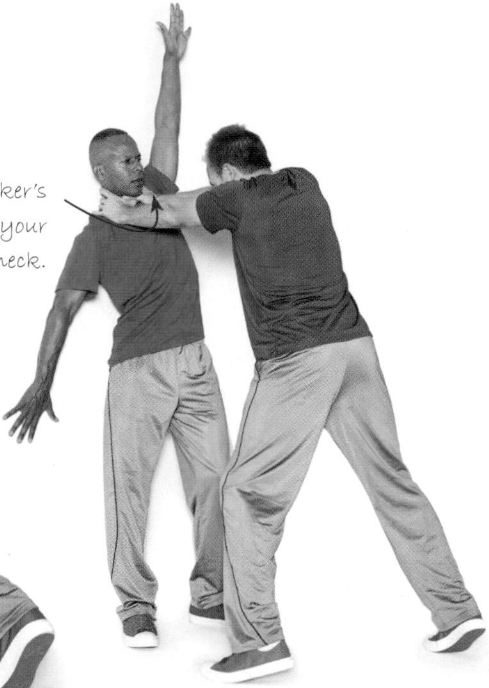

2. Send one arm straight up and touch your hand to the wall above you. Send your other arm straight down and touch your hand to the wall below you.

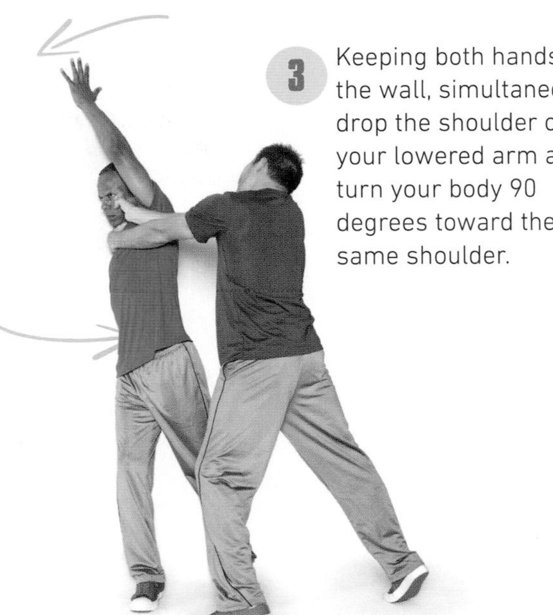

3 Keeping both hands on the wall, simultaneously drop the shoulder of your lowered arm and turn your body 90 degrees toward the same shoulder.

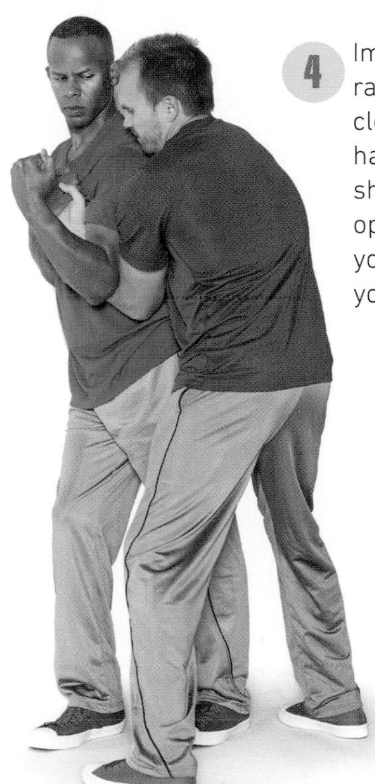

4 Immediately throw your raised arm forward to clear your attacker's hands with your shoulder. Use your opposite hand to trap your attacker's hands to your chest.

5 Turn back toward your attacker and throw an Elbows To the Side.

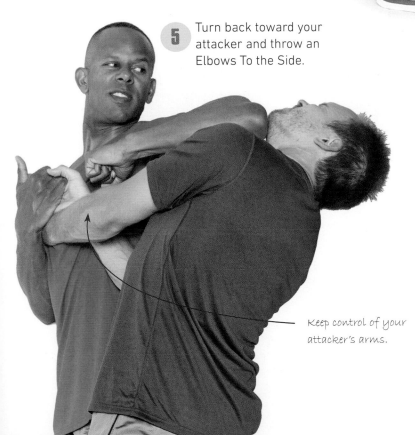

Keep control of your attacker's arms.

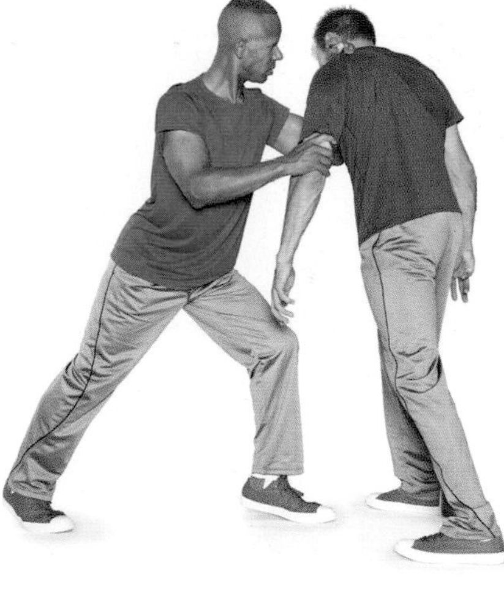

6 Obtain the Control Position and deliver Knees. You can also quickly turn toward your attacker and drive him or her into the wall.

Choke Against the Wall (From Behind)

An attacker might disorient you by spinning your body and choking you face-forward against a wall. Use this turning technique to escape the choke and flee the attack.

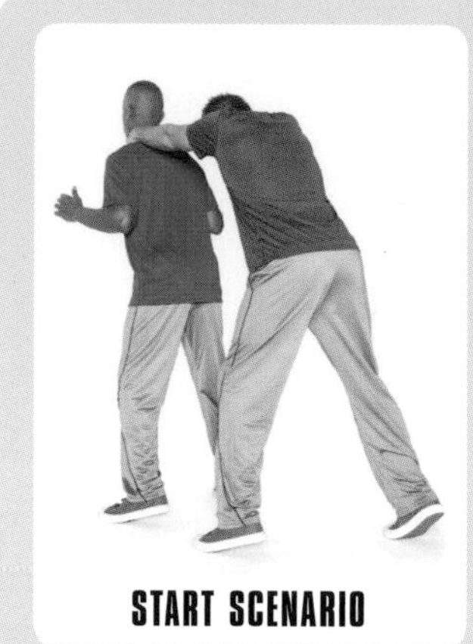

START SCENARIO

Your attacker chokes and pushes you against the wall with a two-handed choke to your throat.

1 On impact, slam your forearms and hands into the wall to minimize the force to your body.

Slam the wall with your hands and forearms.

2 Send one arm straight up and touch your hand to the wall above you. Send your other arm straight down and touch your hand to the wall below you.

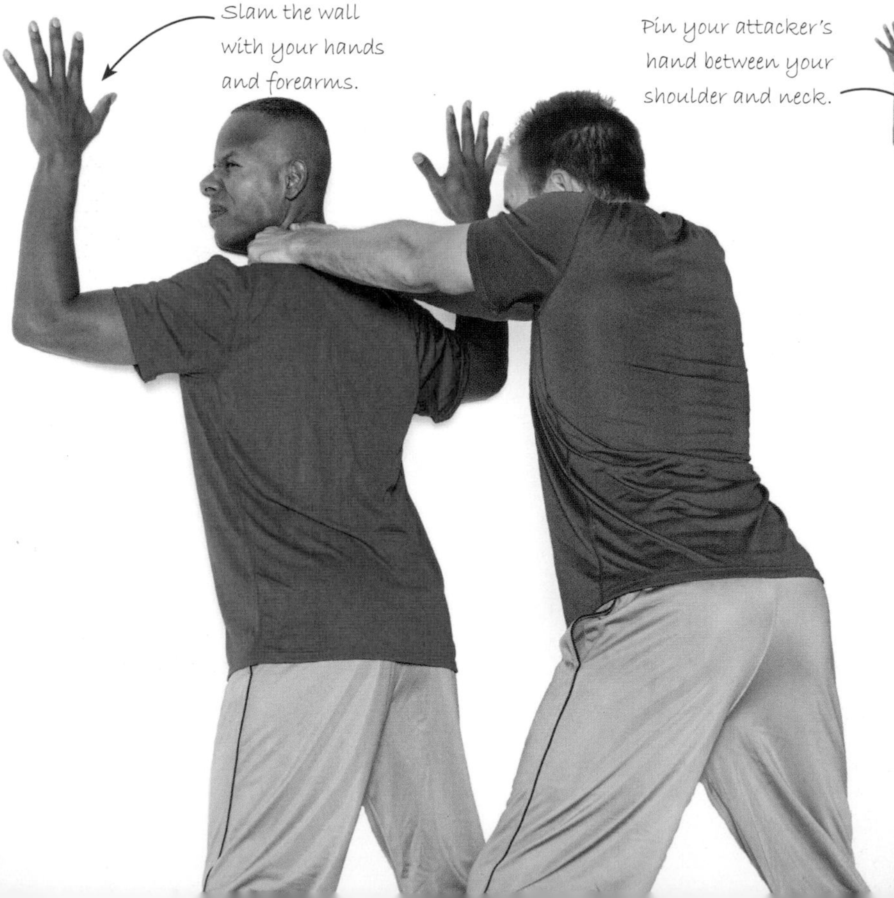

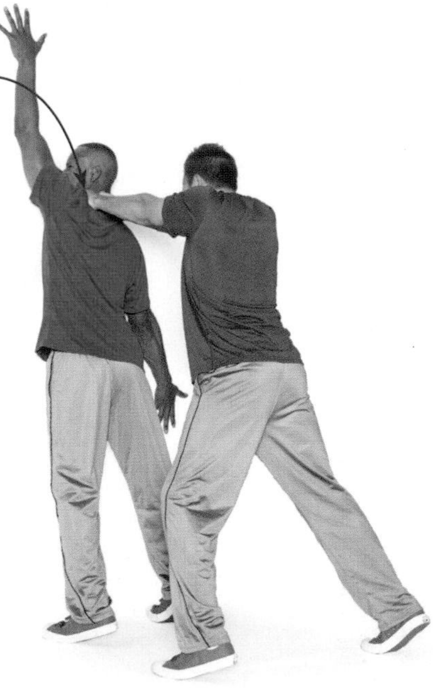

Pin your attacker's hand between your shoulder and neck.

3 Keeping both hands on the wall, simultaneously drop the shoulder of your lowered arm and turn your body 180 degrees toward the same shoulder.

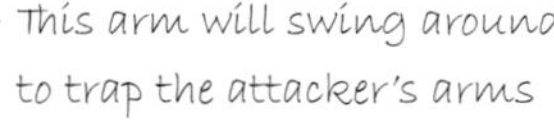
This arm will swing around
to trap the attacker's arms

Turn sharply and drop your shoulder dramatically to lower yourself as much as possible.

DEFENSE TIP

Being thrown face first into a wall can be scary. You can prepare yourself by remembering these steps:

- Turn quickly.
- Clear your attacker's hands.
- Counterattack repeatedly.

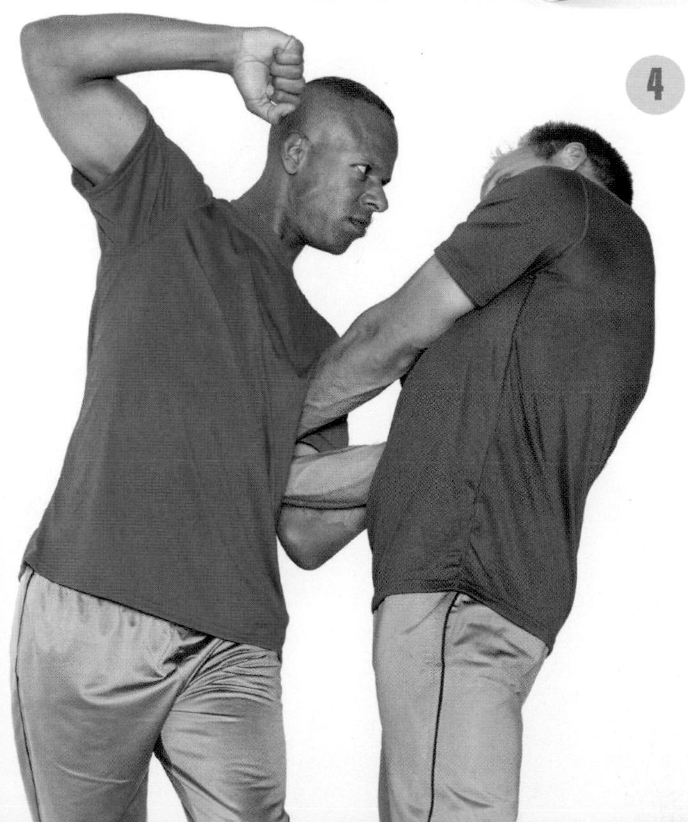

4 Immediately turn 180 degrees and bring your elbow straight down toward your attacker's forearms to clear his or her hands with your shoulder. Use your opposite hand to Hammerfist your attacker's face.

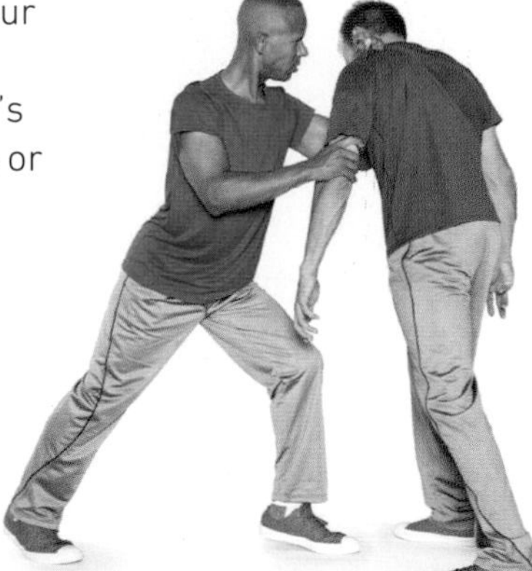

5 Obtain the Control Position and deliver Knees.

Headlock from Behind (Rear Naked Choke)

A headlock and choke from behind is common, especially with the increased popularity of Brazilian jujitsu techniques. This escape uses a pluck to slide your head out of the hold.

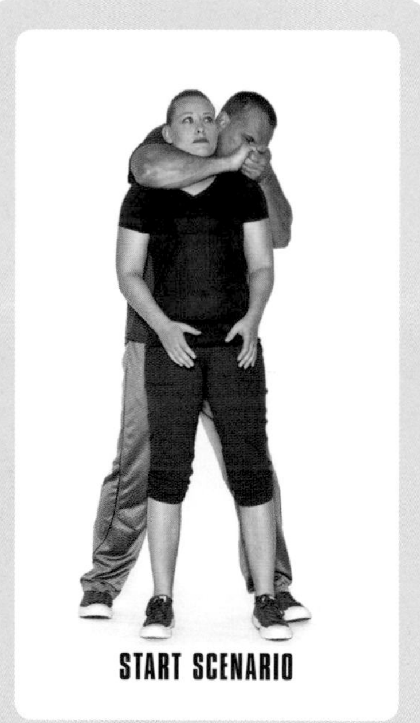

START SCENARIO

The attacker slides an arm under your chin so his or her elbow aligns directly under your chin. The forearm is on one side of your throat, while the bicep on the other side is cutting off your blood supply.

1 As you feel the attack begin, immediately pull your chin downward and turn it toward your attacker, in the opposite direction of his or her elbows. Throw your hands upward and backward, past your attacker's hands.

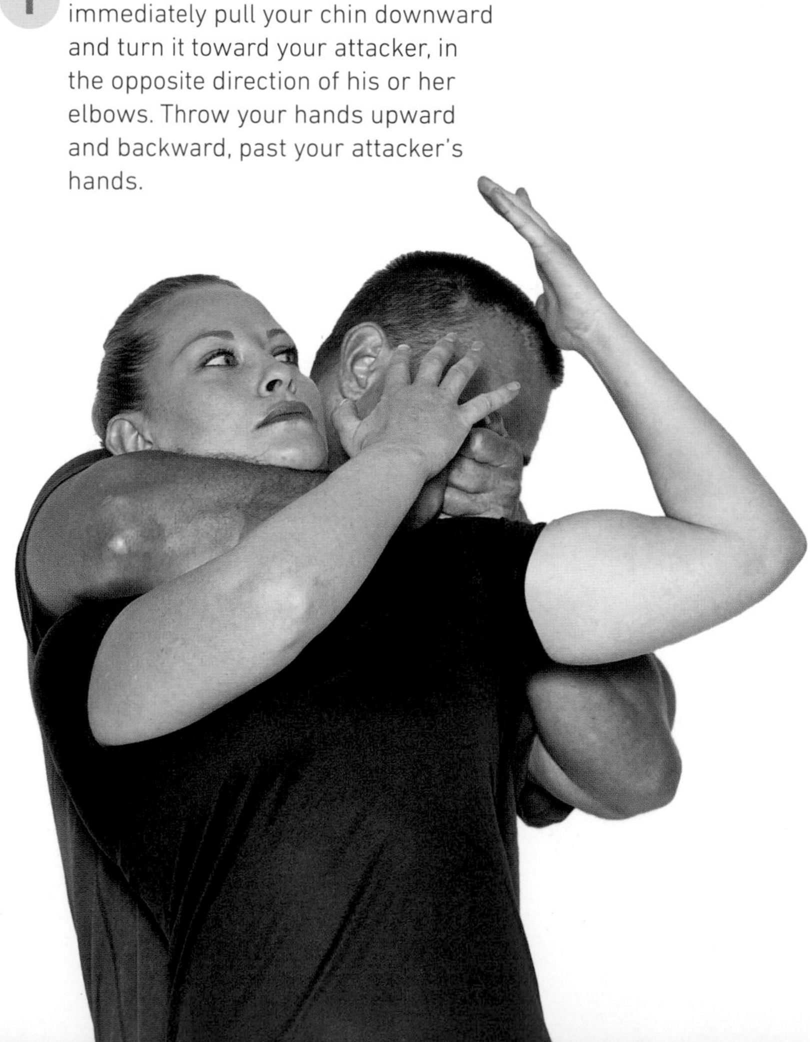

2 Pluck down at a 90-degree angle to your attacker's thumbs, pulling your hands straight down toward your chest.

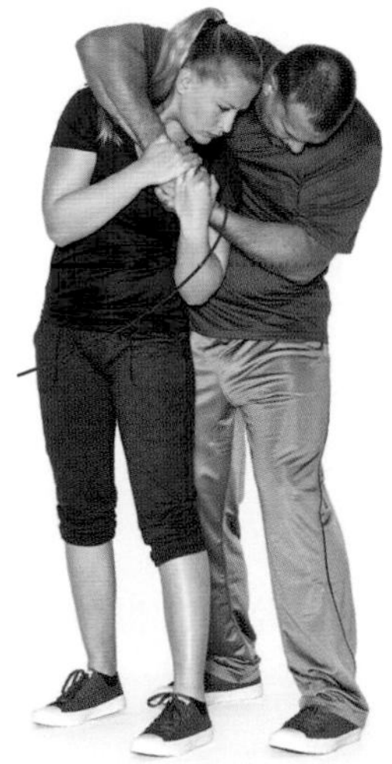

As you turn in toward your attacker, sharply punch your shoulder into your attacker's chest to create space.

3 Maintain your hold on your attacker's hands and slide your head out of the opening.

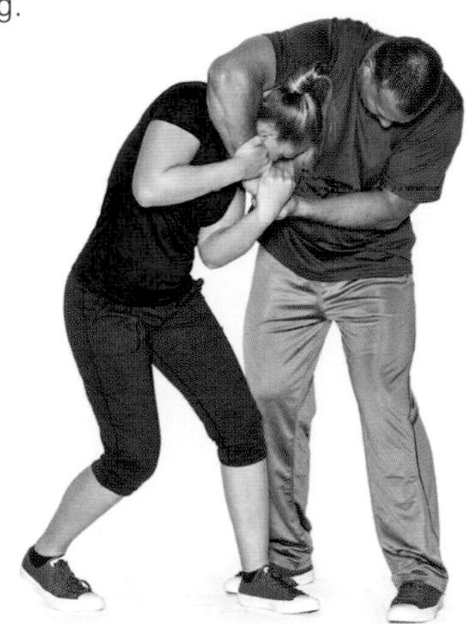

4 As soon as you free your head, assume the Control Position and counterattack.

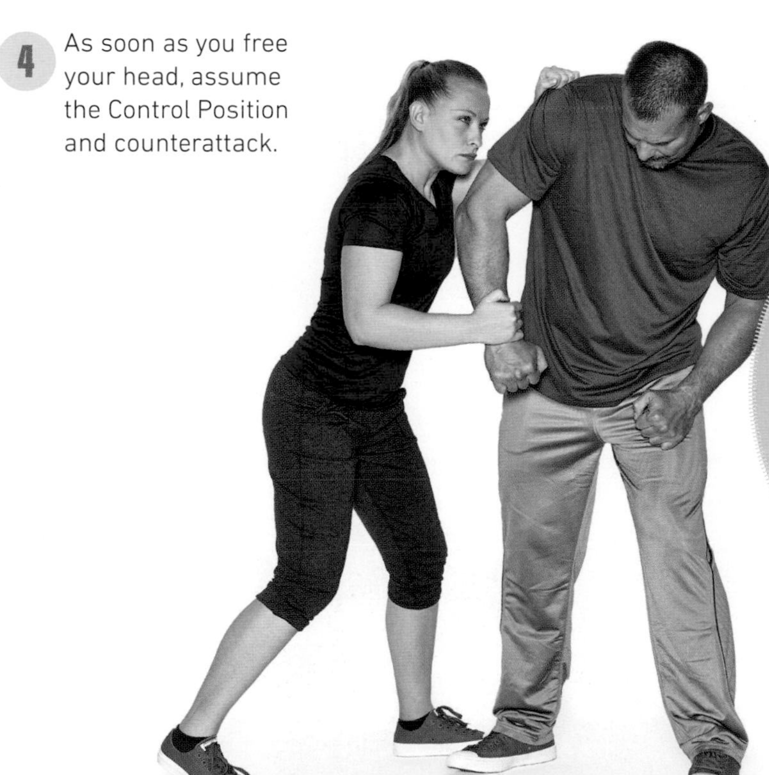

IF IT FAILS

The Headlock from Behind (Rear Naked Choke) blocks blood flow to the brain. By turning your head, you maintain minimal blood flow, which is necessary to escape. If your first pluck fails, continue until you can create enough space to slide out of the headlock.

Headlock from the Side

Often called the *schoolyard attack*, the Headlock from the Side is a common way for attackers to gain control. This escape technique uses the momentum of the attack to assist and enable you to twist out of the headlock and strike.

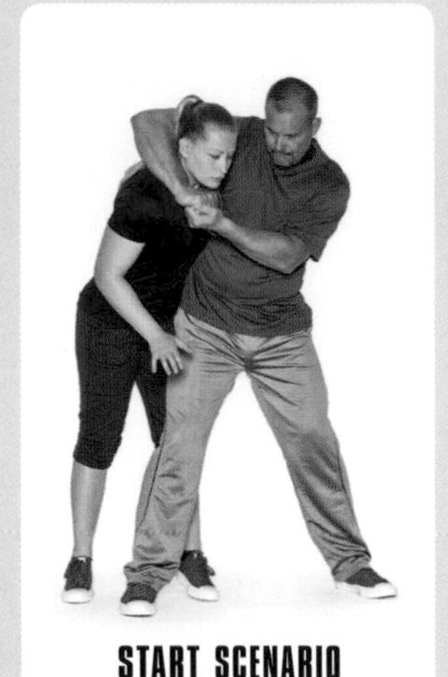

START SCENARIO

Your attacker steps in front of your left side and simultaneously grabs you around your neck, with his or her right arm pulling down and in.

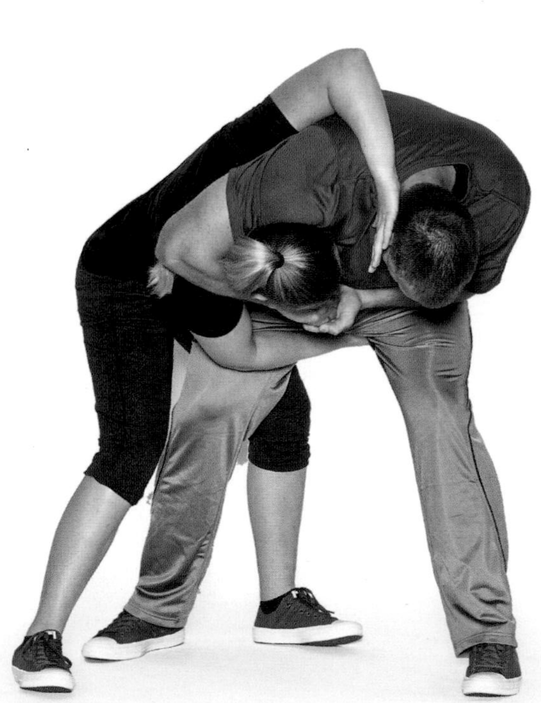

1 With the momentum of your attacker's pull, turn your chin downward and inward toward your attacker. Simultaneously take a large step forward and drop your weight.

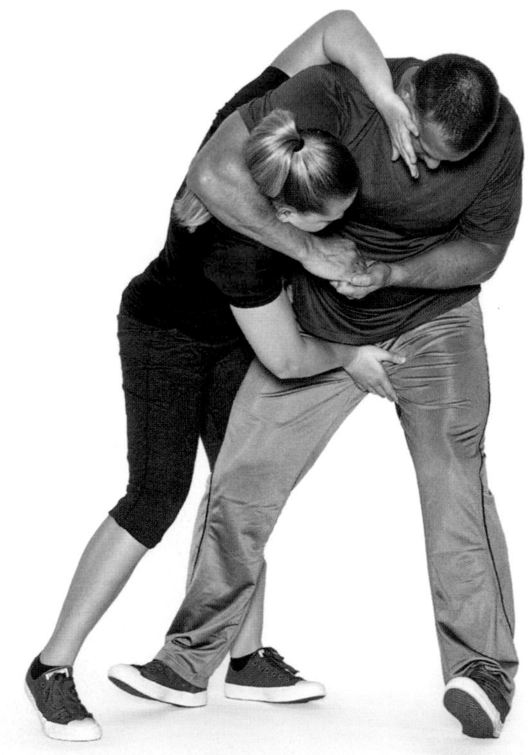

2 As you step, swing your outside arm to perform a Palm Strike to the groin. Take your inside hand and grab a vulnerable part of your attacker's head.

3 Place your thumb under your attacker's chin and your index finger under his or her nose. With your inside hand, pull your inside elbow to your hip, and stand up straight to sharply lift your attacker's chin.

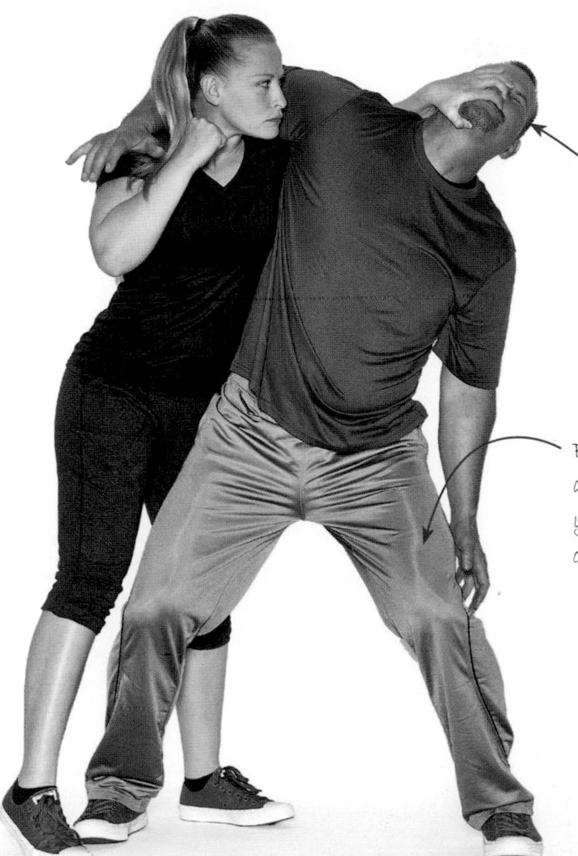

To avoid being bitten, don't place your hand over your attacker's mouth. Instead, grab at eyes, handfuls of hair, or the neck.

By throwing your attacker's head backward, you attempt to disrupt his or her balance.

4 Immediately deliver counterstrikes to your attacker's face or throat.

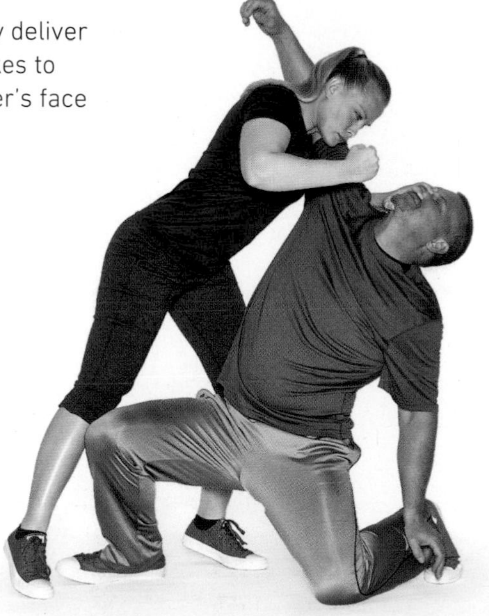

IF IT FAILS

If your escape fails, continue with Palm Strikes to the groin. Deliver repeated counterattacks until you disrupt your attacker's balance or hold. Keep moving until you're in the Control Position.

Bear Hug from the Front (Arms Free)

An attacker may try to carry you away or throw you to the ground by crashing into you and grabbing you in a bear hug. Using this technique to escape, you drop your weight into a stable base and create space between yourself and your attacker.

START SCENARIO

Your attacker attempts to move you to another location by grabbing you in a bear hug around your middle, keeping your arms free.

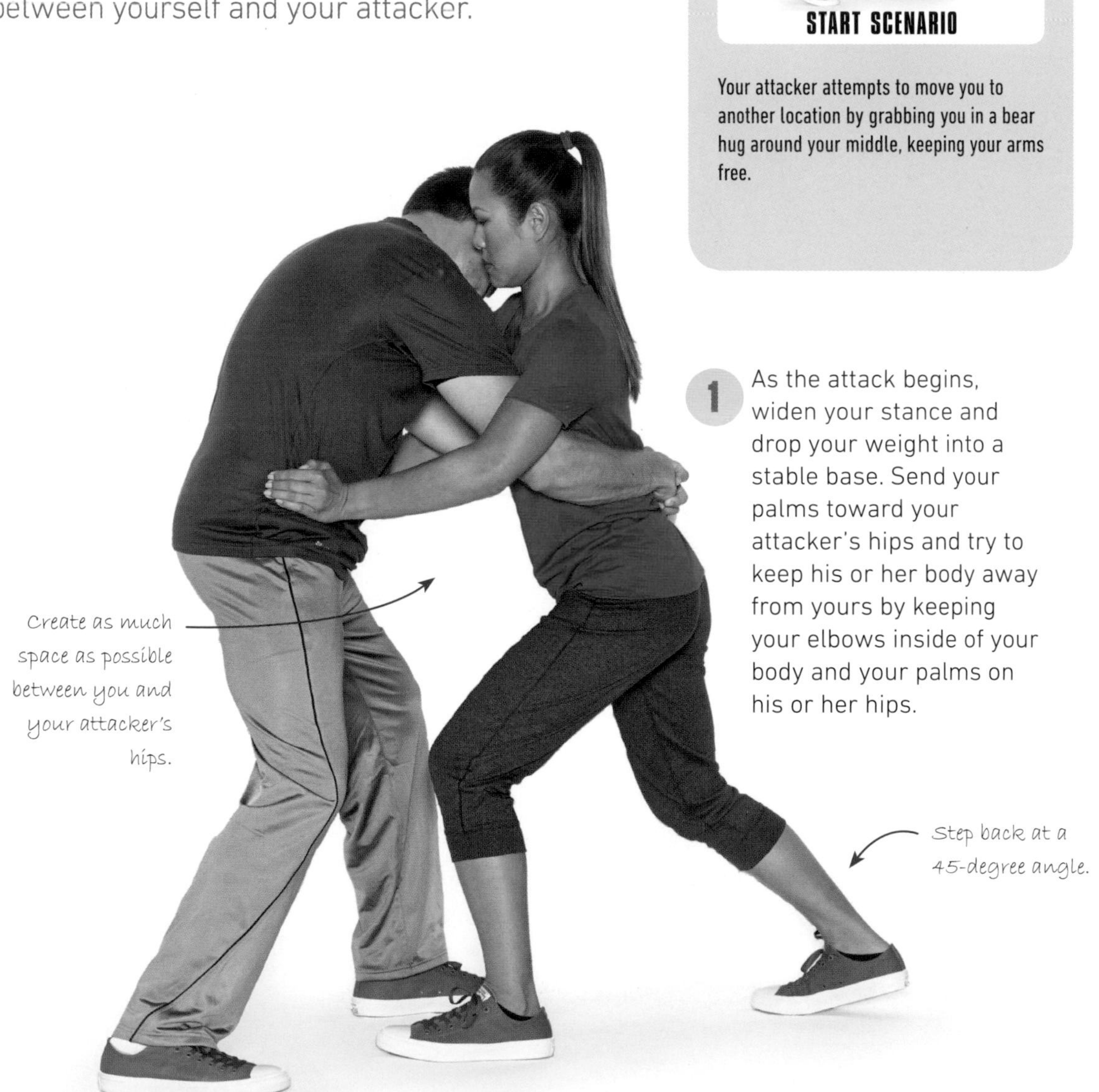

Create as much space as possible between you and your attacker's hips.
Step back at a 45-degree angle.

1. As the attack begins, widen your stance and drop your weight into a stable base. Send your palms toward your attacker's hips and try to keep his or her body away from yours by keeping your elbows inside of your body and your palms on his or her hips.

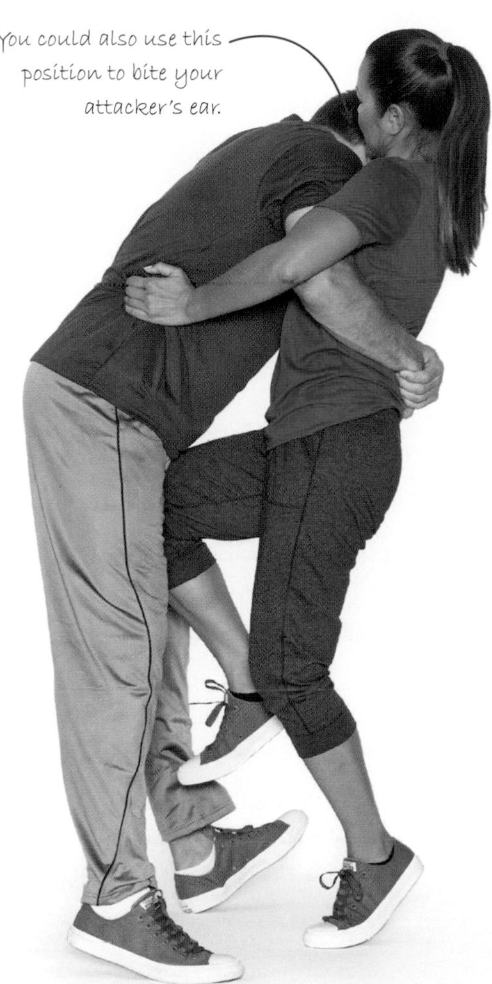

You could also use this position to bite your attacker's ear.

2 Counterattack with repeated Knees to the groin or midsection.

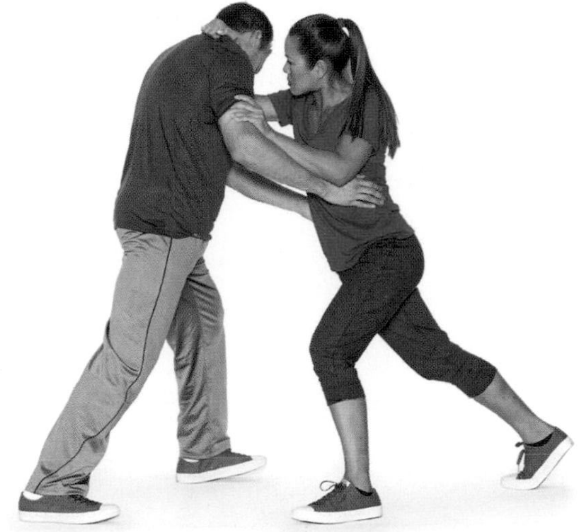

3 Once you have created space, bring your inside arm—the arm that's in the center of his or her body—up into the Control Position.

DEFENSE TIP

While this attack can come quickly, you don't have to wait to be grabbed to begin protecting yourself. If you're aware of the attack early, try delivering strikes on the way in, or go straight to the Control Position and begin counterattacking.

Bear Hug from the Front (Arms Caught)

When an attacker traps you and your arms in a bear hug, you must drop your weight into a stable base and create space between yourself and him or her. This technique then exploits your attacker's most vulnerable area—the groin—to enable your escape.

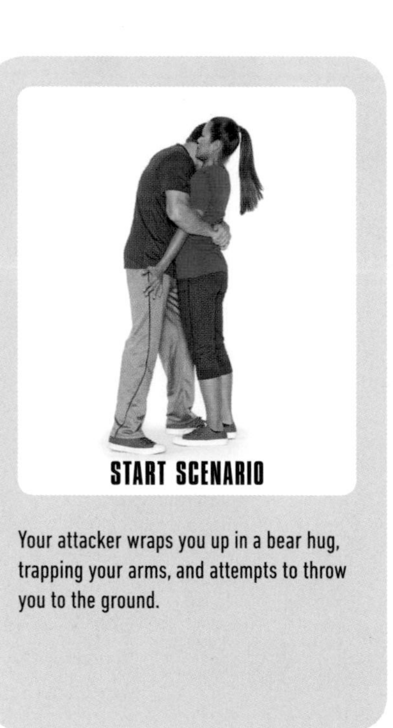

START SCENARIO

Your attacker wraps you up in a bear hug, trapping your arms, and attempts to throw you to the ground.

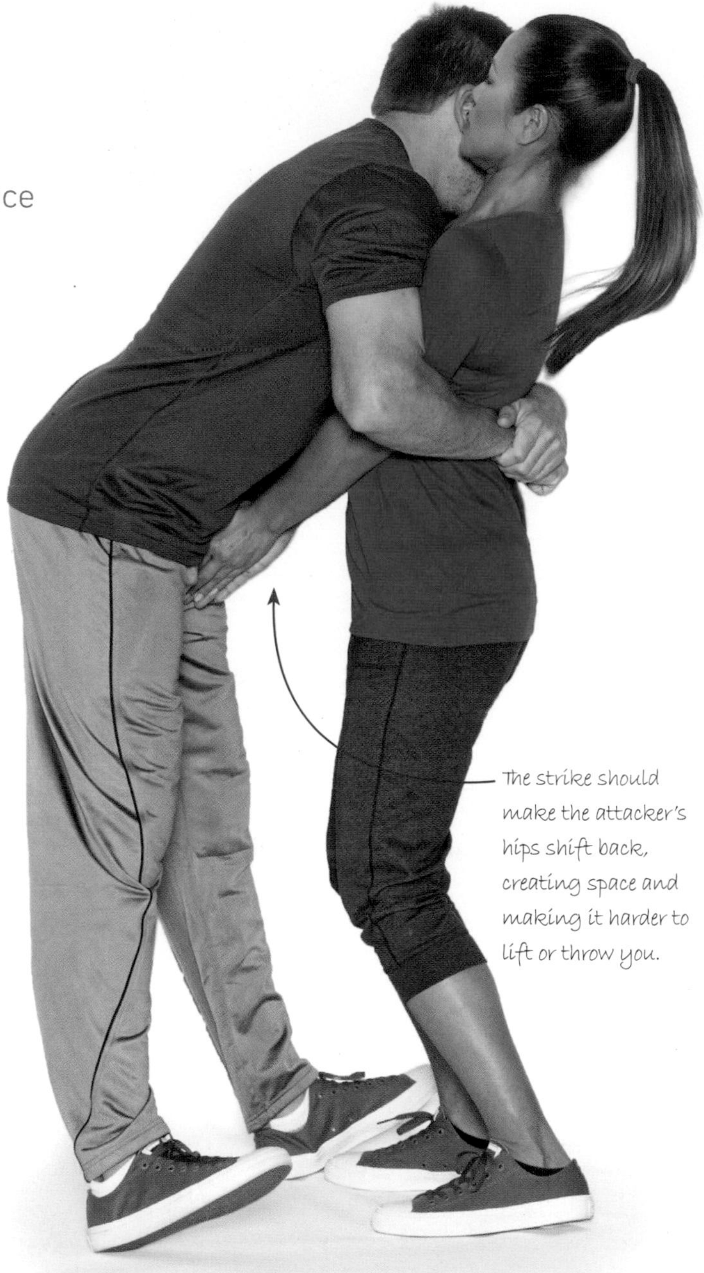

The strike should make the attacker's hips shift back, creating space and making it harder to lift or throw you.

1 As the attack begins, widen your stance and drop your weight into a stable base. Perform a Palm Strike to the groin.

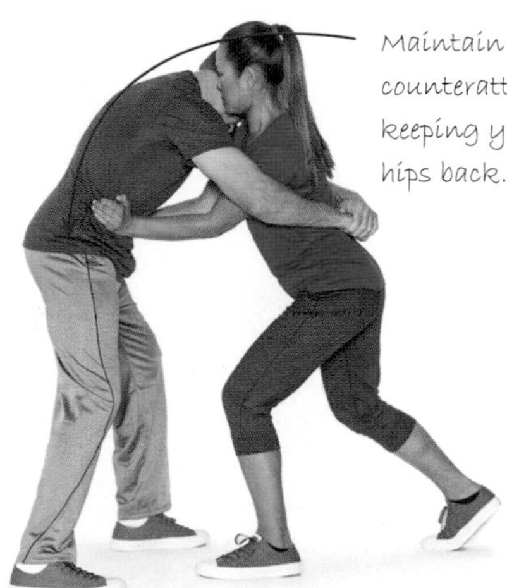
Maintain your counterattack space by keeping your attacker's hips back.

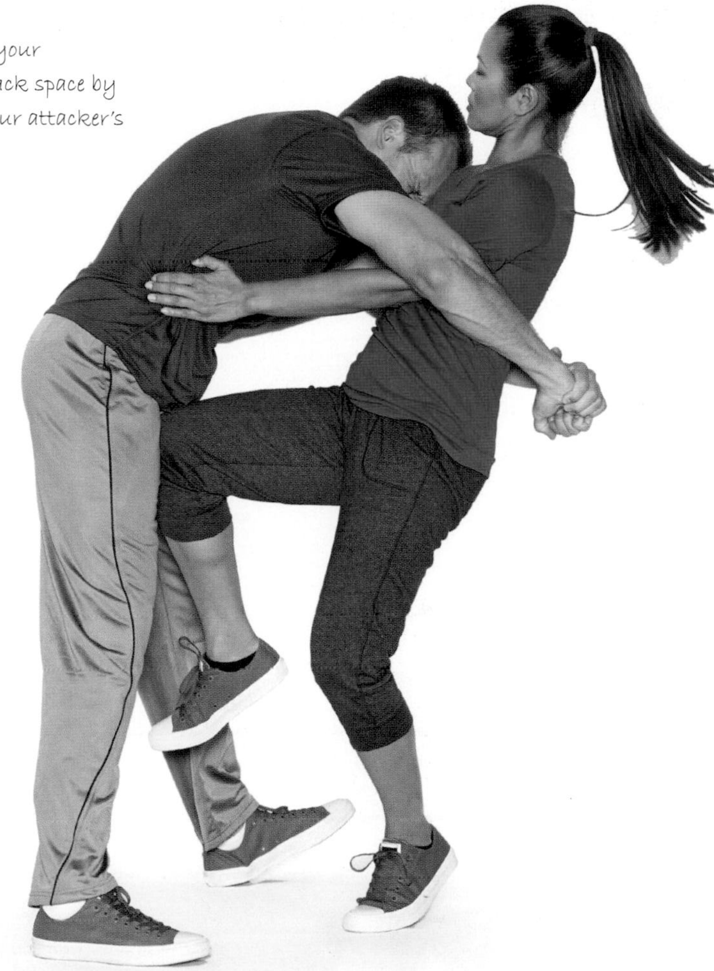

2 Hold your palms at your attacker's hips and deliver multiple Knees to the groin.

DEFENSE TIP

You can also grab, twist, pull, or tear at your attacker's groin. The objective is to create as much space as possible to stop your attacker from carrying or throwing you.

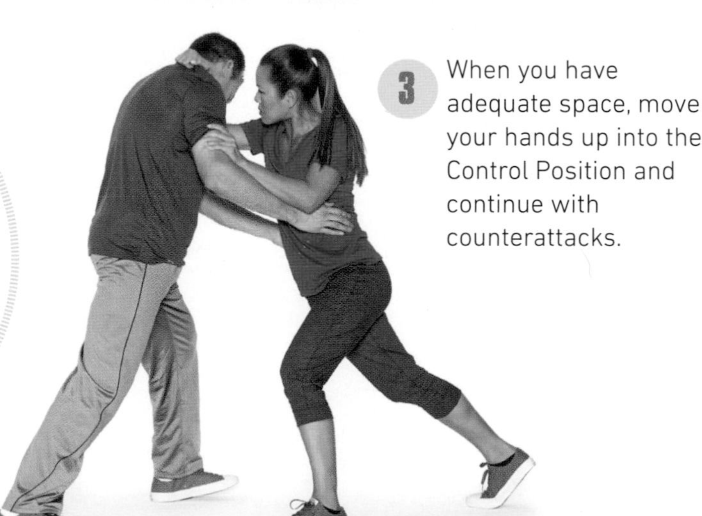

3 When you have adequate space, move your hands up into the Control Position and continue with counterattacks.

Bear Hug from Behind (Arms Free)

To catch you off guard, an attacker might sneak up behind you to carry you away or throw you to the ground. Although this is startling, you can use this "base and space" technique to escape your attacker's hold.

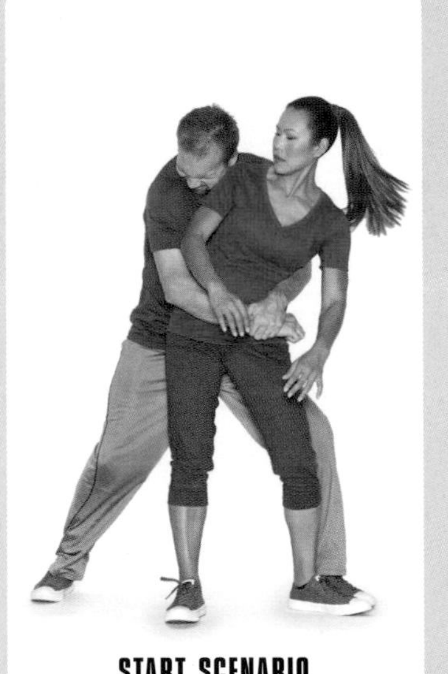

START SCENARIO

Your attacker grabs you from behind by wrapping his or her arms around your waist in a bear hug, keeping your arms free.

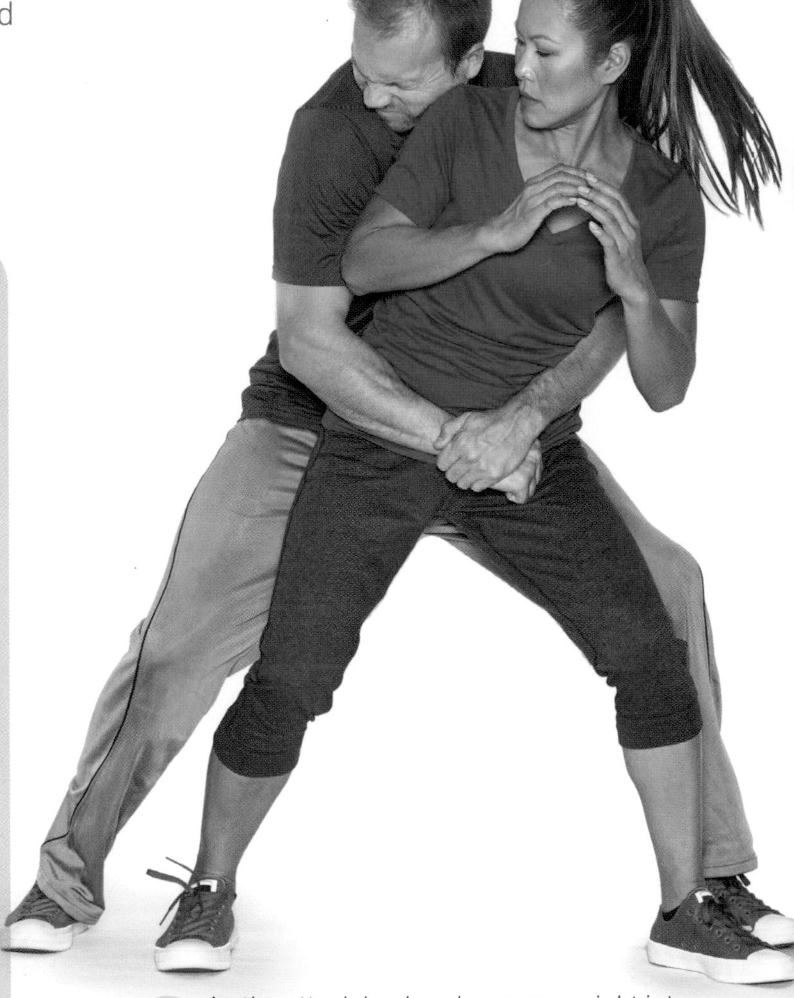

1 As the attack begins, drop your weight into a stable base and bend slightly forward. If your attacker's arms begin to rise up your body, push them down toward your waist. This prevents your attacker from gaining leverage to throw you to the ground.

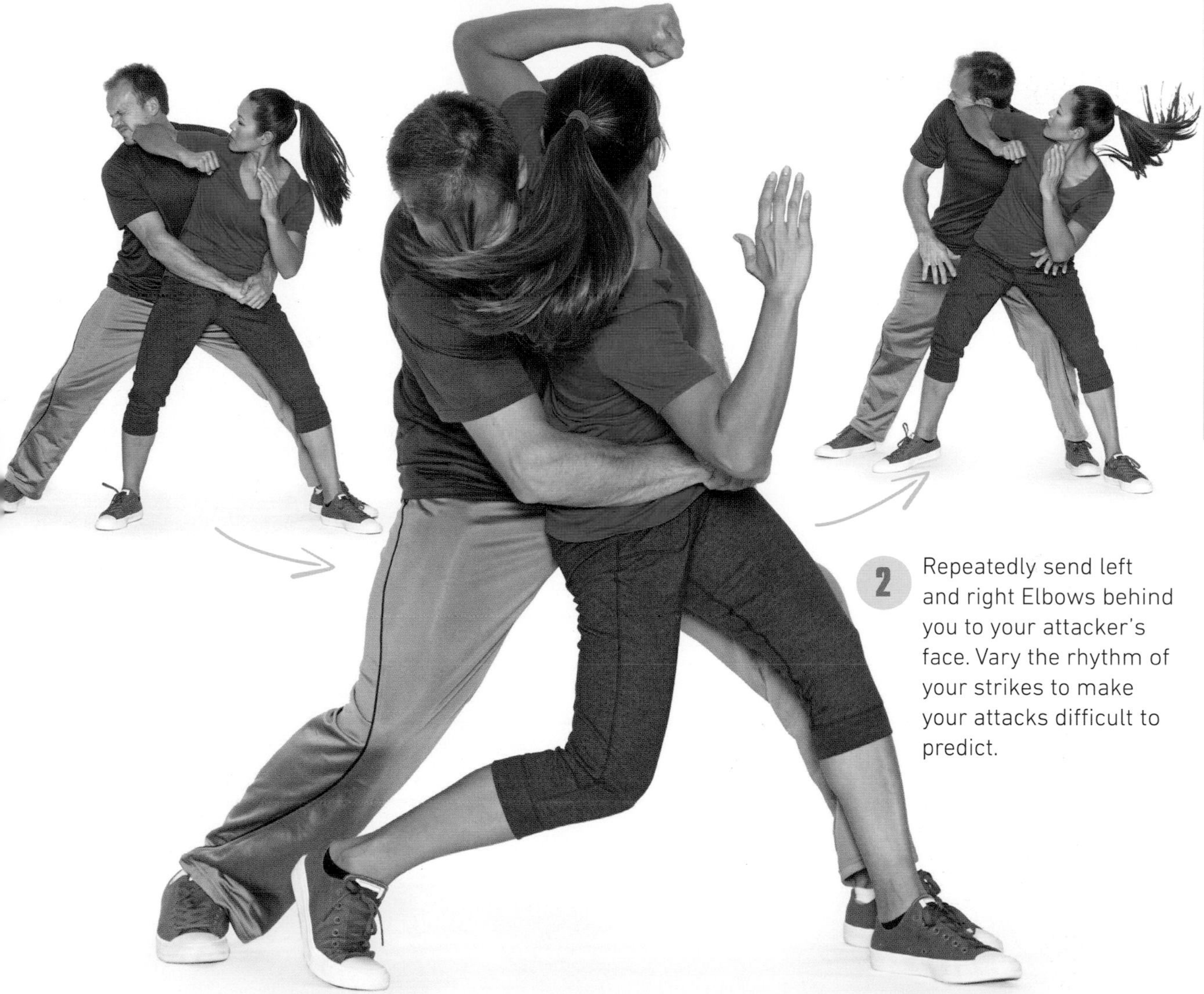

2 Repeatedly send left and right Elbows behind you to your attacker's face. Vary the rhythm of your strikes to make your attacks difficult to predict.

IF IT FAILS

If Elbows aren't working, you can kick your heel back to hit the groin, employ a Stomp Kick, or drag your heel down your attacker's shin.

3 When you create enough space, quickly turn to face your attacker and obtain the Control Position.

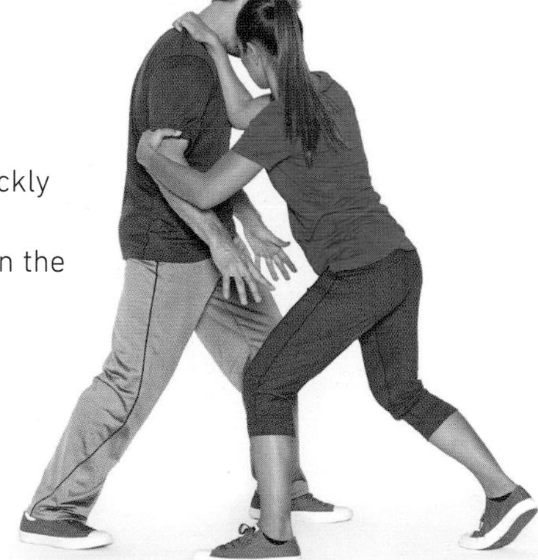

Bear Hug from Behind (Arms Caught)

Although a Bear Hug from Behind with your arms caught can feel intimidating, a quick and aggressive reaction can free you from this kind of attack.

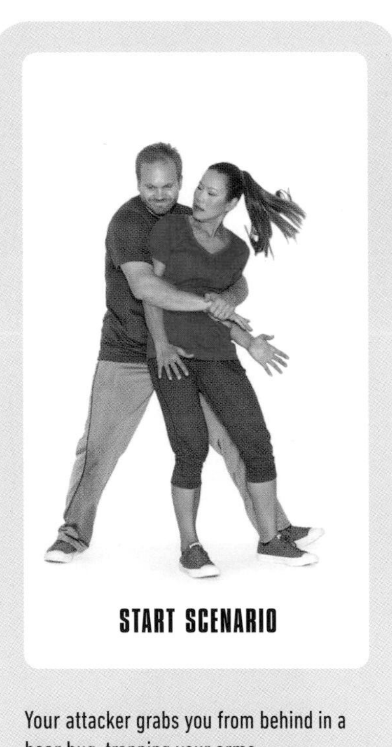

START SCENARIO

Your attacker grabs you from behind in a bear hug, trapping your arms.

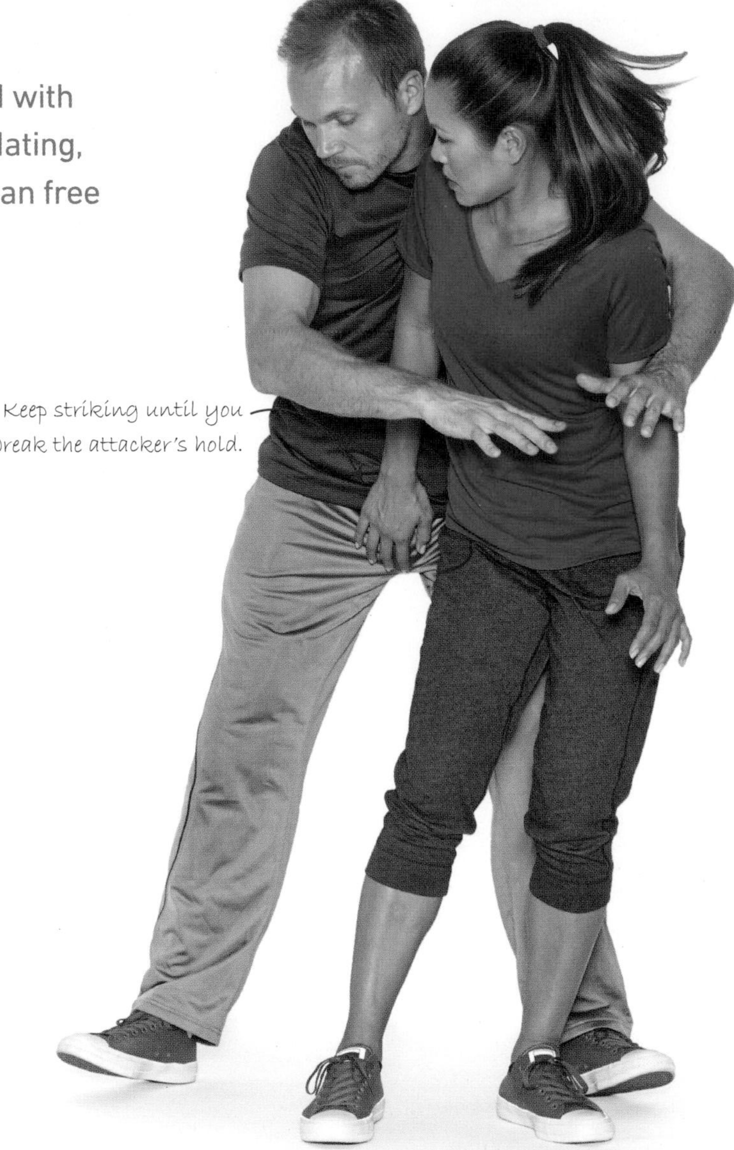

Keep striking until you break the attacker's hold.

1 As the attack begins, drop your weight into a stable base and bend slightly forward. Shift your hips to one side and Palm Strike your attacker's groin repeatedly.

2 When you create enough space, quickly turn to face your attacker and obtain the Control Position.

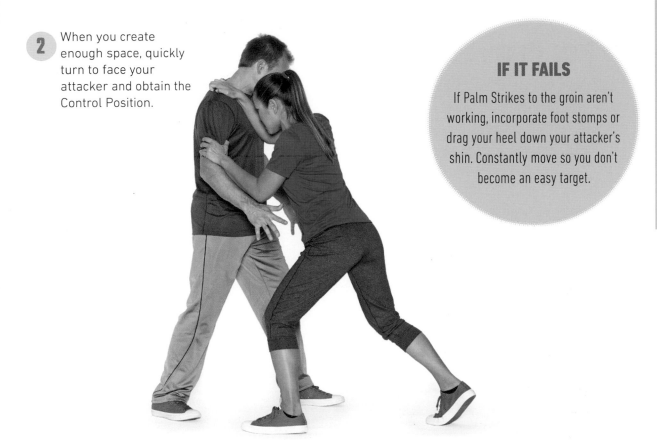

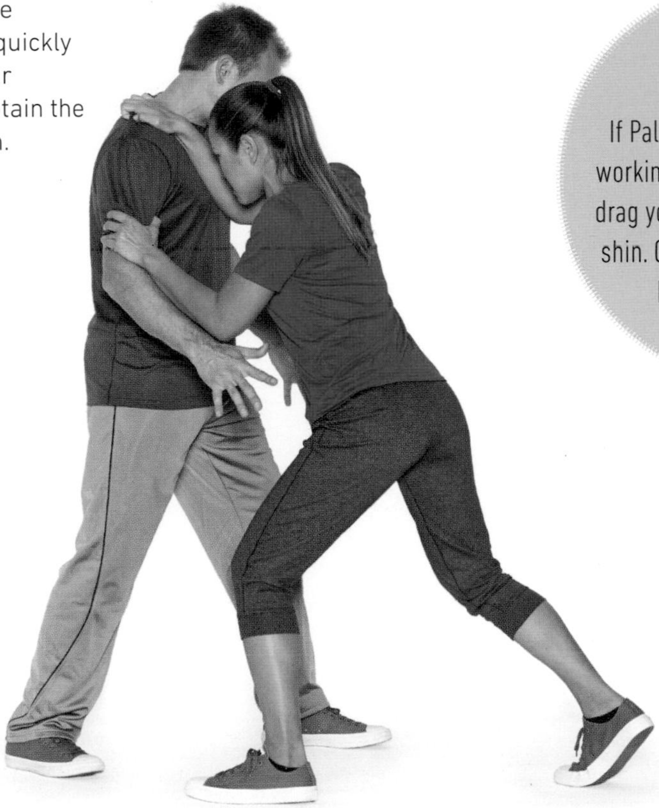

IF IT FAILS

If Palm Strikes to the groin aren't working, incorporate foot stomps or drag your heel down your attacker's shin. Constantly move so you don't become an easy target.

KRAV MAGA PRINCIPLES IN ACTION

Like other defenses in this book, you can see multiple Krav Maga principles in action for this defense. Here are a few:

- **Continuous motion:** This technique involves constant movement, from getting into position to deliver strikes to the final turn into the Control Position, in order to keep the attacker off balance.
- **Instinctive reactions:** With her arms trapped against her body, it's only natural for the defender to want to bring her hand back to hit the attacker. This technique makes use of that innate reaction.
- **Exploitation of vulnerable anatomy:** Delivery of strikes to the groin area causes the attacker to react in pain and slows his reaction to the defender's countermoves.

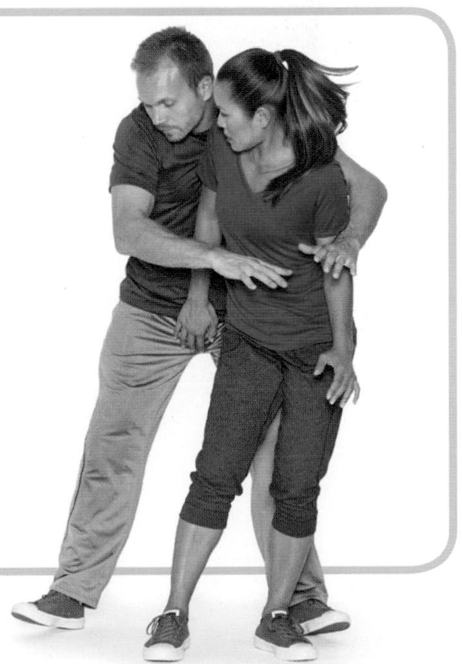

Hair Pulls (Front, Side, and Back)

An attacker might grab your hair and try to pull you to a more secluded location or into a vehicle. With this technique, you burst faster than your attacker's pull to maintain your balance and escape.

START SCENARIO

Your attacker grabs a fistful of your hair and starts to pull.

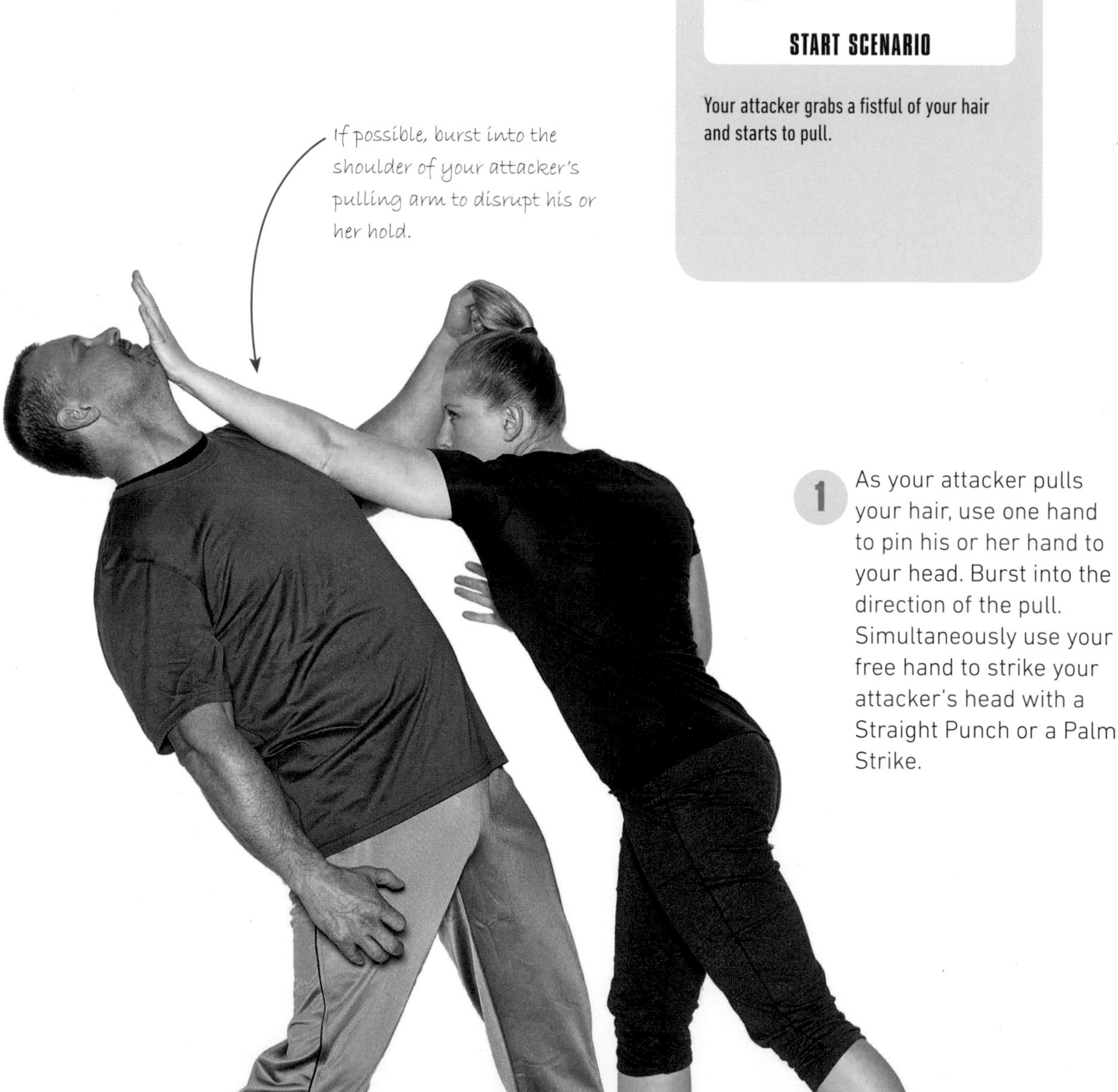

If possible, burst into the shoulder of your attacker's pulling arm to disrupt his or her hold.

1 As your attacker pulls your hair, use one hand to pin his or her hand to your head. Burst into the direction of the pull. Simultaneously use your free hand to strike your attacker's head with a Straight Punch or a Palm Strike.

2 Continue moving into the pull and counterattacking with punches, kicks, Elbows, or Knees.

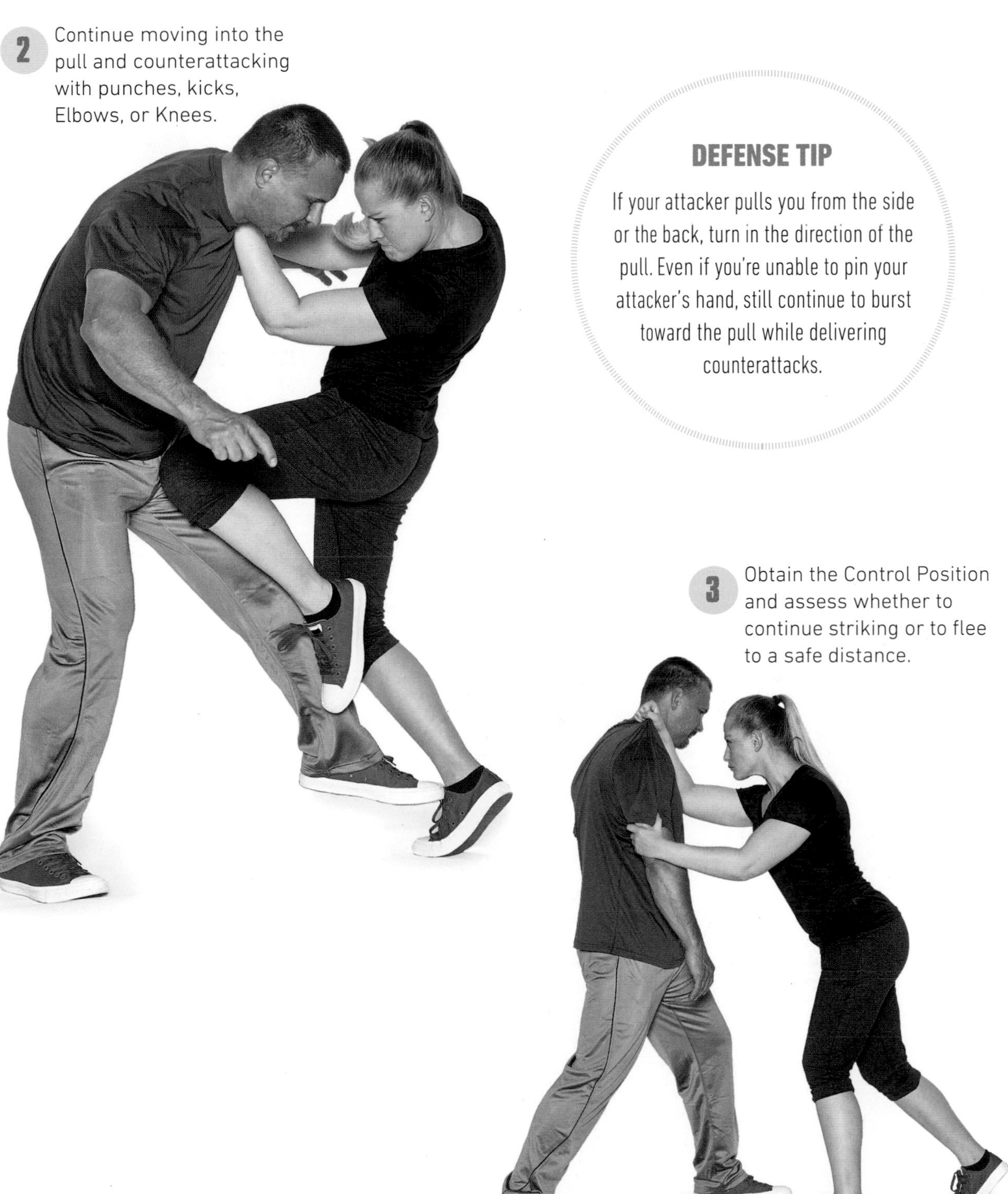

DEFENSE TIP

If your attacker pulls you from the side or the back, turn in the direction of the pull. Even if you're unable to pin your attacker's hand, still continue to burst toward the pull while delivering counterattacks.

3 Obtain the Control Position and assess whether to continue striking or to flee to a safe distance.

Purse or Backpack Snatch

Whether trying to steal your possessions or to pull you to another location, an attacker might grab your purse or your backpack. Similar to the Hair Pulls defense, this technique has you to burst in the direction of the pull either to save your possessions or to escape the attack.

START SCENARIO

Your attacker tries to grab your purse or backpack.

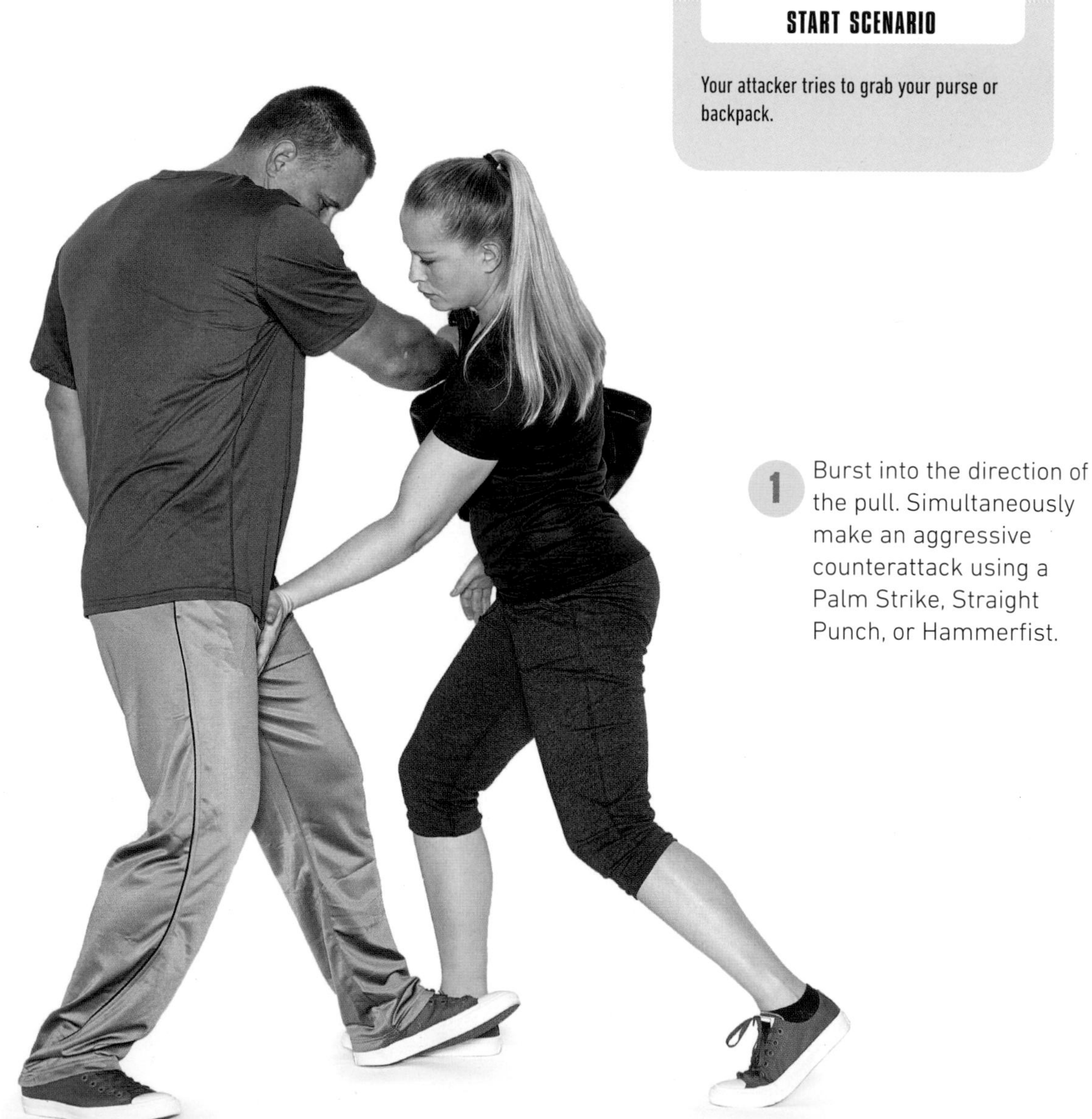

1 Burst into the direction of the pull. Simultaneously make an aggressive counterattack using a Palm Strike, Straight Punch, or Hammerfist.

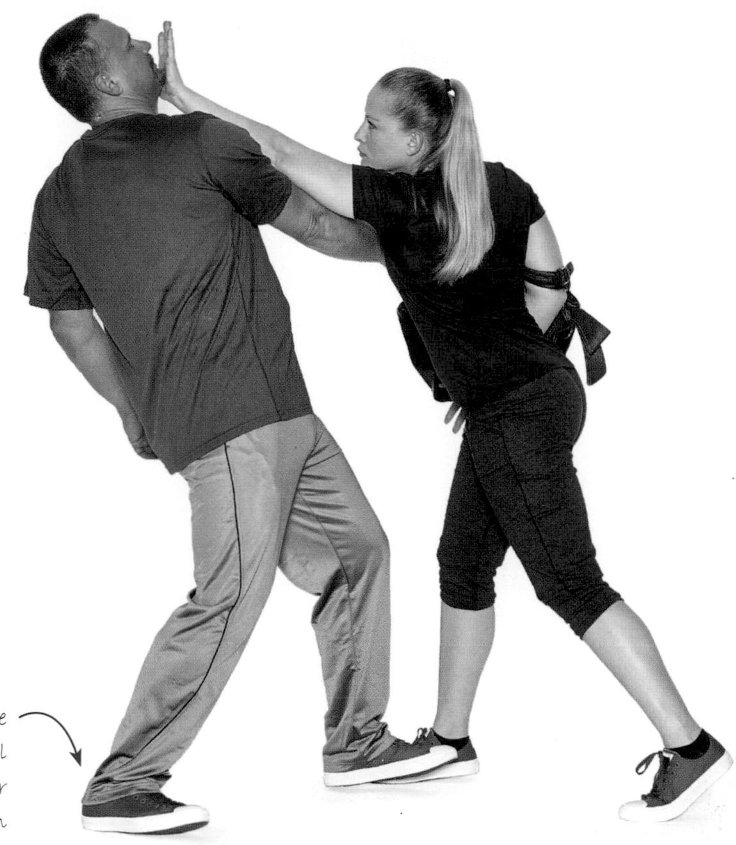

2 Continue with aggressive counterattacks until your attacker lets go of your backpack or purse.

If you continue to strike aggressively, you'll make it difficult for your attacker to maintain balance and fight.

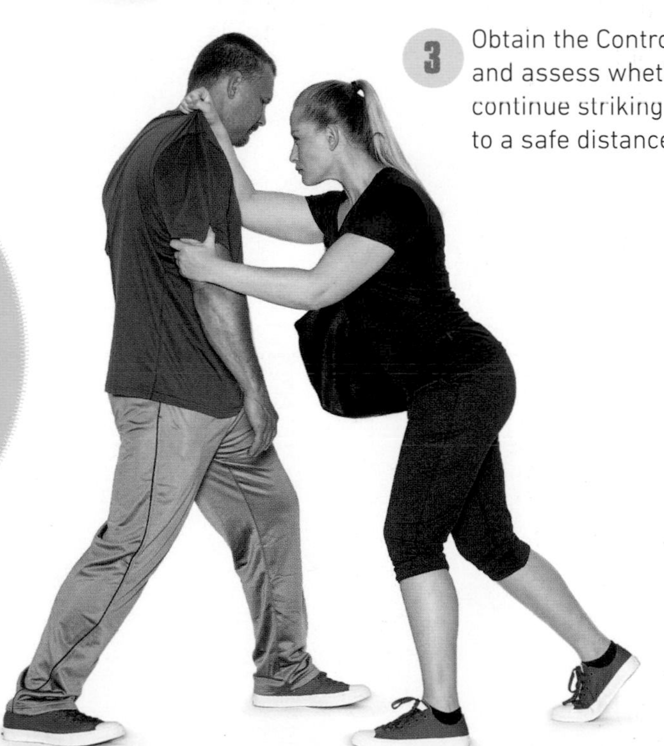

3 Obtain the Control Position and assess whether to continue striking or to flee to a safe distance.

WARNING

You must decide your attacker's intention. If he or she is trying to steal your purse or backpack, you must determine if the contents warrant protecting. Conversely, if your attacker is after you, always defend yourself against this life-threatening danger.

Multiple-Attacker Situation

Sometimes more than one attacker will confront you. So you don't have to fight all of them at the same time, you can first use movement to stack the attackers and then deal with the closest attacker first.

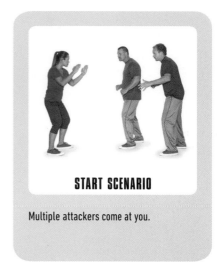

START SCENARIO

Multiple attackers come at you.

1. Use movement to stack your attackers in front of or behind each other. As your first attacker closes the distance, strike out with a kick.

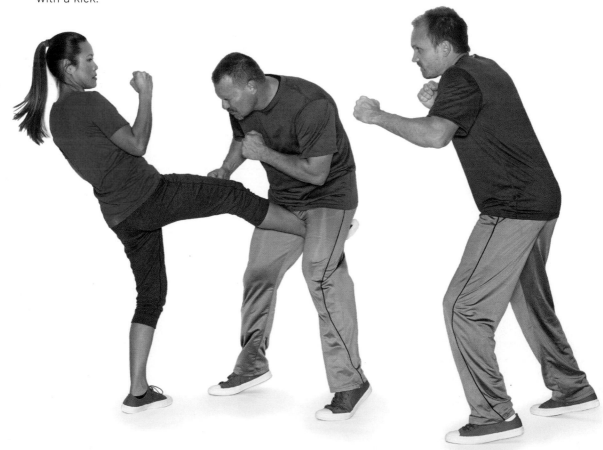

DEFENSE TIP

A Multiple-Attacker Situation can seem intimidating. This is where having good situational awareness is key. Use your surroundings to your advantage, whether it's to stack your attackers or to improvise a weapon. Most of all, keep calm, and think and react aggressively.

2 While maintaining your Control Position, bring your first attacker into position to be used as a shield.

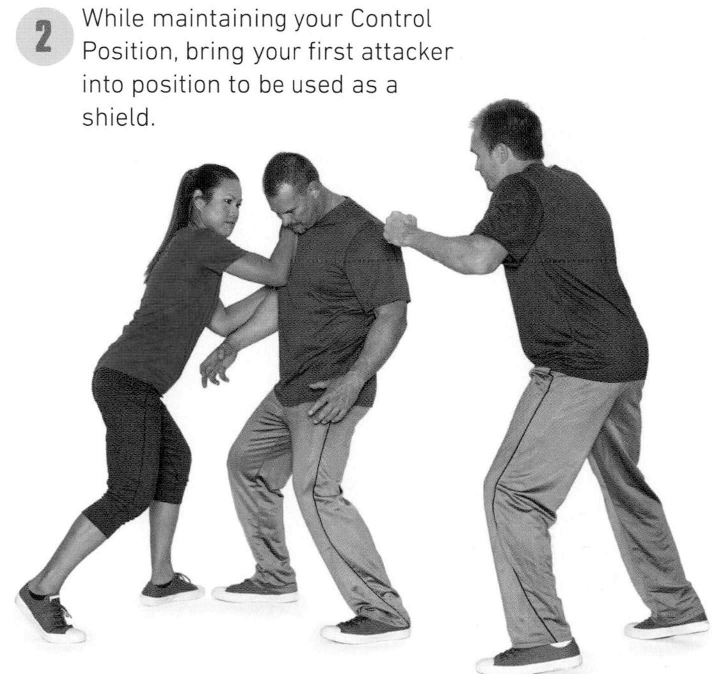

3 With your first attacker in place as a shield, kick your second attacker as he or she approaches.

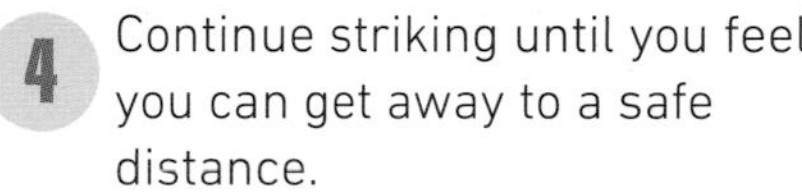

4 Continue striking until you feel you can get away to a safe distance.

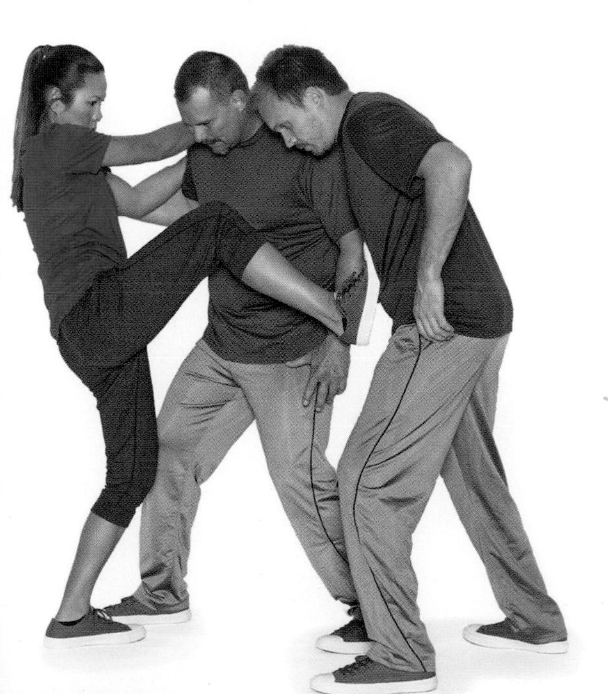

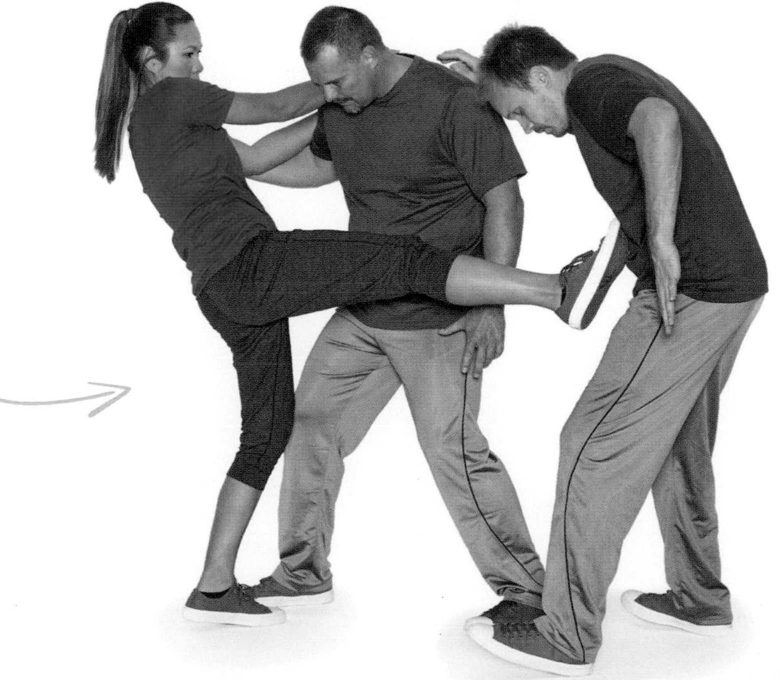

FROM THE GROUND

Learning to defend yourself even when in a position of disadvantage is key in Krav Maga. These techniques teach you different actions you can take when on the ground.

Buck, Trap, and Roll

If you're lying on the ground with an attacker mounted on top of you, use this swift and forceful technique to escape—the Buck, Trap, and Roll.

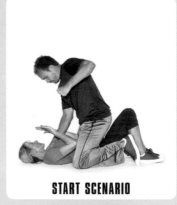

START SCENARIO

Your attacker straddles you while you're in a prone position and prepares to deliver a srike.

1 Buck your hips explosively upward, causing your attacker to fall forward onto his or her hands.

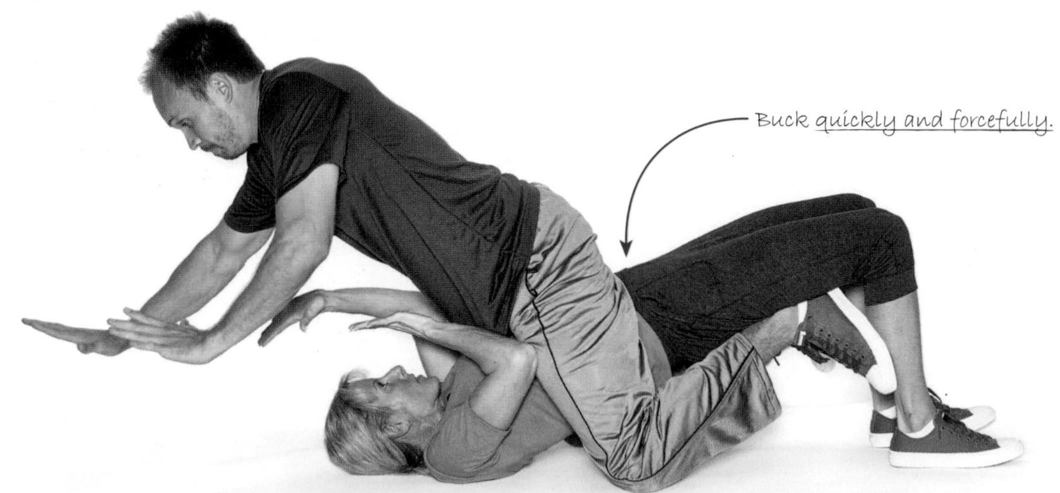

Buck quickly and forcefully.

2 Wrap one arm around your attacker's arm, and then quickly pull it down and pin it to the side of your body. On the same side, move your foot to the outside of your attacker's leg, trapping it to the ground with your leg.

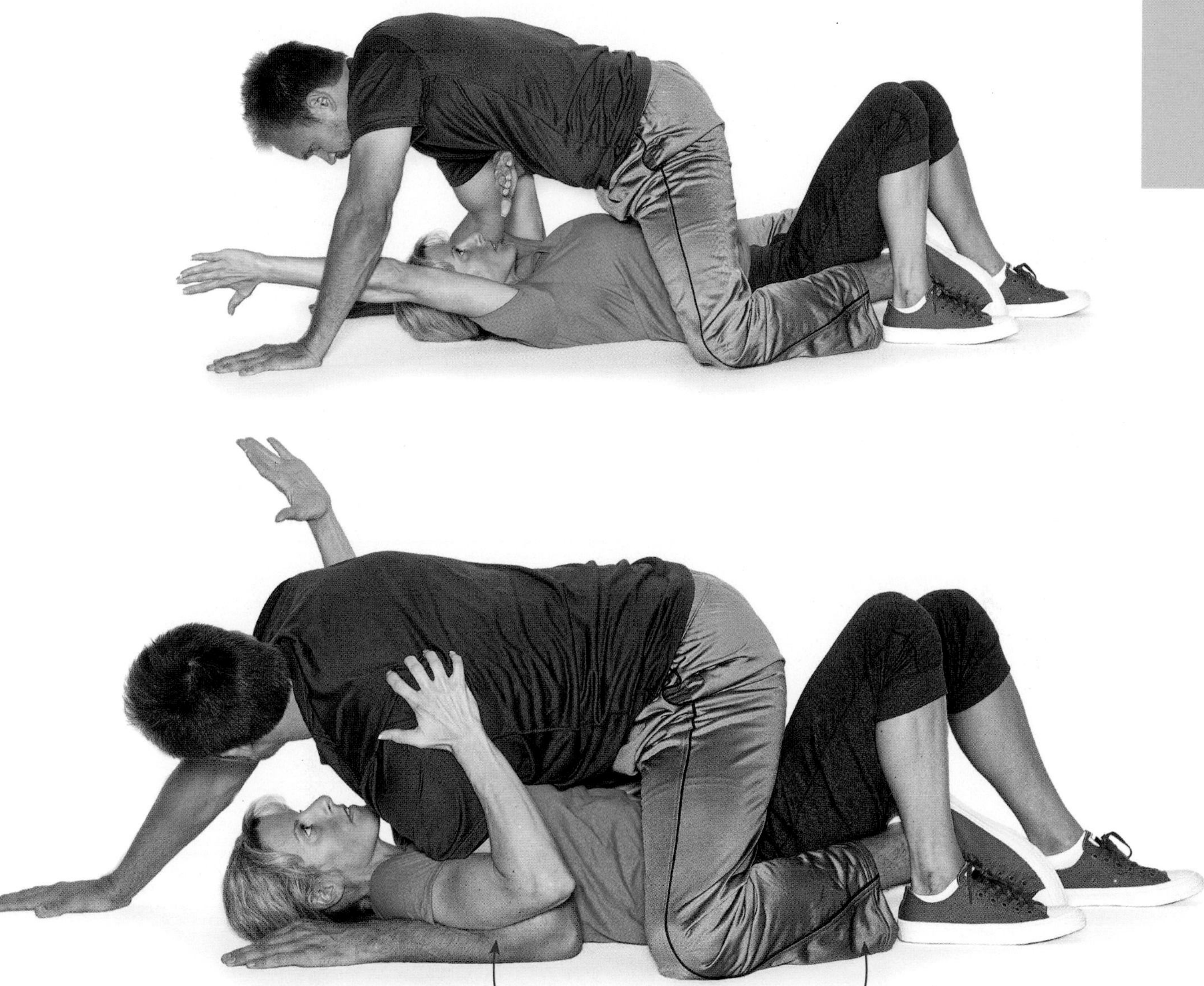

Hold your elbow and foot tightly to your body to securely trap your attacker's arm and leg.

3 Continue to buck your hips upward and sideways toward your attacker's pinned arm and leg.

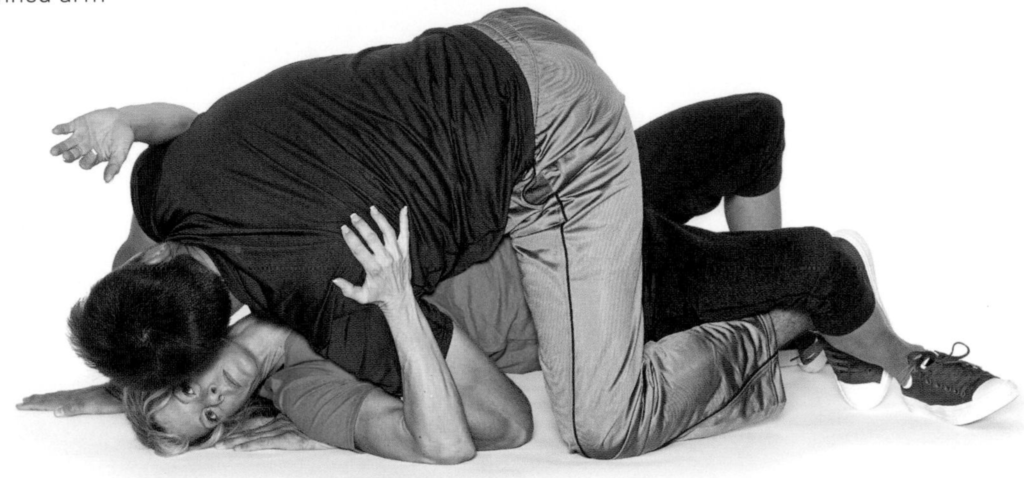

4 Use the momentum to roll over until you're on top of your attacker.

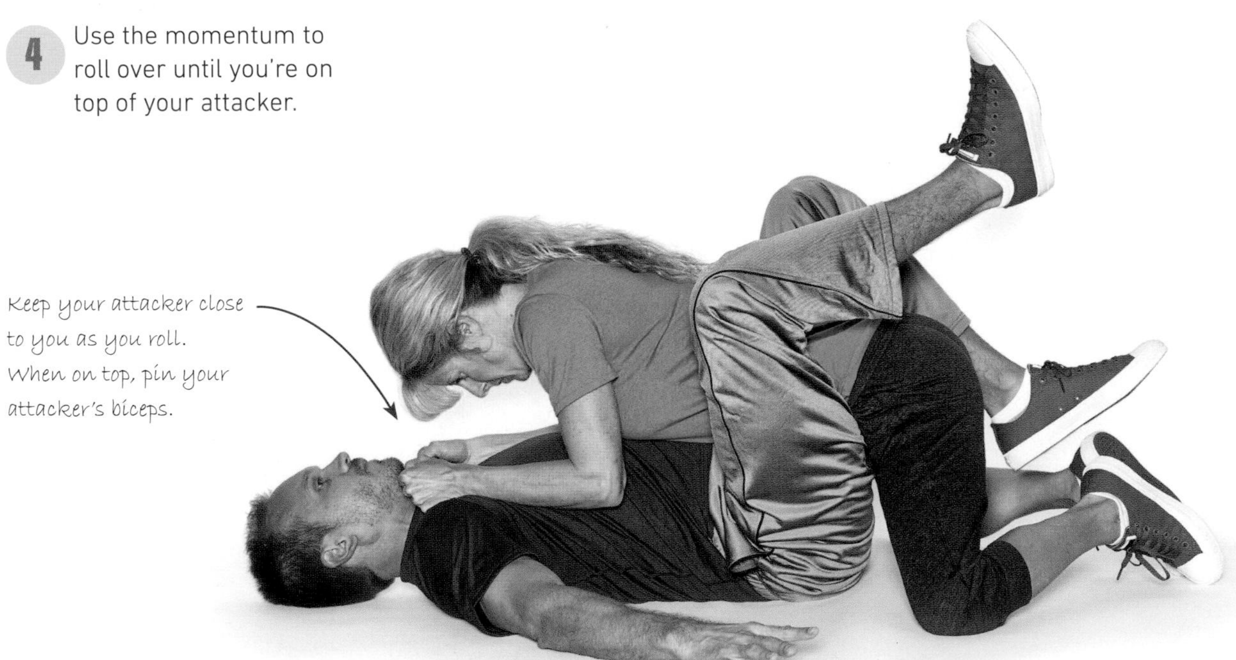

Keep your attacker close to you as you roll. When on top, pin your attacker's biceps.

5 Sit back on your attacker and deliver strikes to the face or groin, such as Straight Punches, Elbows, Hammerfists, and Palm Strikes.

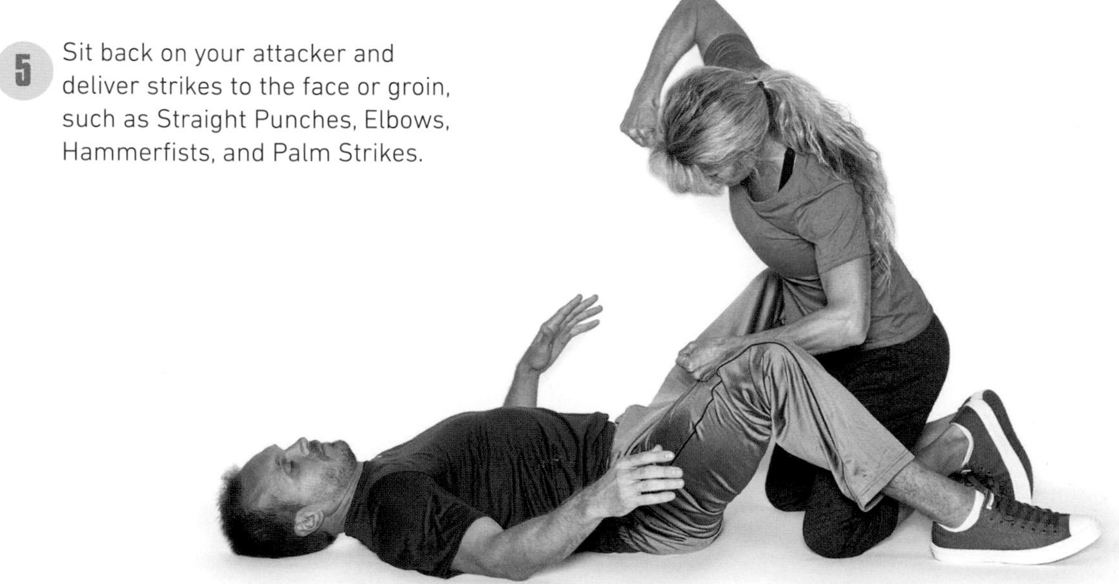

IF IT FAILS

You may need to buck several times if your first buck doesn't cause your attacker to fall forward. Deliver punches and Elbows to the face or bite and Eye Strike your attacker—anything to unpin yourself from the ground.

6 Stand upright by pushing down on your attacker's knees as you back up and out of your crouch.

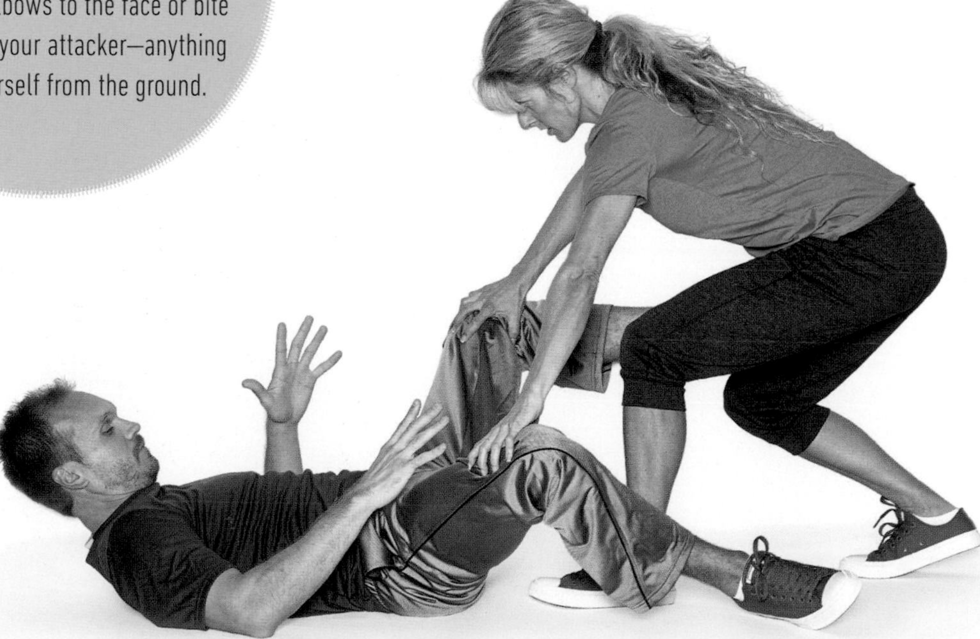

Choke on the Ground

An aggressive attacker might pin you to the ground and choke you to cut off blood and oxygen to your head. This pluck-and-buck technique will help you escape.

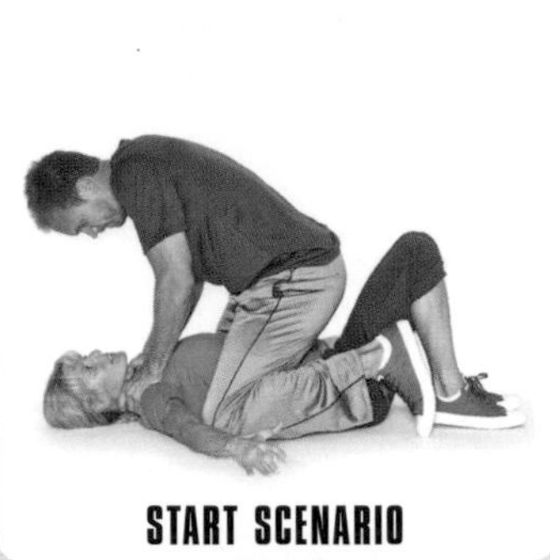

START SCENARIO

Your attacker straddles you while you're in a prone position on the ground. His or her hands are around your throat, making a wringing motion.

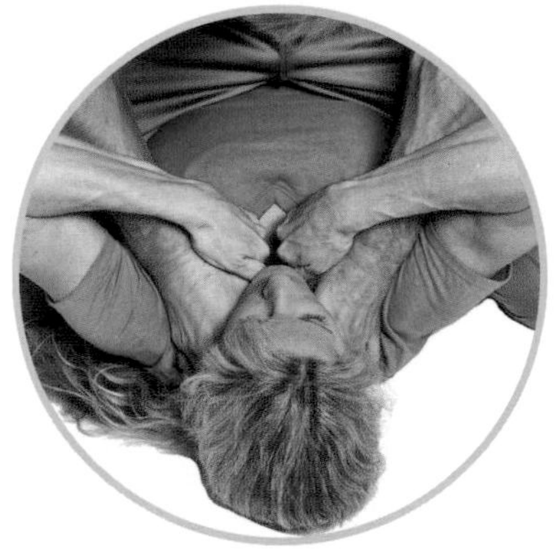

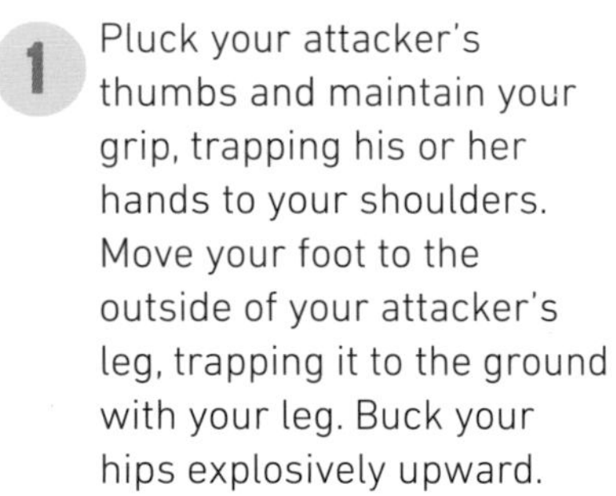

1 Pluck your attacker's thumbs and maintain your grip, trapping his or her hands to your shoulders. Move your foot to the outside of your attacker's leg, trapping it to the ground with your leg. Buck your hips explosively upward.

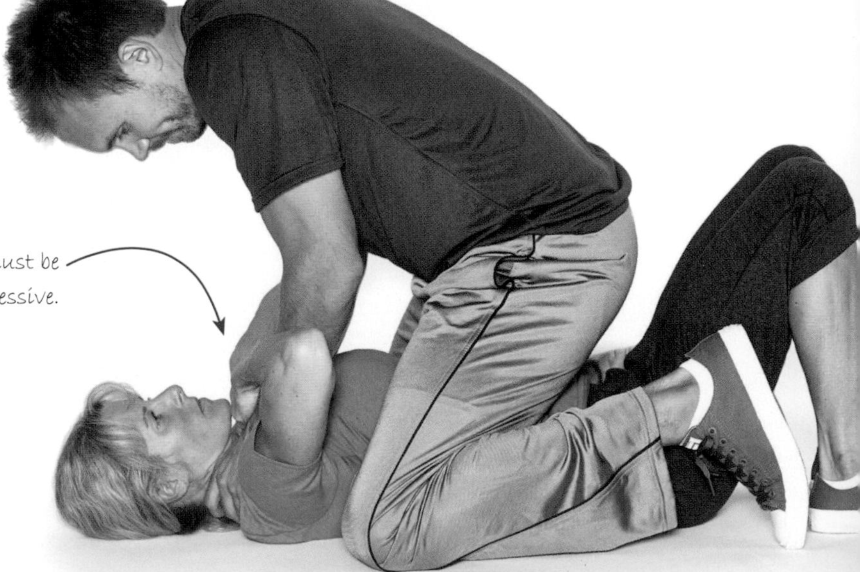

Your movements must be speedy and aggressive.

2 Continue to buck your hips upward and sideways toward your attacker's pinned arm and leg while maintaining control of your attacker's hands.

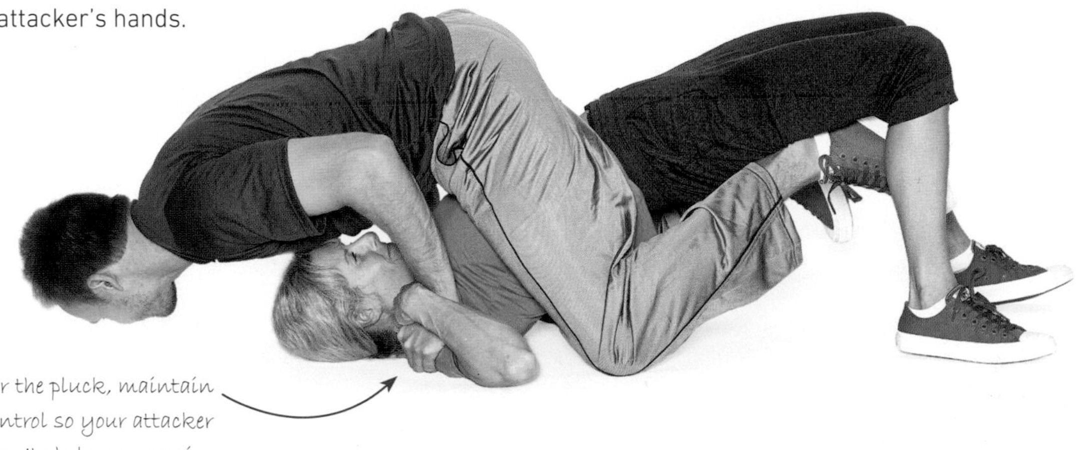

After the pluck, maintain control so your attacker doesn't choke you again.

3 Use the momentum to roll over until you're on top of your attacker.

Keep your attacker close to you as you roll, so he or she can't counterattack.

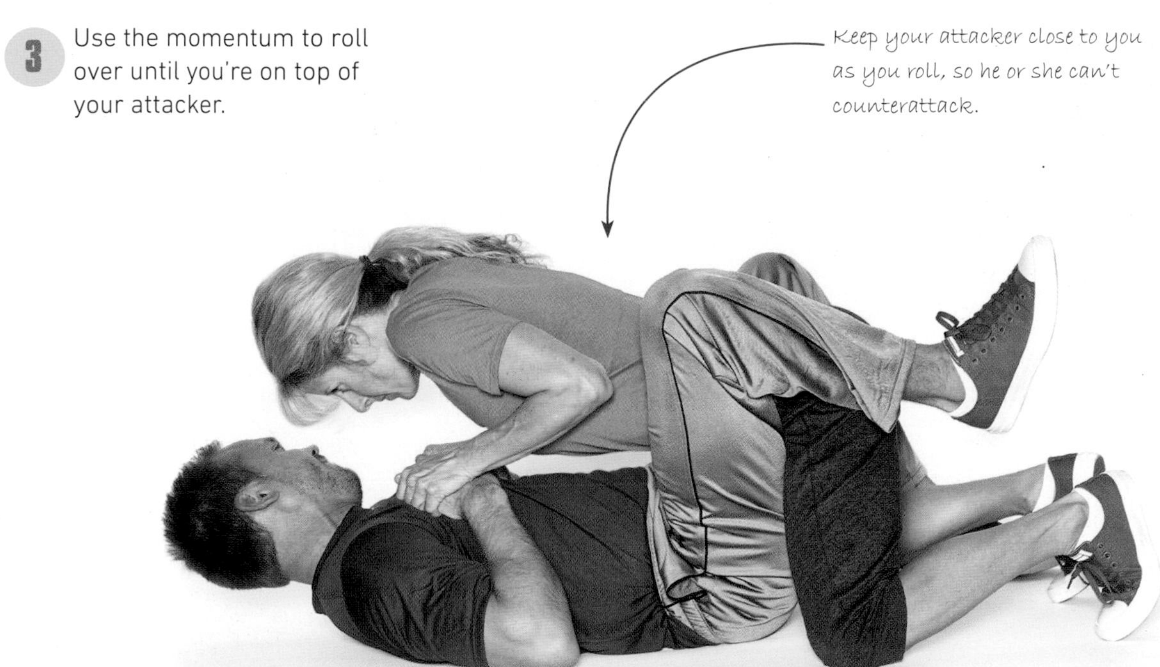

4 Sit back on your attacker and deliver strikes to the face or groin, such as Straight Punches, Elbows, Hammerfists, and Palm Strikes.

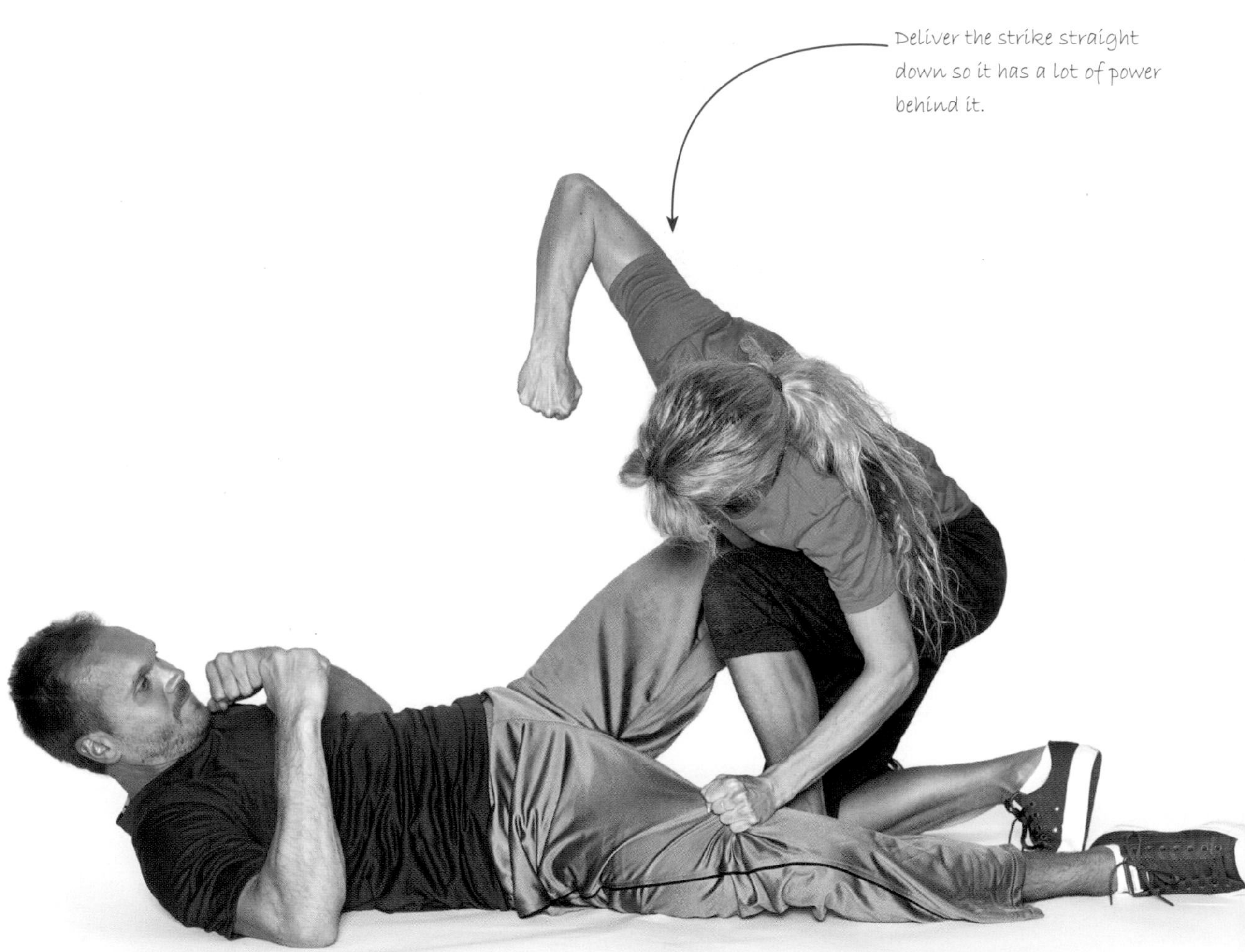

Deliver the strike straight down so it has a lot of power behind it.

5 Stand upright by pushing down on your attacker's knees as you back up and out of your crouch.

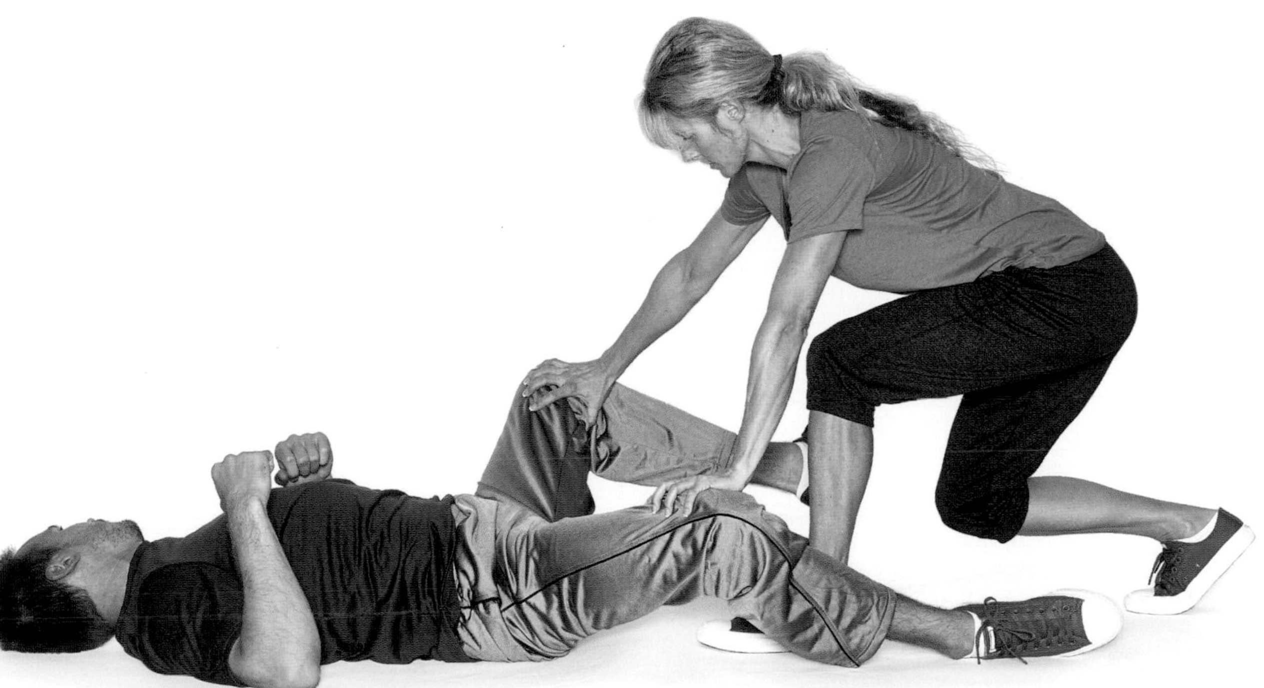

DEFENSE TIP

Relieving the pressure of the choke must be your immediate goal. Pluck and buck persistently until you unsettle your attacker's balance and escape the hold.

Headlock While Mounted

The Headlock While Mounted is common in sexual assaults, and the close proximity of an attacker's face can make you particularly vulnerable to degradation. This tecnique helps you aggressively buck and counterattack to escape safely.

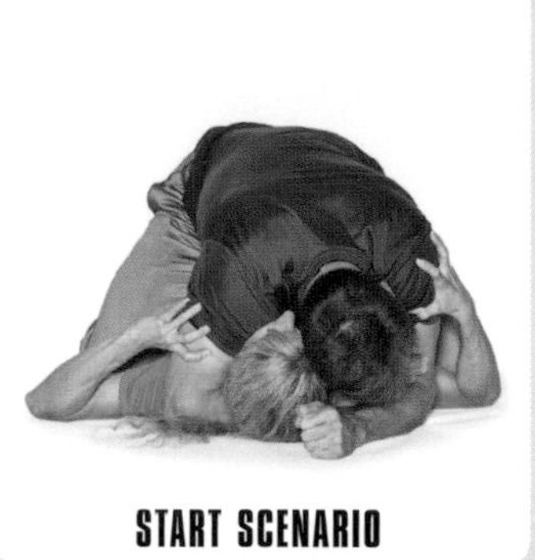

START SCENARIO

Your attacker straddles you while you're in a prone position and puts one of his or her arms around your neck in a headlock.

1. Reach up to the arm placing the chokehold and pin it to your head. On the same side, move your foot to the outside of your attacker's leg, trapping it on the ground with your leg. Buck your hips explosively upward.

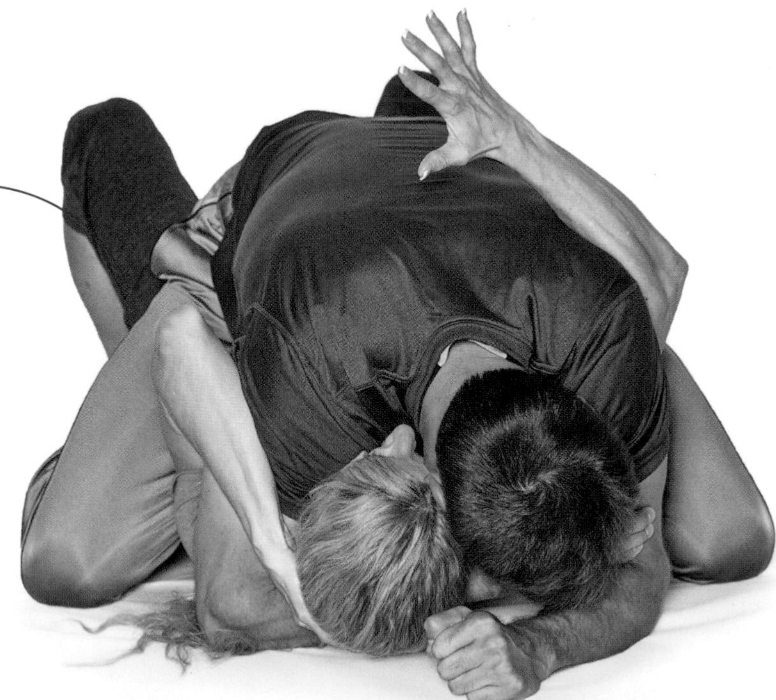
Buck quickly and forcefully.

2 Continue to buck your hips upward and at a 45-degree angle over your shoulder toward your attacker's pinned arm and leg.

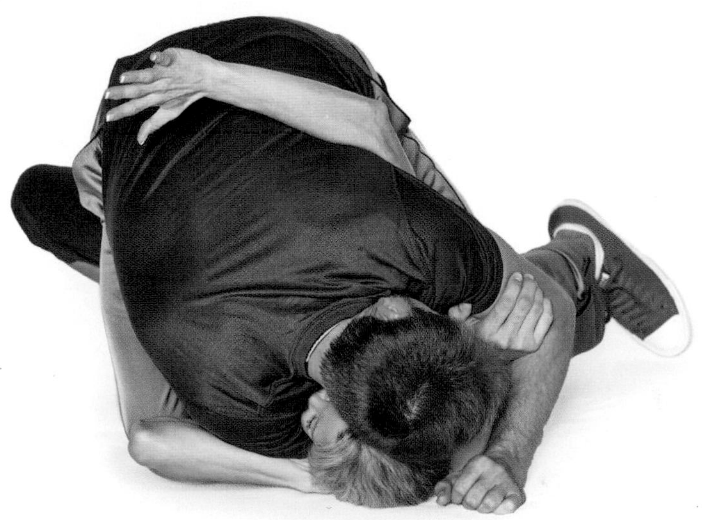

3 Use the momentum to ride the attacker over until you are on top of him or her.

As you sit up, push your attacker's face to the side and deliver strikes.

4 Sit back on your attacker and deliver strikes to the face or groin, such as Straight Punches, Elbows, Hammerfists, and Palm Strikes.

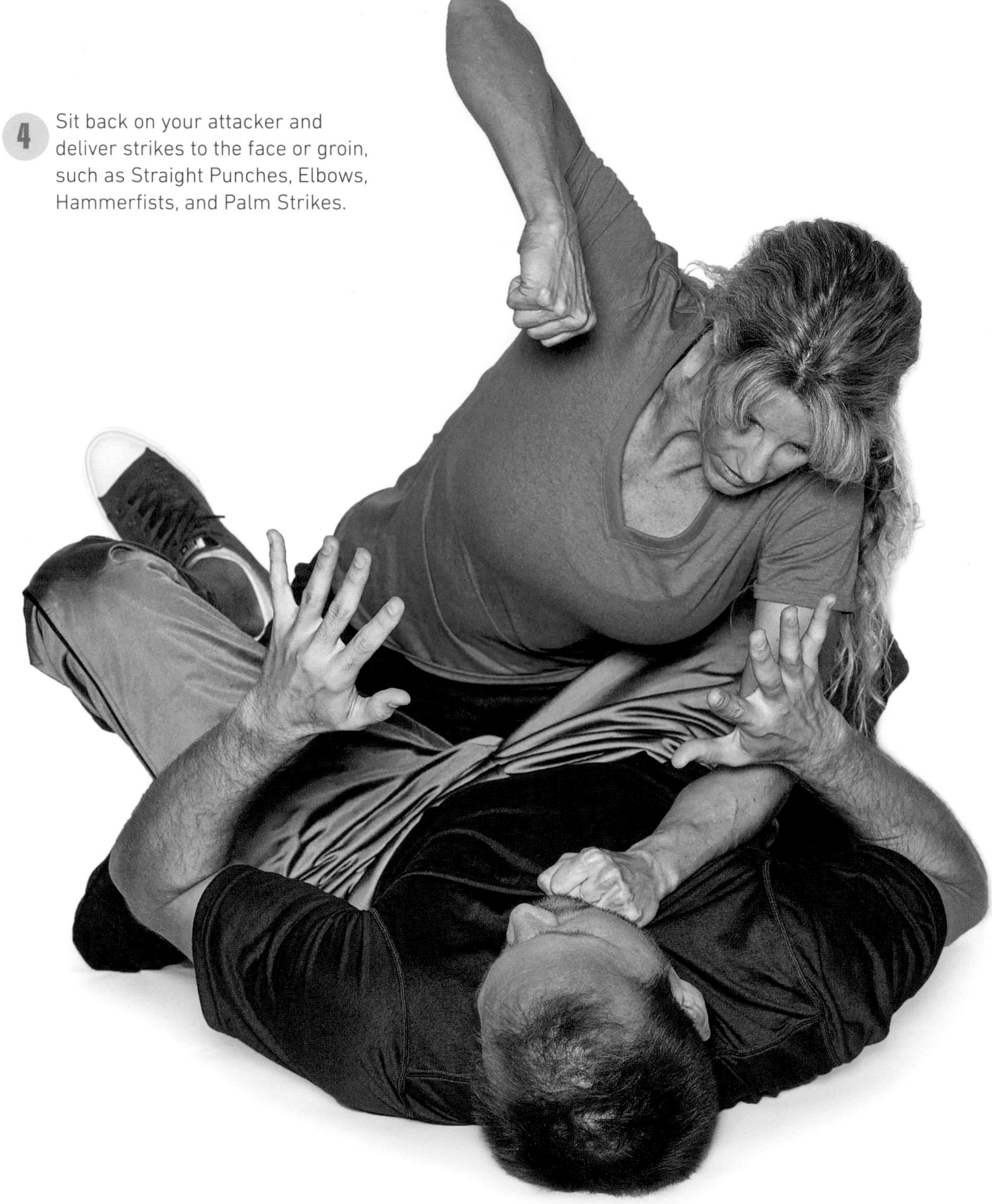

IF IT FAILS

If you can't escape (whether on top or below), you must disrupt your attacker's thought process. Scratch, claw, and bite at your attacker until you can safely get away.

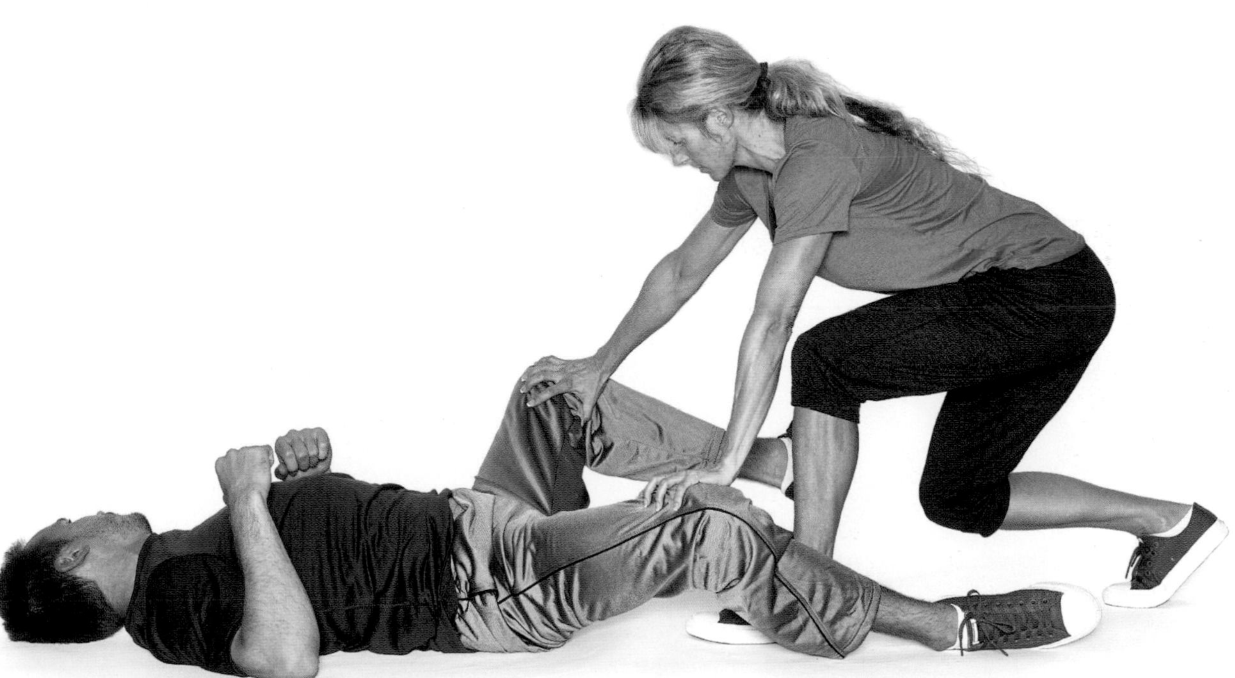

5 Stand upright by pushing down on your attacker's knees as you back up and out of your crouch.

Kick Off from the Guard

In a sexual attack, your attacker may end up in your guard position–between your legs while you're on your back. Kicking is an effective way to create space to escape.

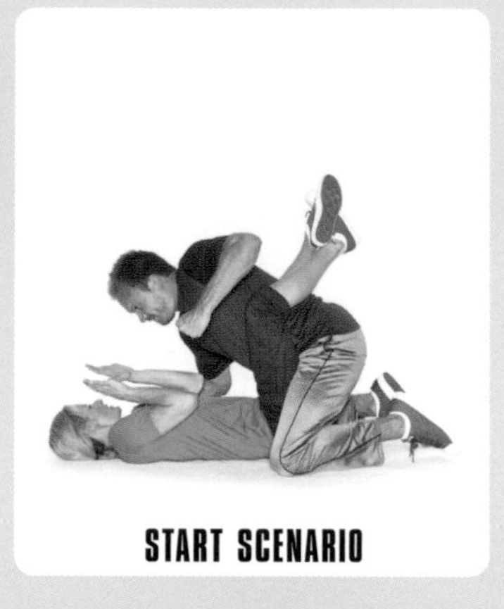

START SCENARIO

Lie on your back with the attacker between your legs, acting sggressively.

1 Grab your attacker's striking arm with both hands. Shift your weight onto one hip and force your raised knee against your attacker's chest.

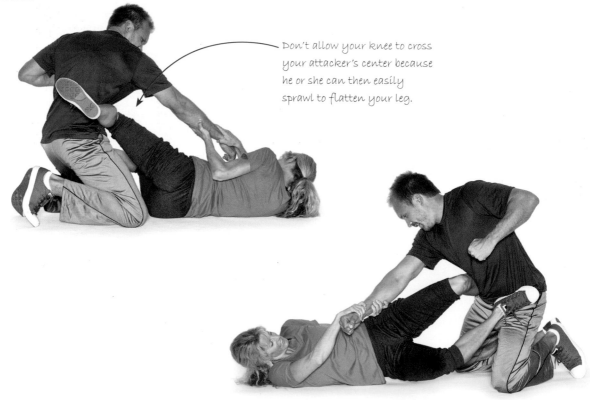

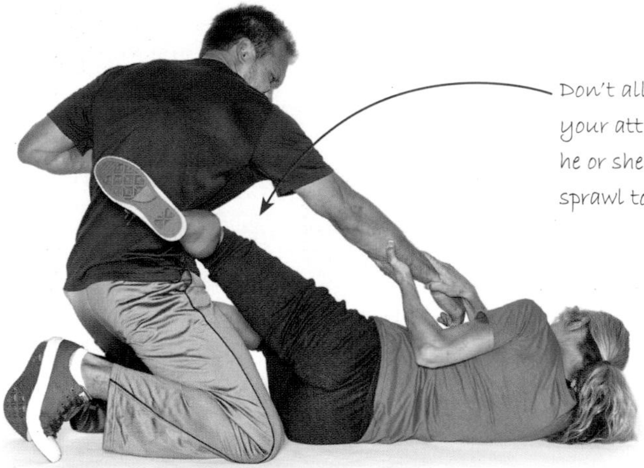

Don't allow your knee to cross your attacker's center because he or she can then easily sprawl to flatten your leg.

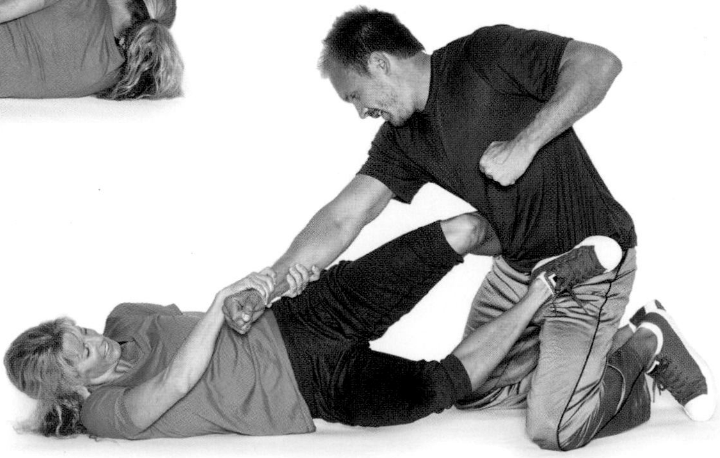

2 Hold your opposite foot against your attacker's hip and push off to create space to kick.

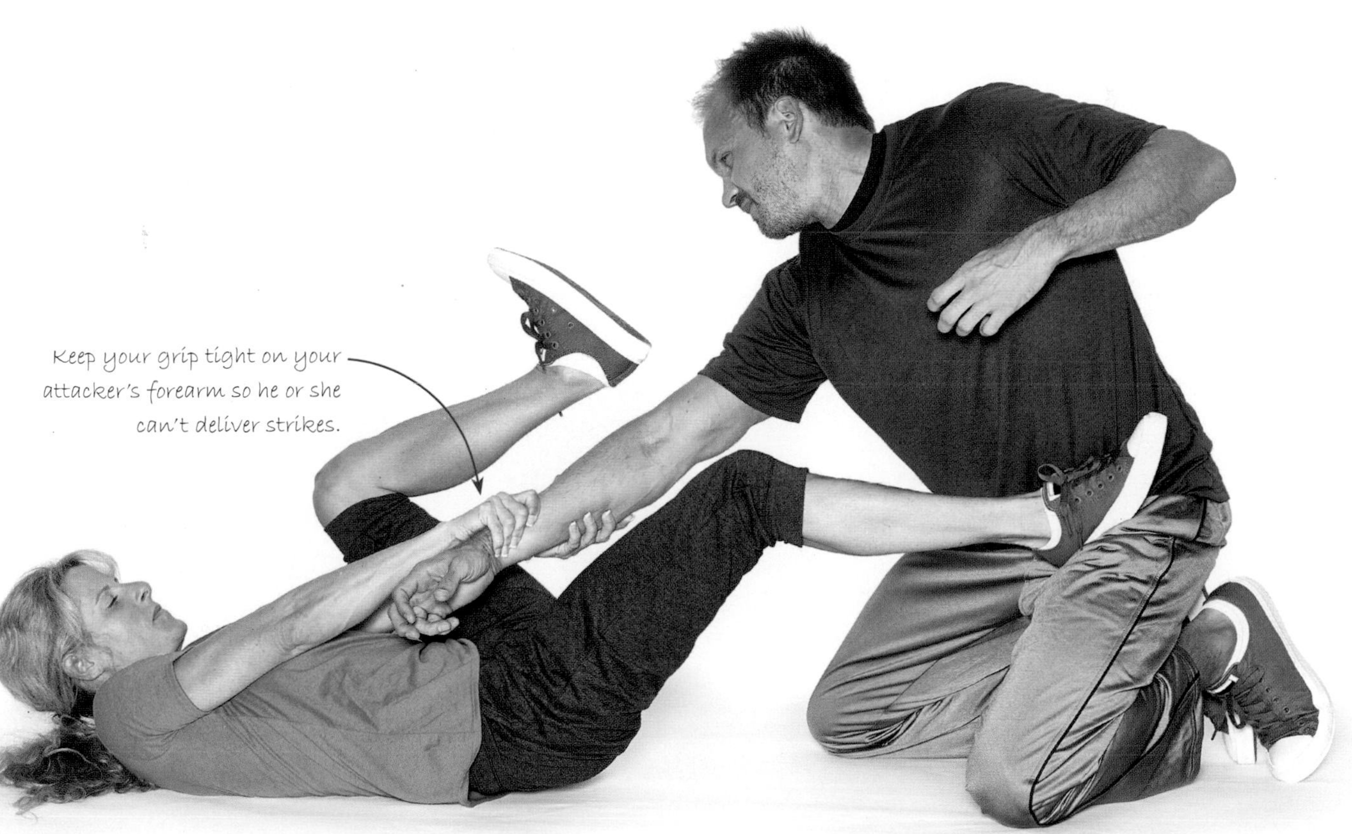

Keep your grip tight on your attacker's forearm so he or she can't deliver strikes.

3 Keeping your foot against his or her hip, use your raised leg to Stomp Kick your attacker's chest or face.

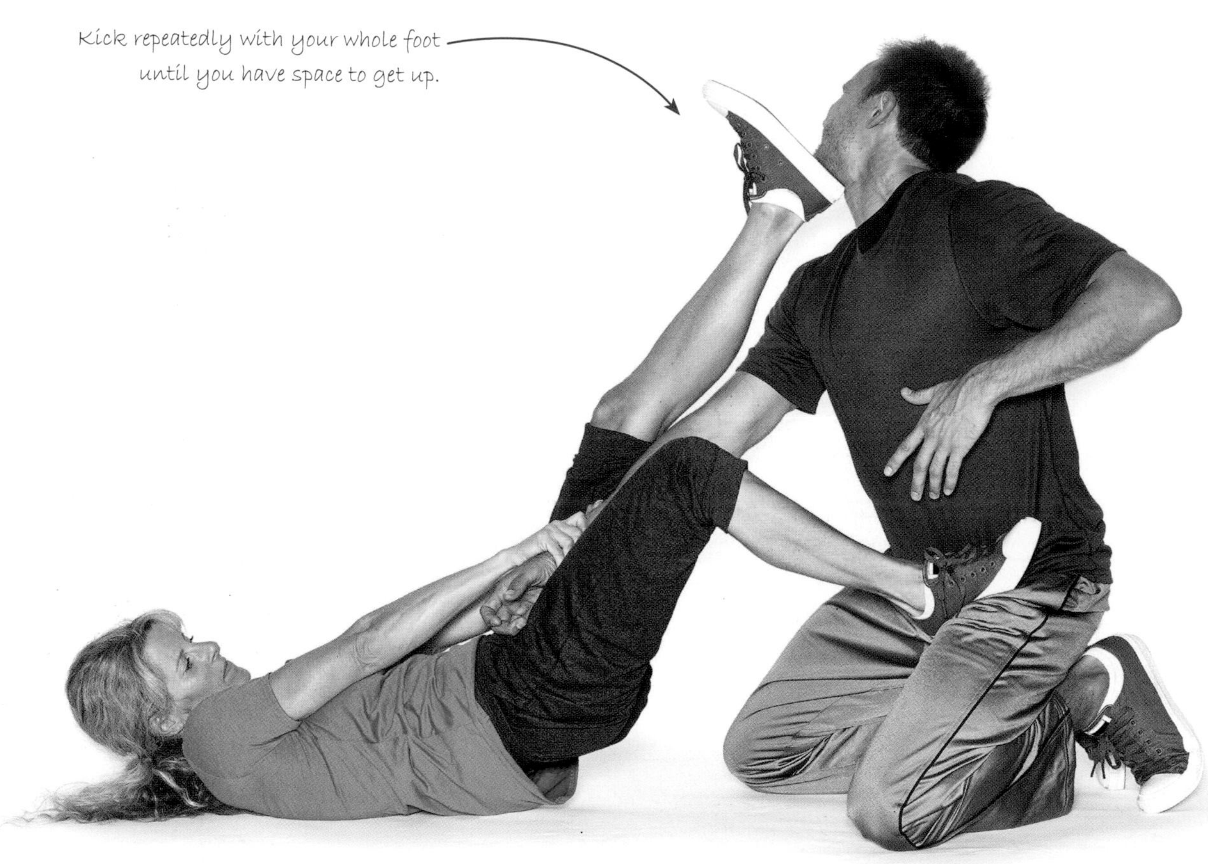

Kick repeatedly with your whole foot until you have space to get up.

4 When you have enough space from kicking, immediately get up.

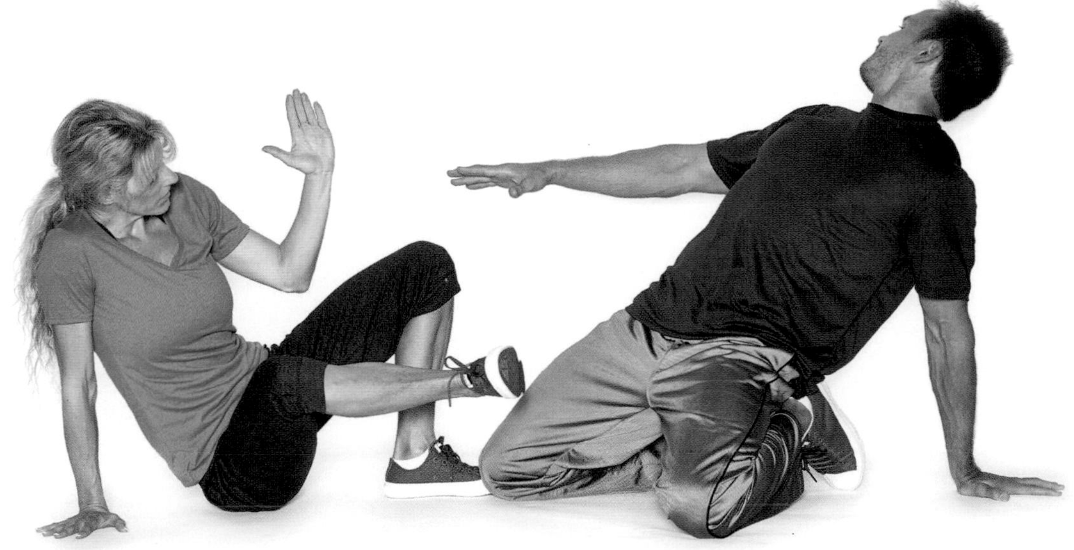

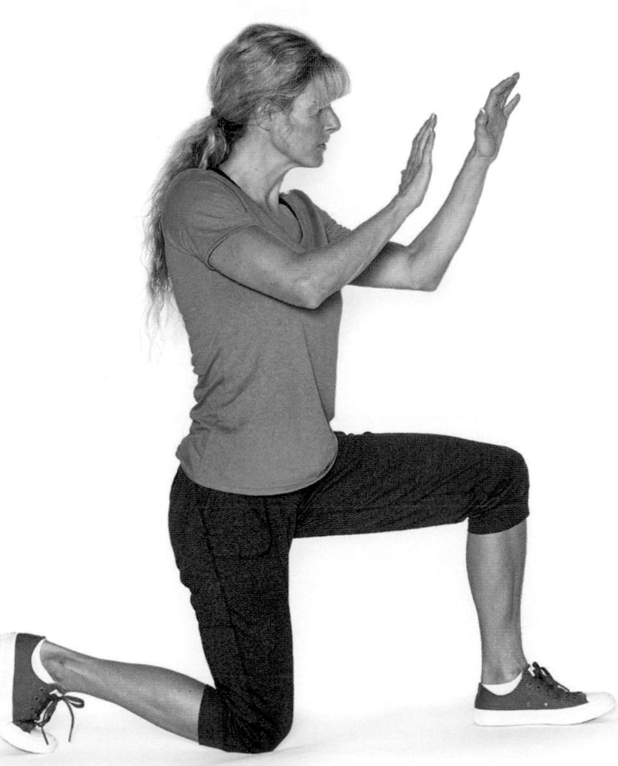

DEFENSE TIP

Although it's more difficult, you can still use this technique when your attacker is leaning forward onto your body. Strike at the eyes or throat until your attacker sits up. With this space, you can properly position your knee on your attacker's chest.

Escape from the Guard and Getting Up

You may find yourself trapped in your attacker's guard position—on the ground between his or her legs. Your goal is to strike your attacker's groin until you're able to escape and get off the ground safely.

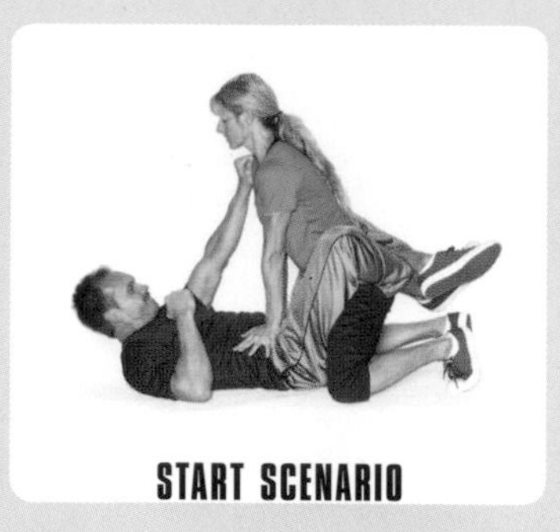

START SCENARIO

Your attacker traps you on the ground between his or her legs.

1. With an upright posture—head up, knees wide, and hips forward—strike your attacker's groin with both hands together. Use your elbows to then dig into your attacker's thighs to further break the guard.

Maintain control of your attacker's legs to avoid getting kicked in the face.

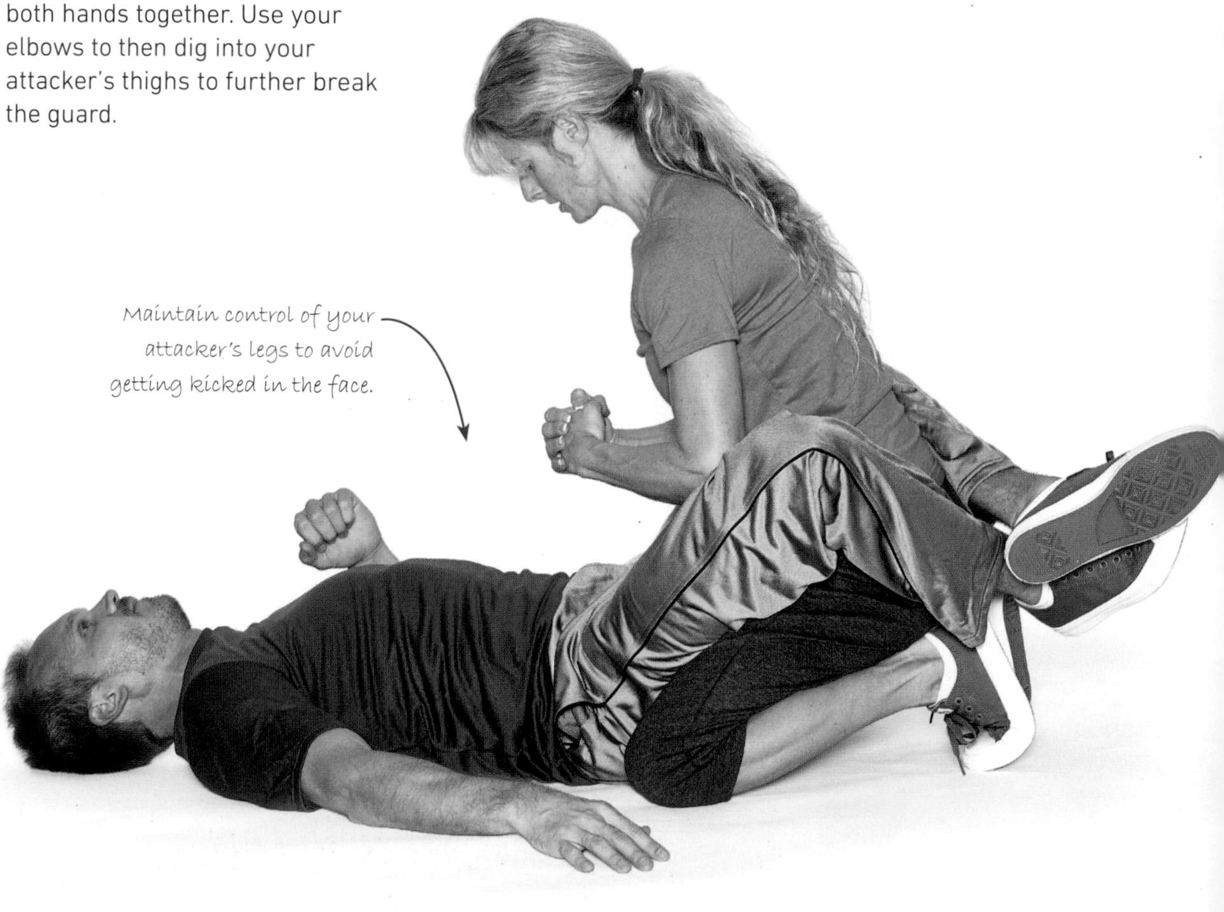

2 When your attacker's legs open, secure the inside one of his or her knees with one hand. Bring yourself to a kneeling position and deliver strikes.

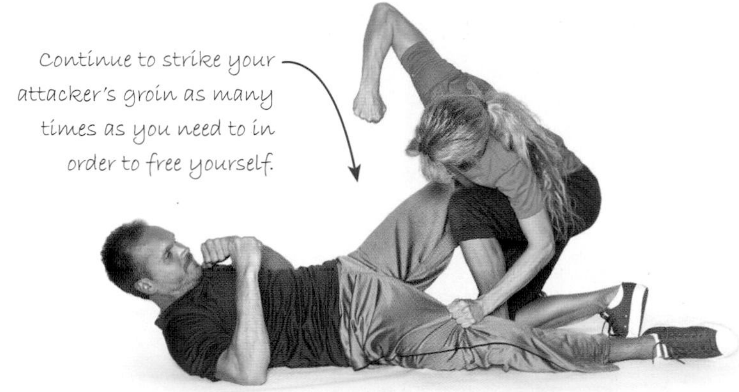
Continue to strike your attacker's groin as many times as you need to in order to free yourself.

3 Explosively pop out your attacker's guard by pushing out on the insides of his or her legs and bursting backward off your base foot. Maintain contact by tracing your attacker's legs as long as possible to avoid getting kicked.

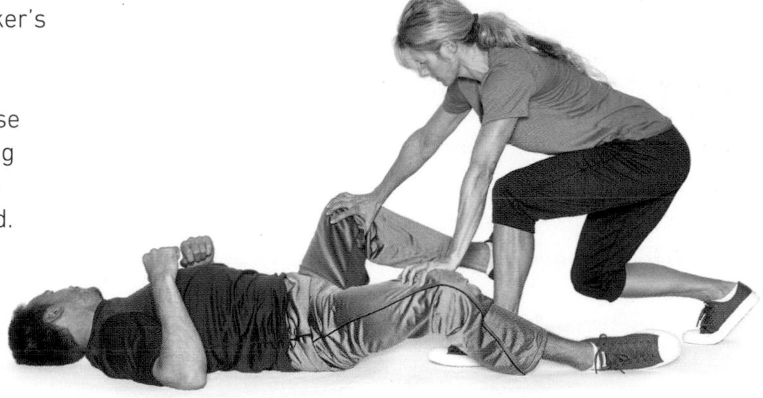

DEFENSE TIP

Sometimes an attacker will also pull you inward and trap your upper body. In this case, position your hands on his or her hips, keeping your elbows inward. Next, assume an upright posture and drive your knees into your attacker's groin until the hold loosens.

4 When completely free, get to your feet in Fighting Stance and counterattack or make your escape, depending on whether your attacker is still fighting back.

WEAPONS DEFENSE

Sometimes you may not simply be confronted by an attacker in hand-to-hand combat. Instead, he or she might wield a weapon, such as a knife, baseball bat, or gun. This section teaches you how to defend against these weapons safely so you can disarm your attacker and escape.

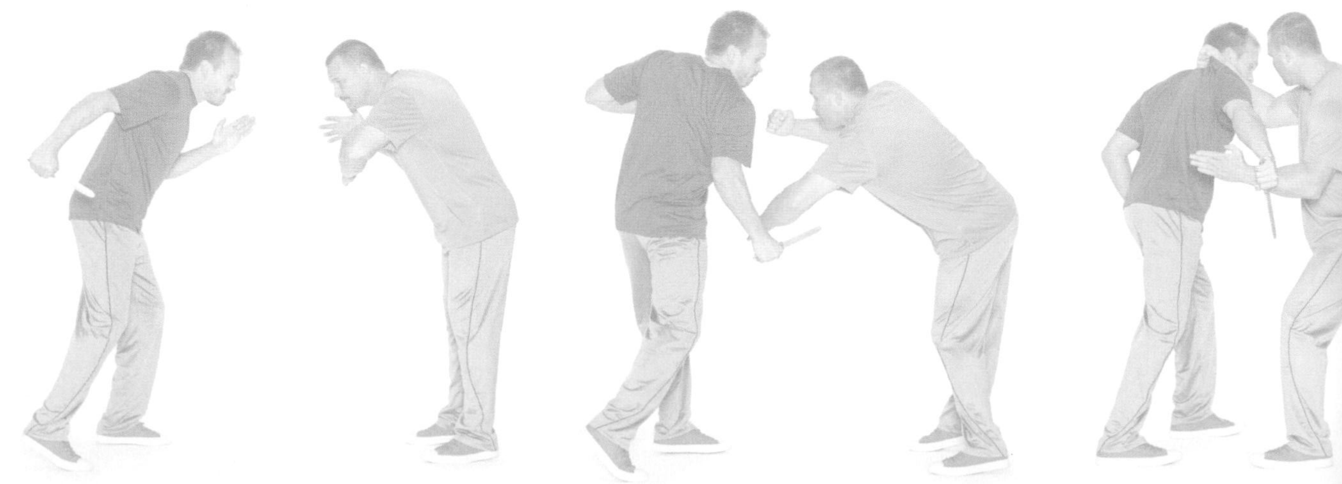

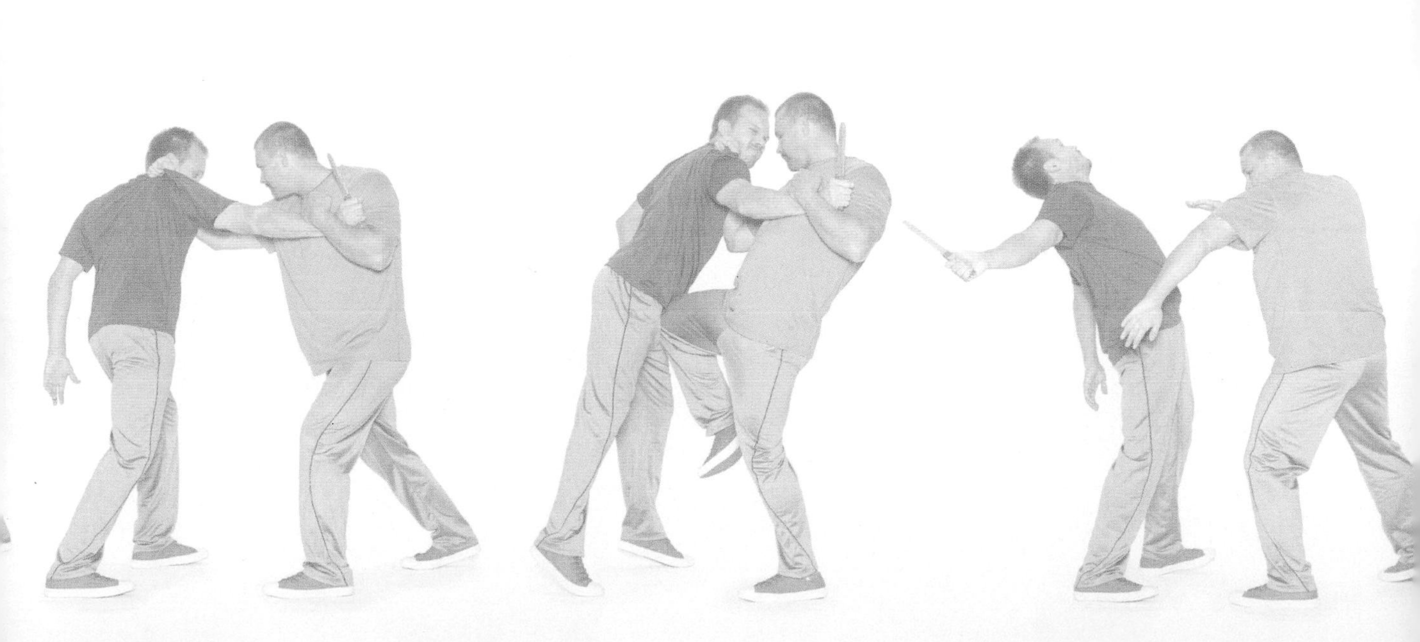

EDGED WEAPONS

These types of weapons may be used by your attacker to stab or slash at you, or simply to threaten. Two techniques using a knife can help you defend against overhead and underhand attacks.

Overhead Knife Attack

Use this defense if an attacker tries to stab your head, face, or neck from above with a knife or other edged weapon.

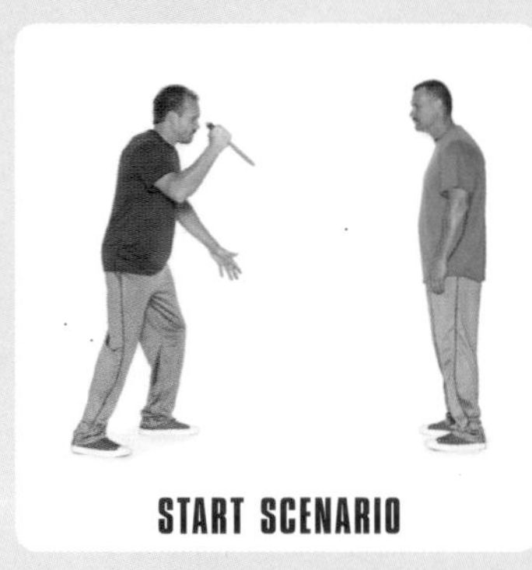

START SCENARIO

Begin in the Passive Stance, with your attacker holding a knife vertically.

1. As your attacker begins the stabbing motion, bring one arm up, bent at a 90-degree angle, to defend. Bring your other hand up in front of your face for protection.

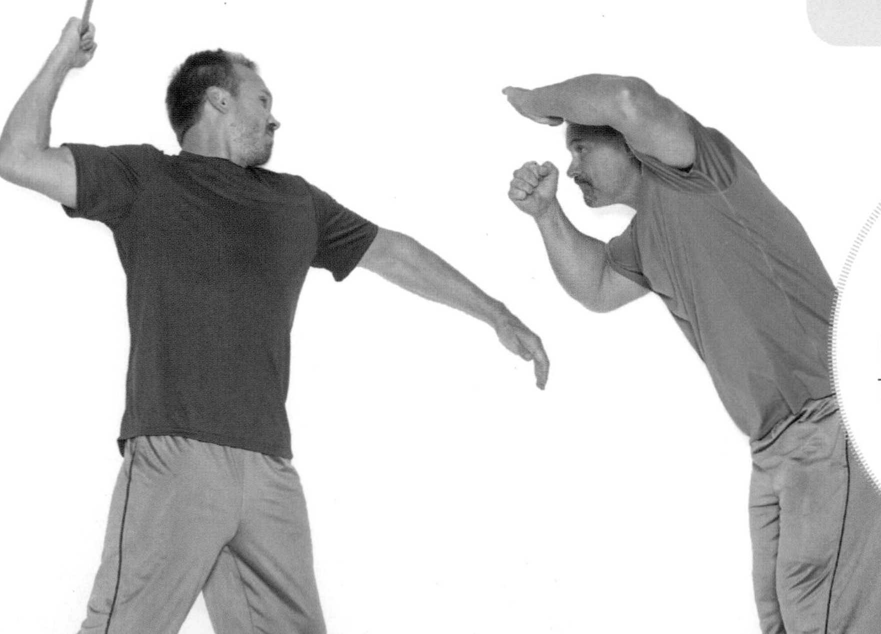

DEFENSE TIP

You must aggressively try to disrupt your attacker's thought process and balance with repeated counterattacks. The point is to gain control of the knife as quickly as possible and then flee.

2 Burst toward the inside of your attacker's arm holding the knife. Use the wrist of your defending arm to make contact with his or her stabbing arm. With your protecting hand, Straight Punch your attacker's face and quickly recoil.

Raise your defending arm before bending at the waist and bursting forward.

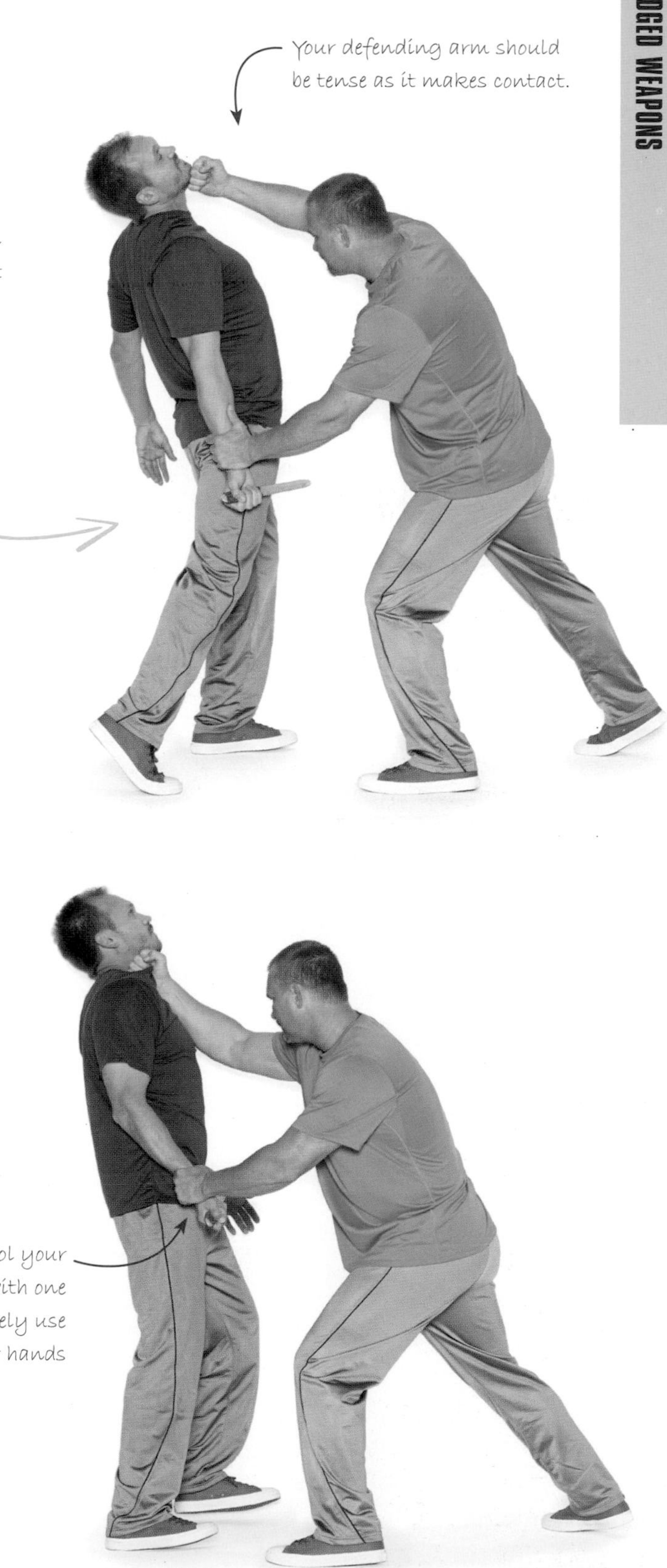

Your defending arm should be tense as it makes contact.

3 After making contact, slide your defending hand down to your attacker's wrist to gain control. Use your protecting hand to obtain a modified Control Position. Repeatedly deliver counterattacks until you disarn your attacker or are able to escape safely.

If you can't control your attacker's wrist with one hand, immediately use both of your hands

Underhand Knife Attack

Because an underhand knife attack is difficult to detect until a fight has begun, you must use this aggressive attack-against-the-attack technique—a simultaneous defense and counterattack.

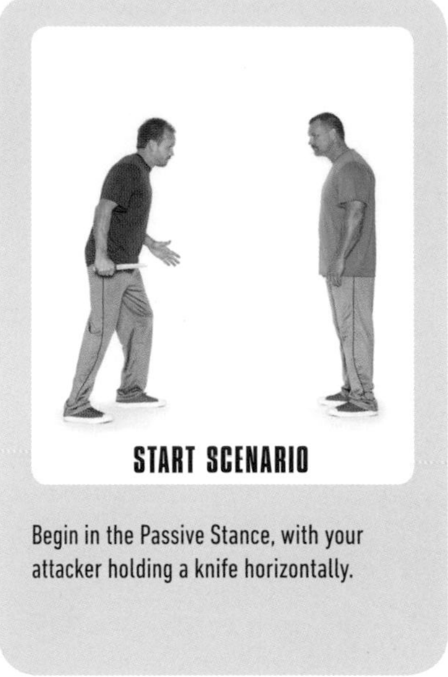

START SCENARIO

Begin in the Passive Stance, with your attacker holding a knife horizontally.

1 As your attacker begins the stabbing motion, send one arm down in front of your chest, bent at a 90-degree angle, to defend. Bring your other hand up in front of your face for protection.

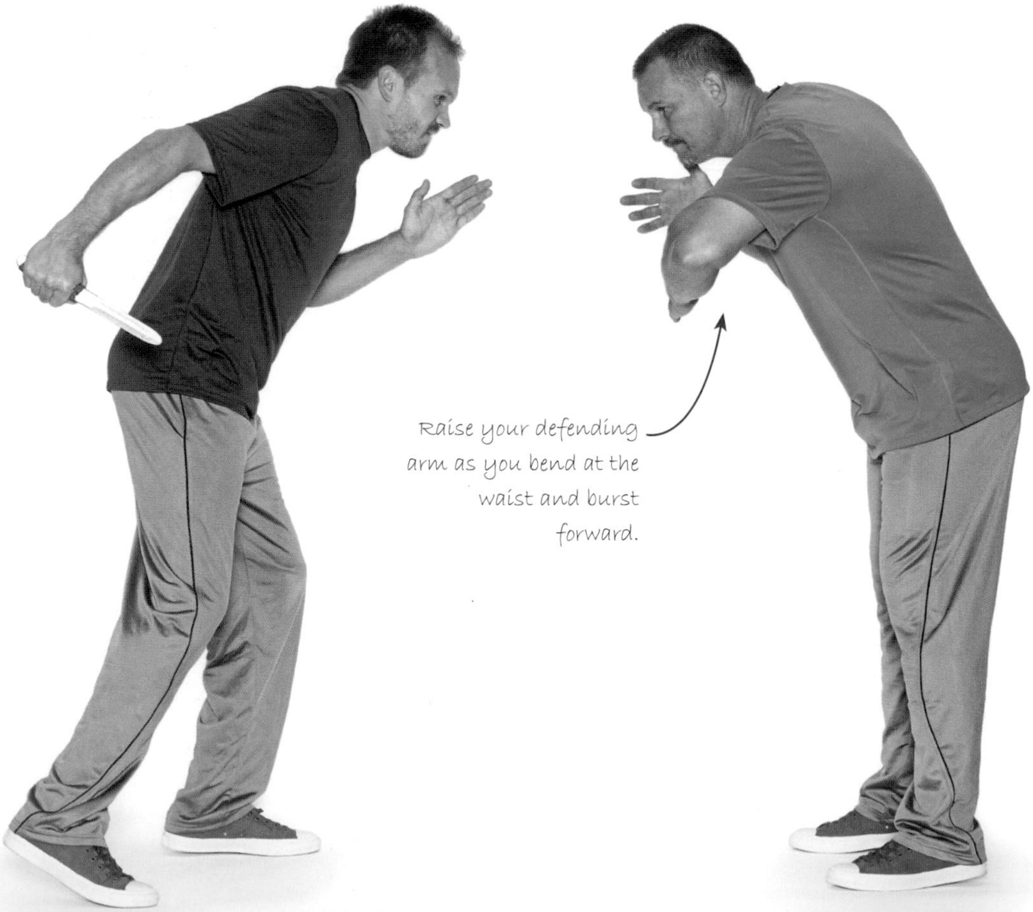

Raise your defending arm as you bend at the waist and burst forward.

2 Burst toward the inside of your attacker's arm holding the knife. Use the wrist of your defending arm to make contact with his or her wrist on the stabbing arm. With your opposite hand, Straight Punch your attacker's face and quickly recoil.

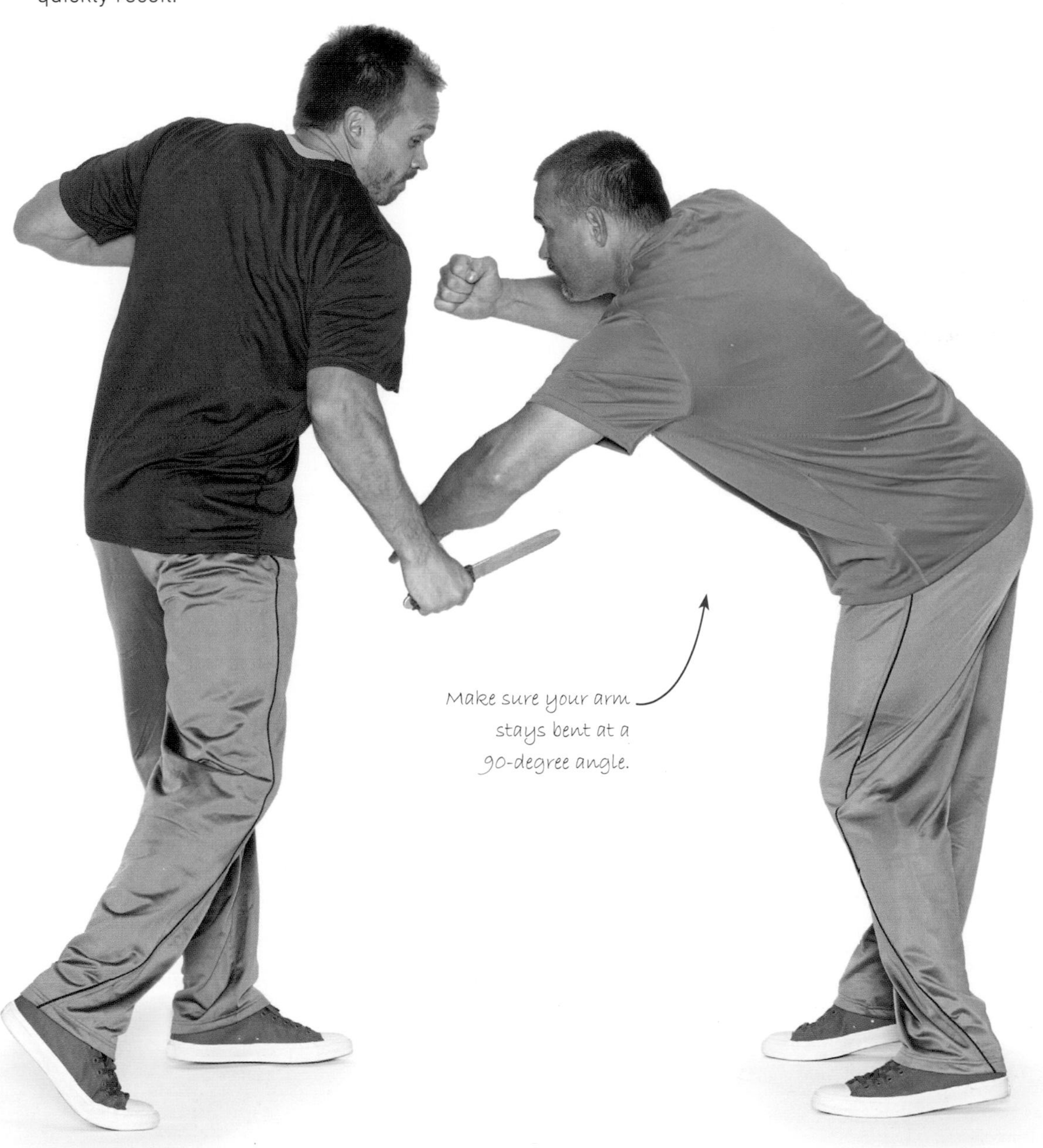

Make sure your arm stays bent at a 90-degree angle.

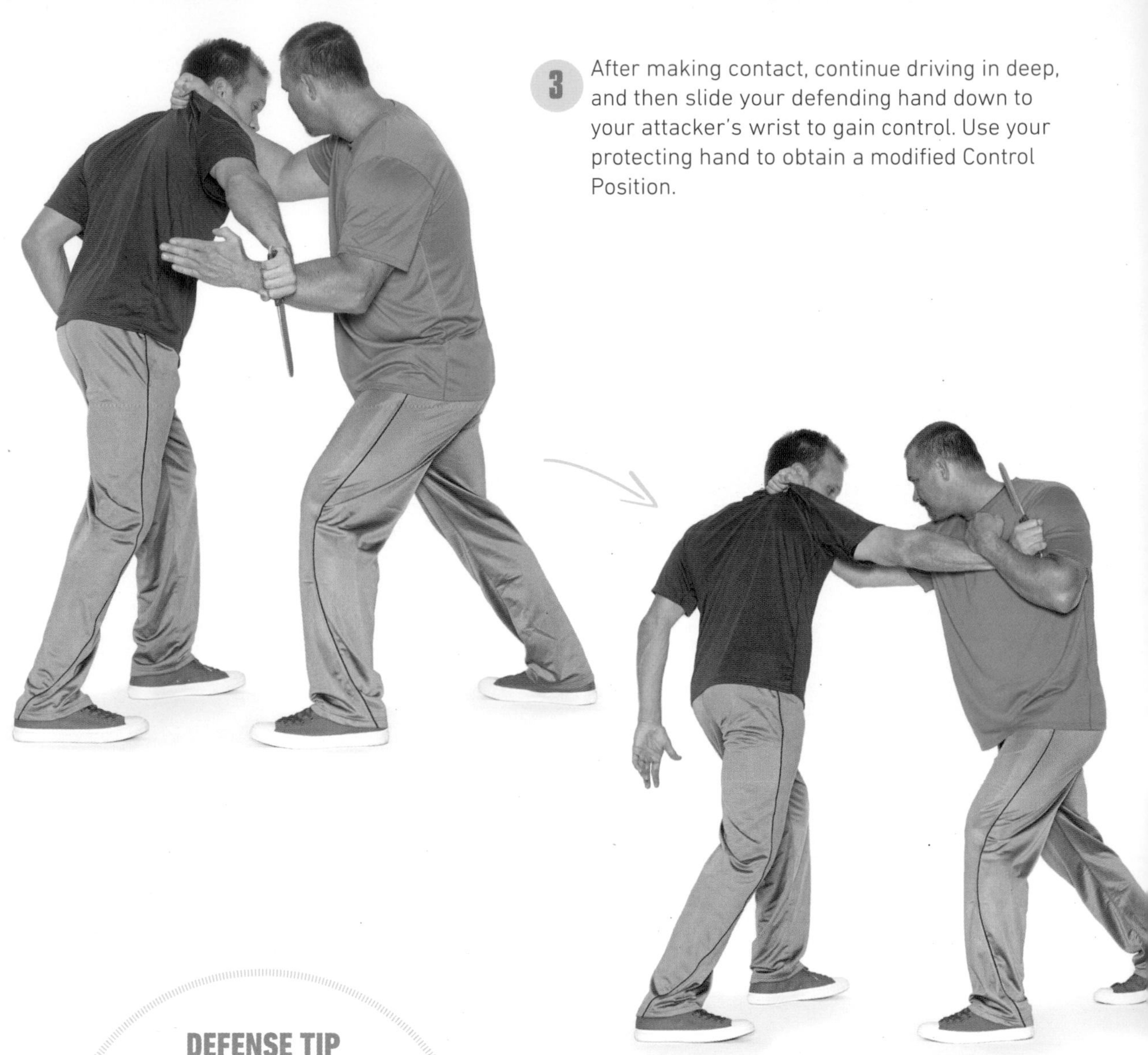

3 After making contact, continue driving in deep, and then slide your defending hand down to your attacker's wrist to gain control. Use your protecting hand to obtain a modified Control Position.

DEFENSE TIP

After your simultaneous defense and counterattack, obtain the Control Position as quickly as possible. As with all serious threats, you must strike until your attacker loses control of the weapon or you feel you can safely disengage.

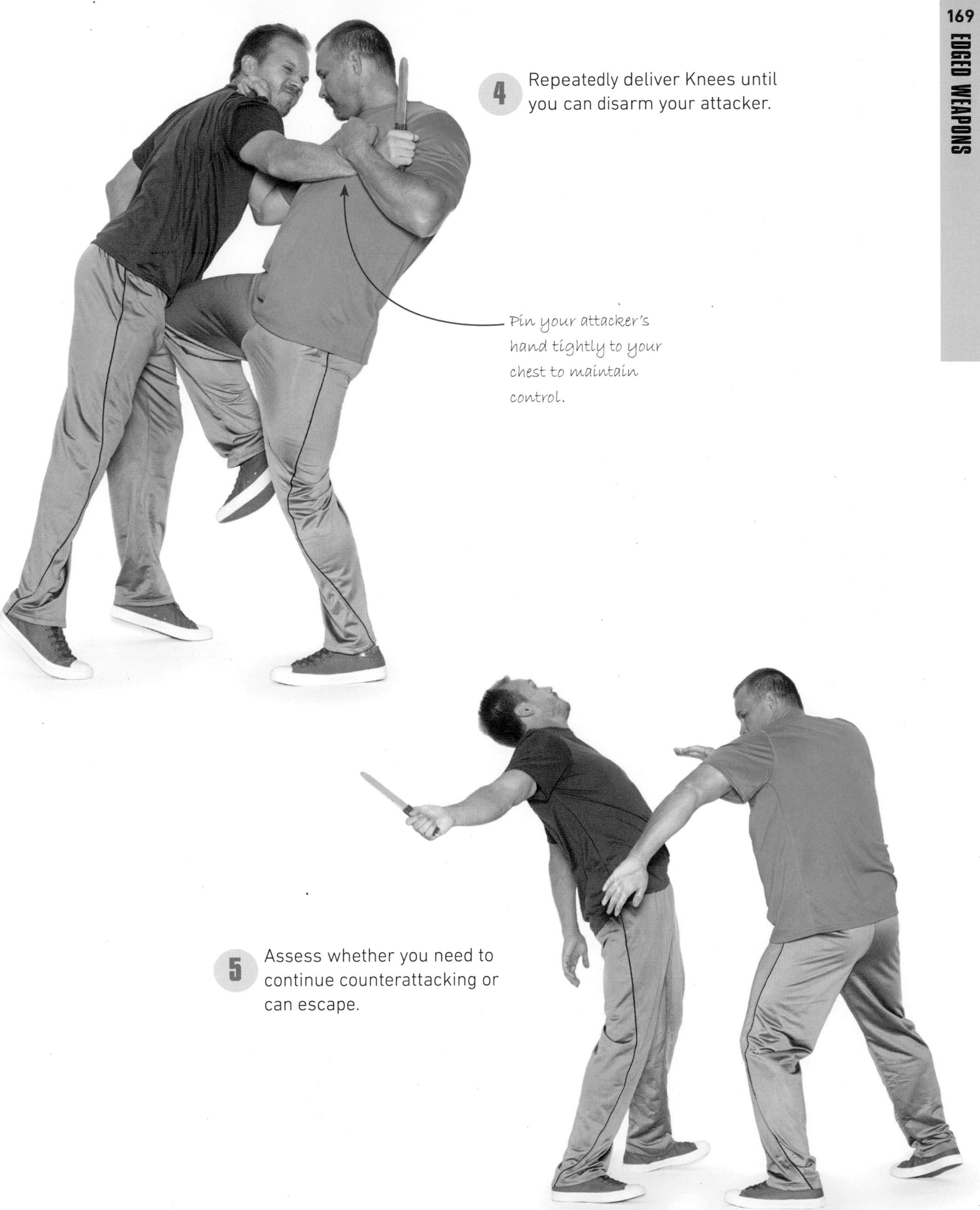
4
Repeatedly deliver Knees until you can disarm your attacker.
Pin your attacker's hand tightly to your chest to maintain control.
5
Assess whether you need to continue counterattacking or can escape.

IMPACT WEAPONS

Your attacker may also wield an impact weapon to incapacitate you, such as a baseball bat. These techniques show you how to defend against attacks from the side and overhead.

Side Baseball Bat Attack

Because the front ends are the fastest and most dangerous parts of impact weapons, you're safest when you move close to your attacker and the weapon.

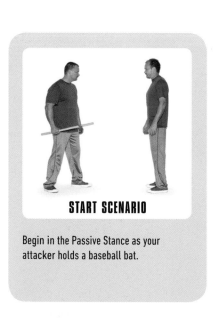

Begin in the Passive Stance as your attacker holds a baseball bat.

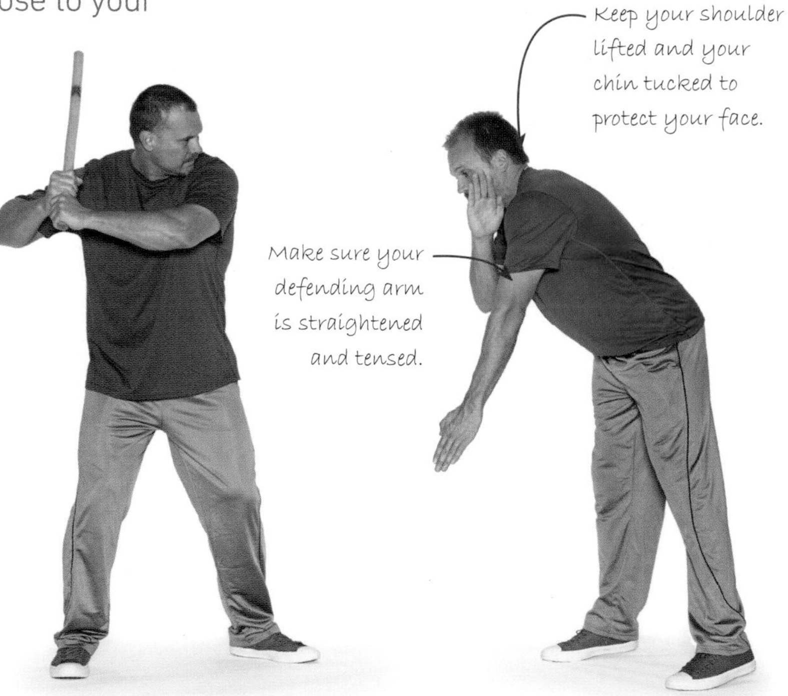

Keep your shoulder lifted and your chin tucked to protect your face.
Make sure your defending arm is straightened and tensed.

1 As your attacker begins the swing, turn your shoulder on the same side as the bat in toward your attacker's swinging arm. Hold up your outside hand to protect your face.

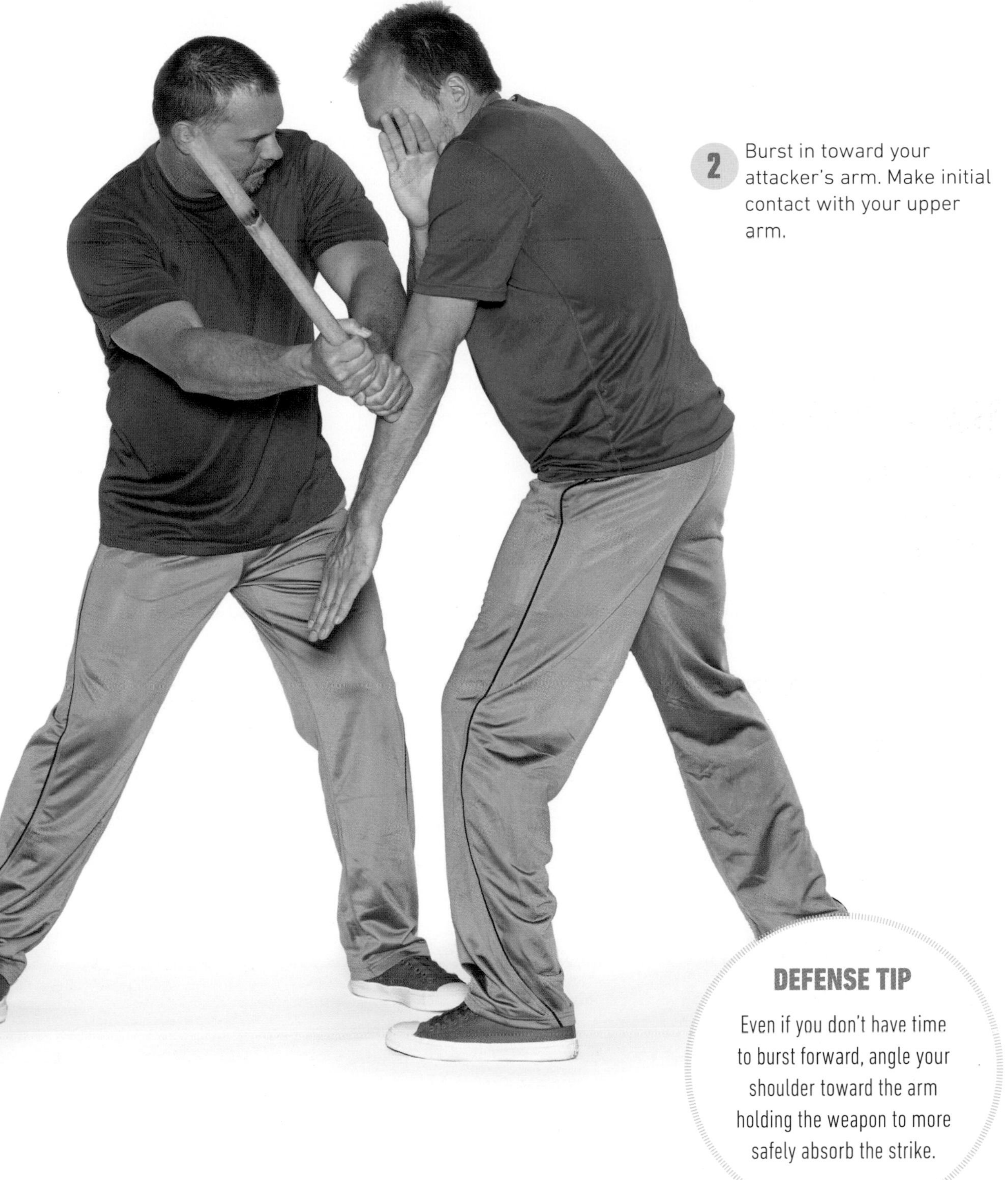

2 Burst in toward your attacker's arm. Make initial contact with your upper arm.

DEFENSE TIP

Even if you don't have time to burst forward, angle your shoulder toward the arm holding the weapon to more safely absorb the strike.

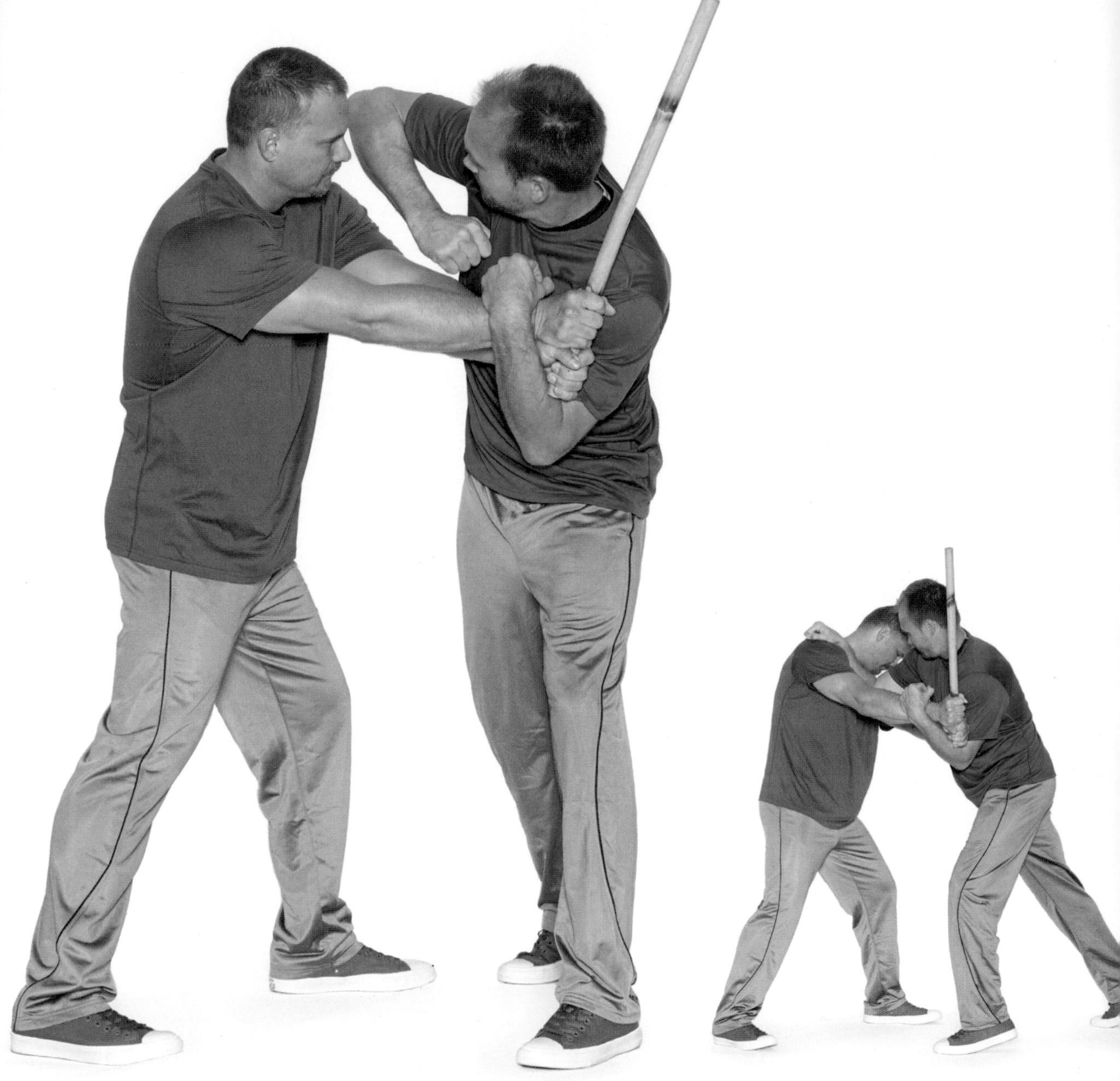

3 To trap the attacking arm, wrap your outside arm around your attacker's arm by bringing your hand to your shoulder. Simultaneously use your opposite arm to send an Elbow to his or her face.

4 Obtain a modified Control Position.

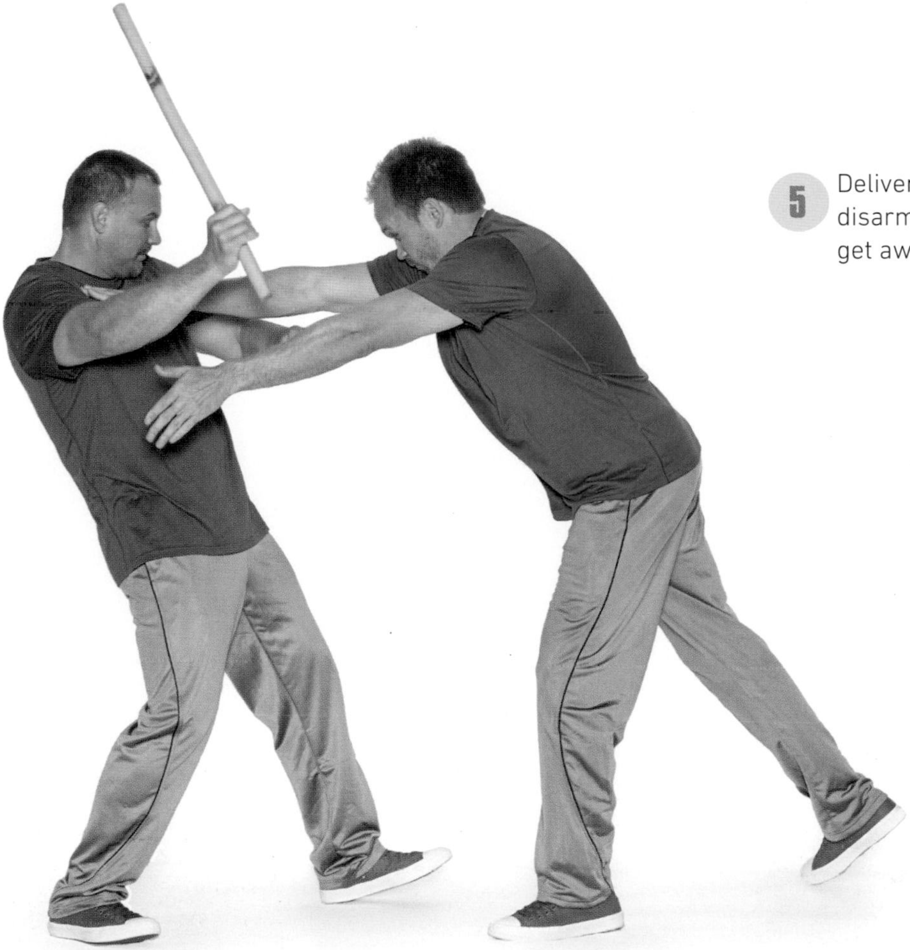

5 Deliver strikes until you disarm your attacker or can get away.

DEFENSE TIP

Even when you're unable to burst into the attacker right away, angling your body minimizes the force. As soon as you can, burst in and trap his or her arm. Send Knees until you can obtain the Control Position.

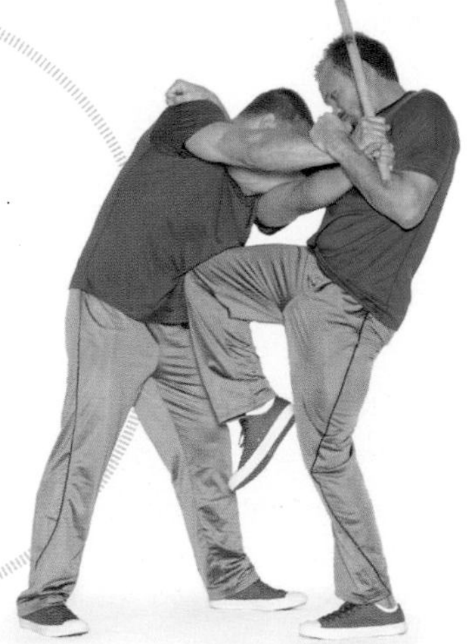

Overhead Baseball Bat Attack

If your attacker uses an impact weapon to assault you with a swing from above, your goal is to minimize the force to vulnerable parts of your body. By bending at the waist and bursting in with your hand up, you defend more quickly and lessen the chance of the weapon hitting your head.

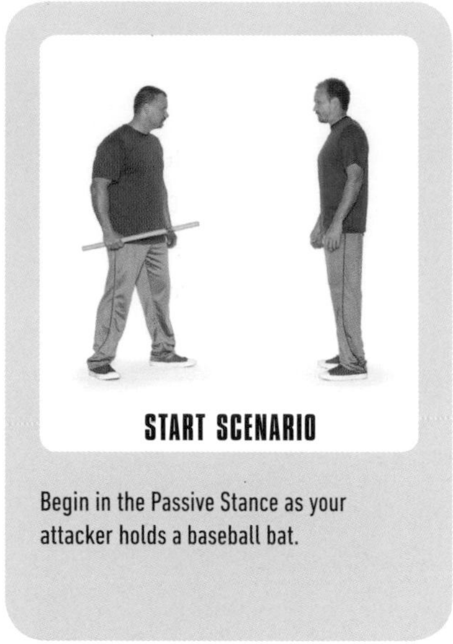

START SCENARIO

Begin in the Passive Stance as your attacker holds a baseball bat.

Always throw up your hand in defense before making a move toward your attacker.

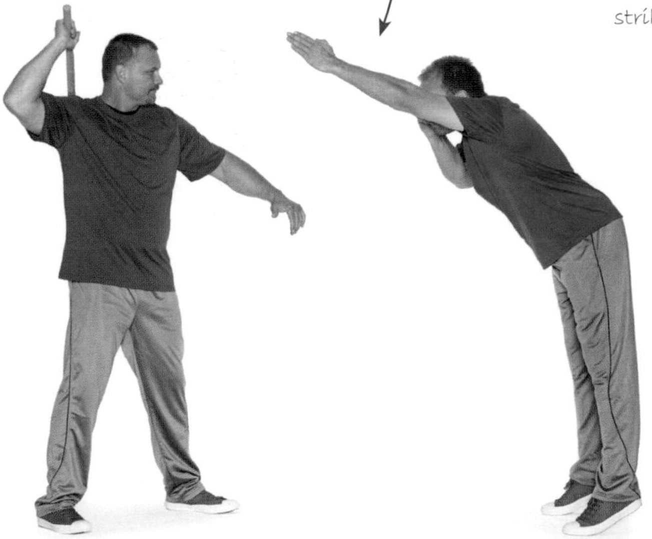

Your defending arm should be straight and tense when you make contact. As soon as you strike, quickly recoil.

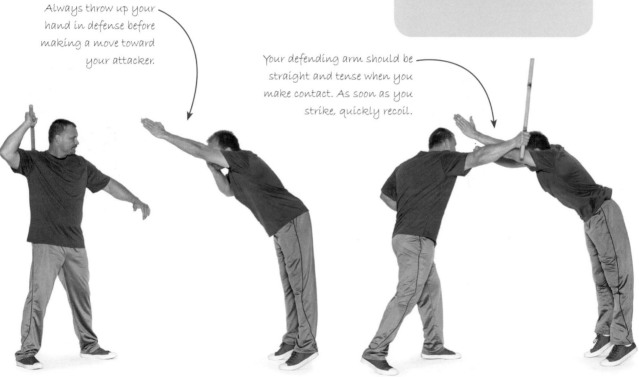

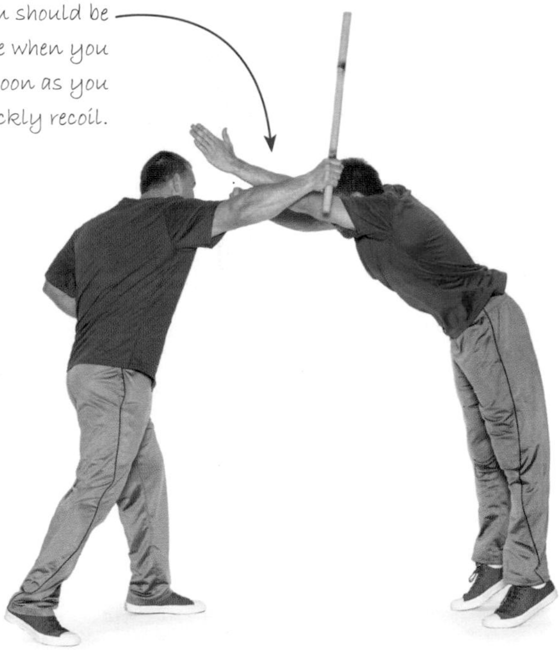

1. As your attacker begins to swing, send one hand straight up and out to defend while bringing your other hand up to your face for protection.

2. Bend at the waist and burst toward your attacker's swinging arm. Use your defending arm to defend against your attacker's hand, wrist, or arm while simultaneously striking his or her face with your other hand.

DEFENSE TIP

To protect your head, you may have to take some of the force from the strike and then keep fighting and moving forward to close the distance. That way, the attacker loses the advantage the reach of the weapon provides.

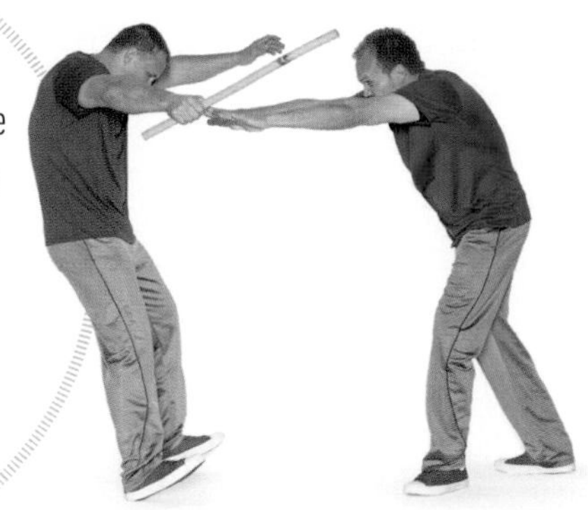

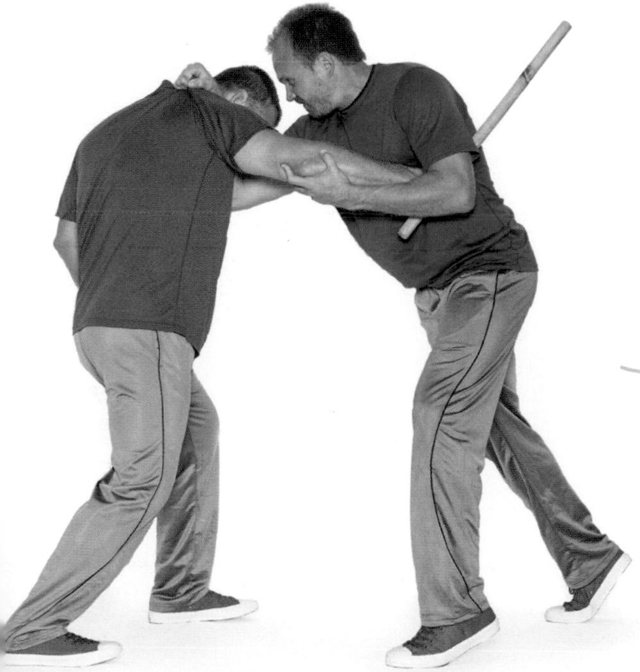

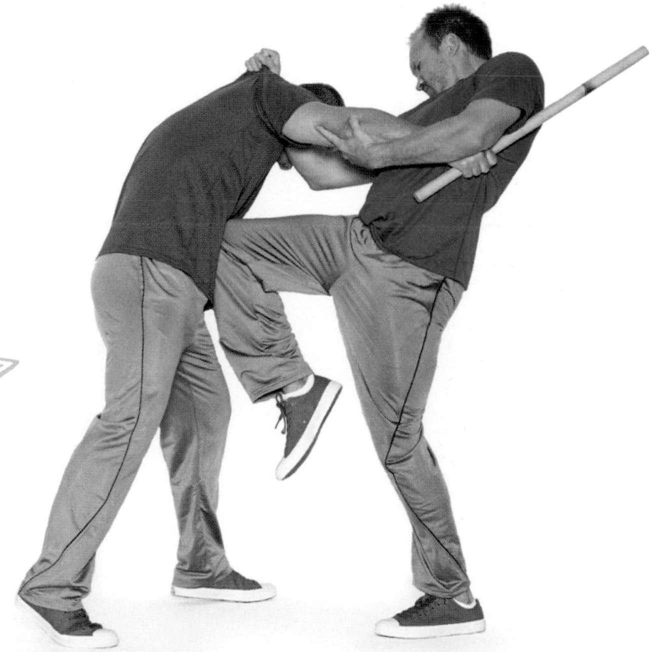

3 After impact, tuck your defending arm to your side by dropping your elbow. Simultaneously use your opposite hand to obtain a modified Control Position.

4 Repeatedly deliver Knees until you disarm your attacker or can get away. Because disarming your attacker doesn't guarantee defeat, continue striking until you can escape.

HANDGUNS

While encountering a handgun can be a scary prospect, you can protect yourself and make your escape using certain defenses.

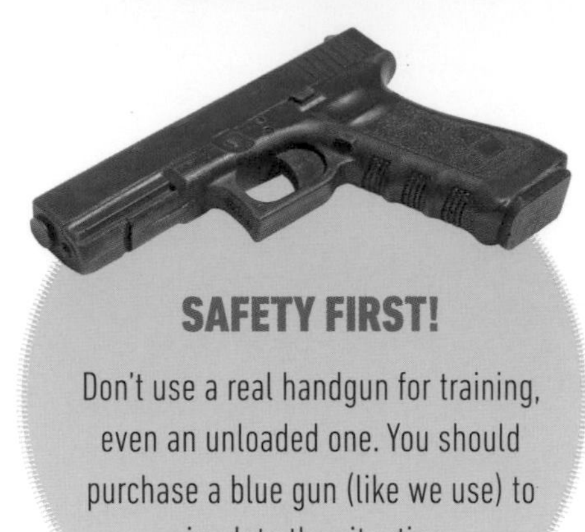

SAFETY FIRST!

Don't use a real handgun for training, even an unloaded one. You should purchase a blue gun (like we use) to simulate the situation.

Handgun from the Front

If someone threatens you with a handgun from the front to scare you, rob you, or force you to another location, you can redirect the gun using this technique.

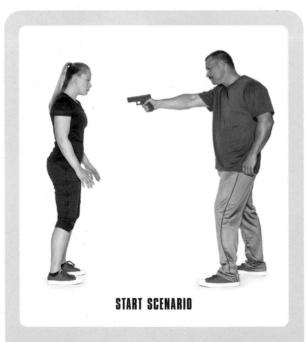

START SCENARIO

Begin in the Passive Stance, with your attacker pointing the gun at your chest.

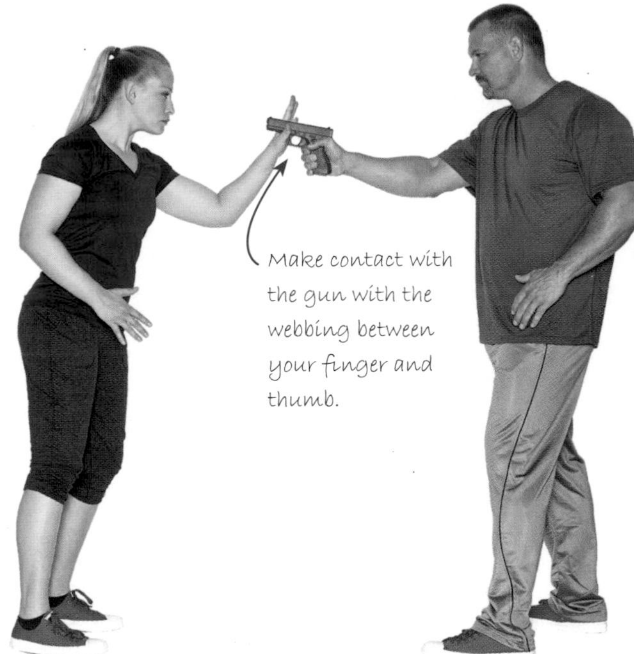

Make contact with the gun with the webbing between your finger and thumb.

1. With the arm closest to the gun, send your hand directly up along the side of the weapon. Rotate this shoulder toward your attacker to defend your body while simultaneously tracing your opposite hand up and close to your own body.

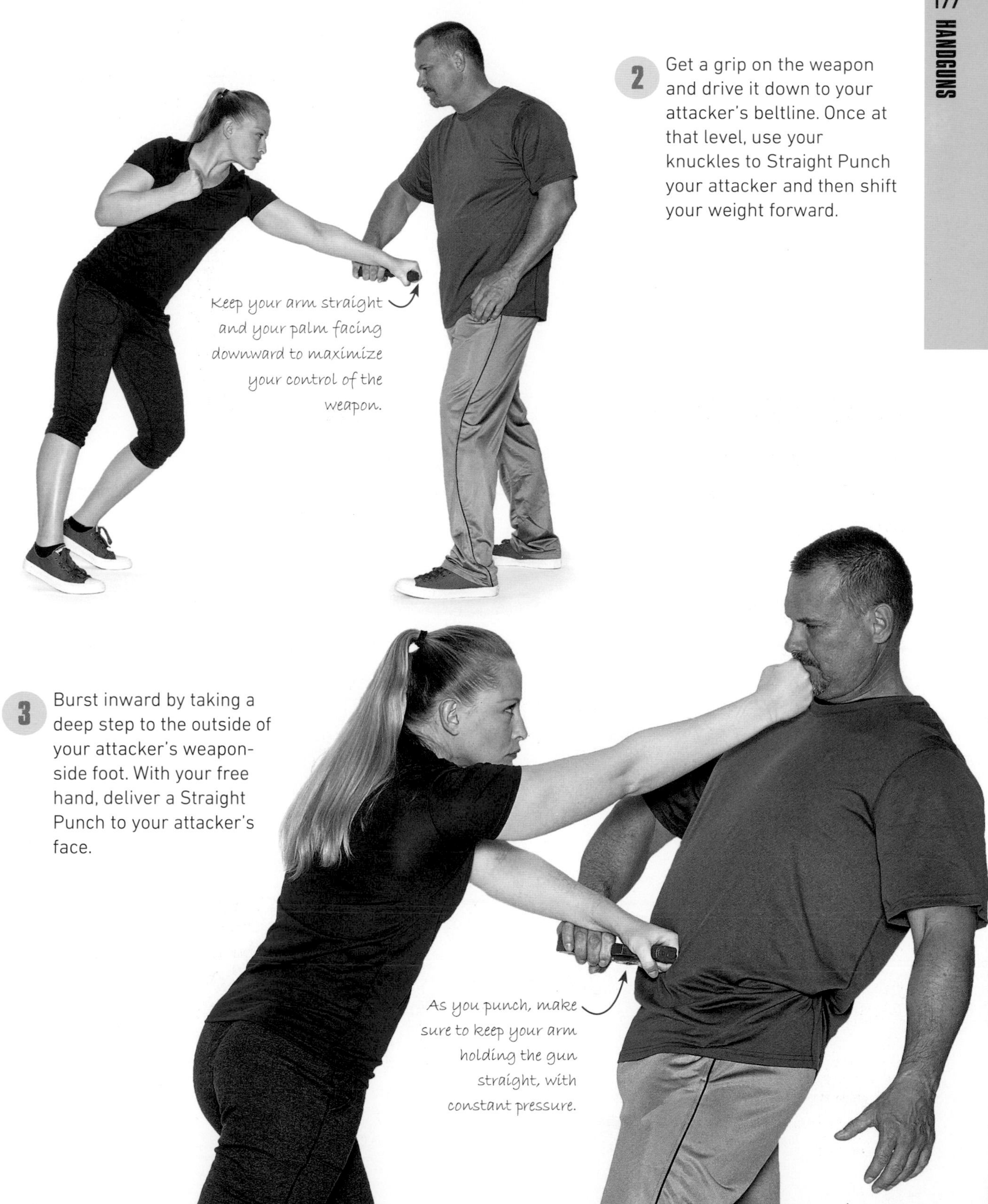

Keep your arm straight and your palm facing downward to maximize your control of the weapon.
As you punch, make sure to keep your arm holding the gun straight, with constant pressure.

2 Get a grip on the weapon and drive it down to your attacker's beltline. Once at that level, use your knuckles to Straight Punch your attacker and then shift your weight forward.

3 Burst inward by taking a deep step to the outside of your attacker's weapon-side foot. With your free hand, deliver a Straight Punch to your attacker's face.

4 Recoil your punching arm and trace that hand down your opposite arm to the back underside of the gun.

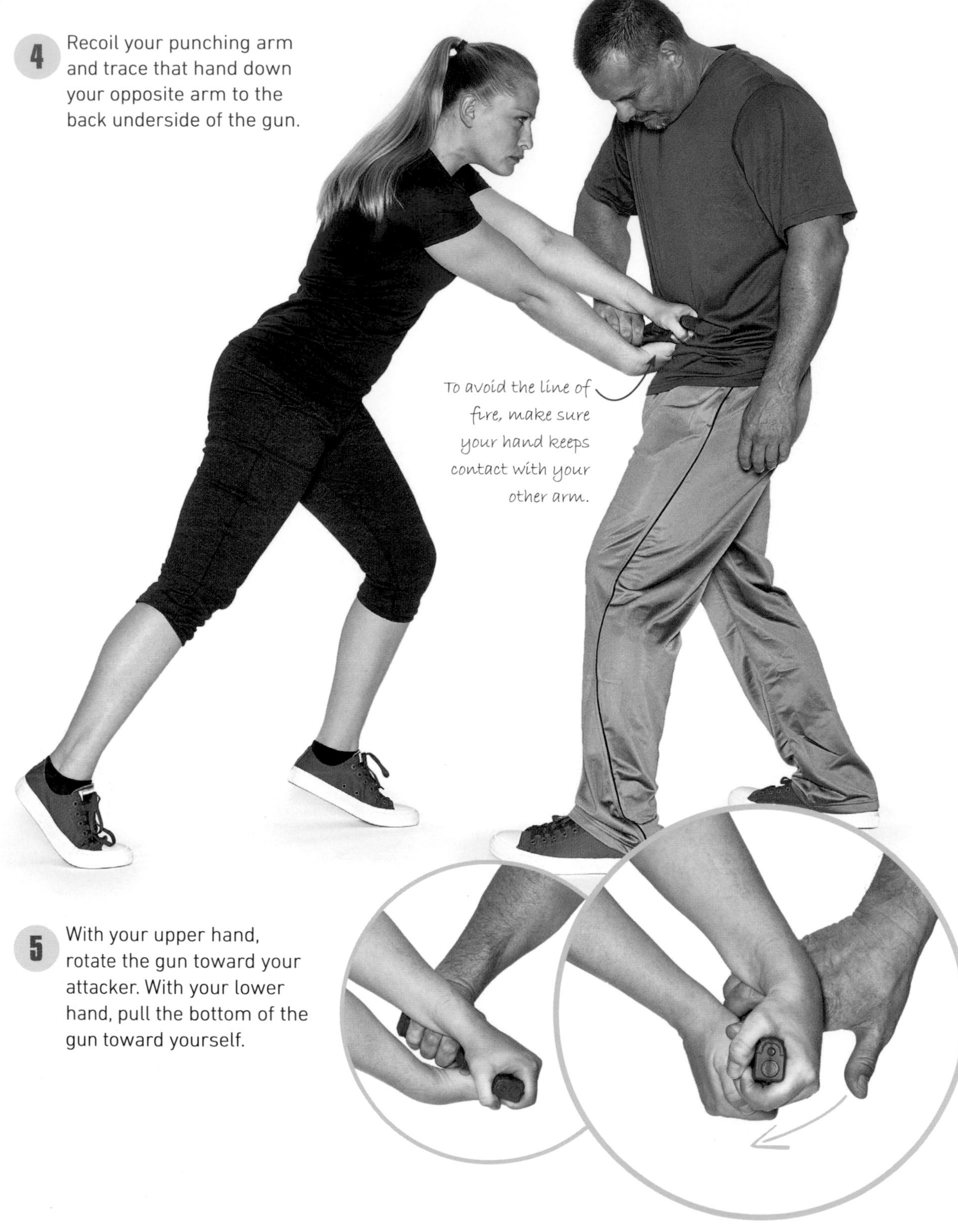
To avoid the line of fire, make sure your hand keeps contact with your other arm.

5 With your upper hand, rotate the gun toward your attacker. With your lower hand, pull the bottom of the gun toward yourself.

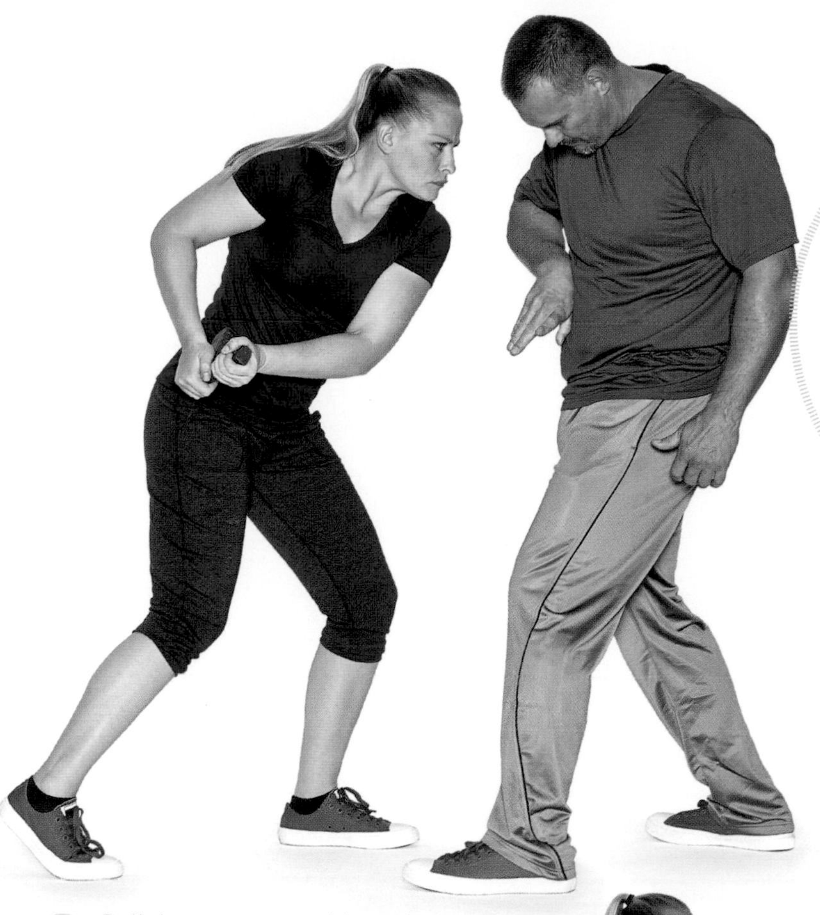

DEFENSE TIP

If at any point you feel the attacker really struggling to get the gun away from you, return to a two-handed control of the weapon. This way, you can avoid any chance of crossing the line of fire.

6 Pull the gun to your hip and then burst backward, removing it from your attacker's grasp.

7 Raise your free arm defensively to create a distance barrier between you and your attacker.

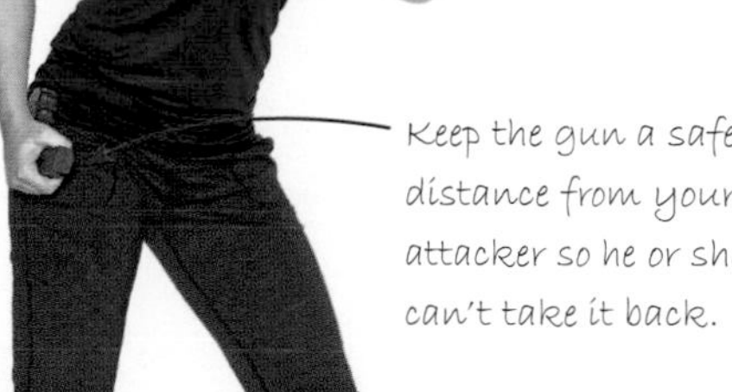

Keep the gun a safe distance from your attacker so he or she can't take it back.

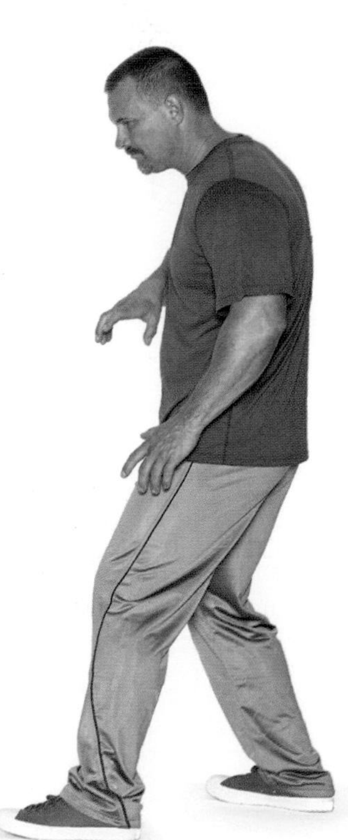

Handgun from the Back

An armed attacker may approach you from behind with a surprise attack. When this happens, you can redirect the gun and counterattack to escape safely.

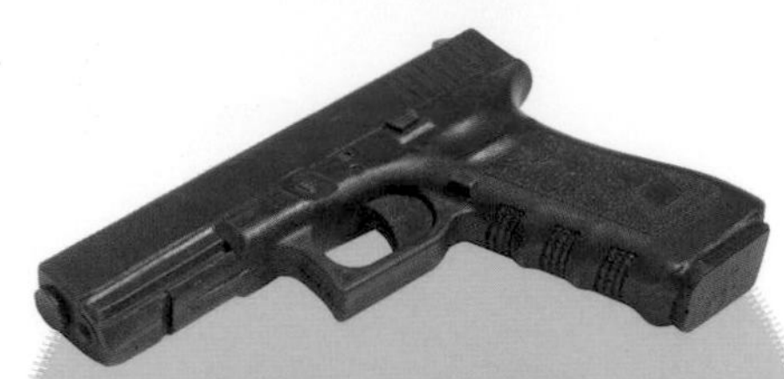

SAFETY FIRST!

Practice these techniques in a safe environment using only rubber training weapons. Never use a real gun for practice, even if it's unloaded.

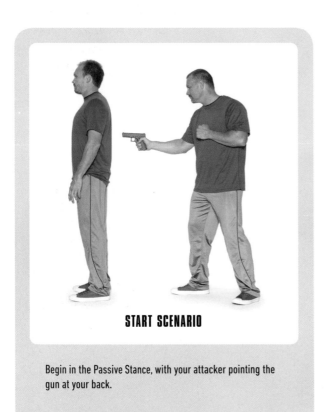

START SCENARIO

Begin in the Passive Stance, with your attacker pointing the gun at your back.

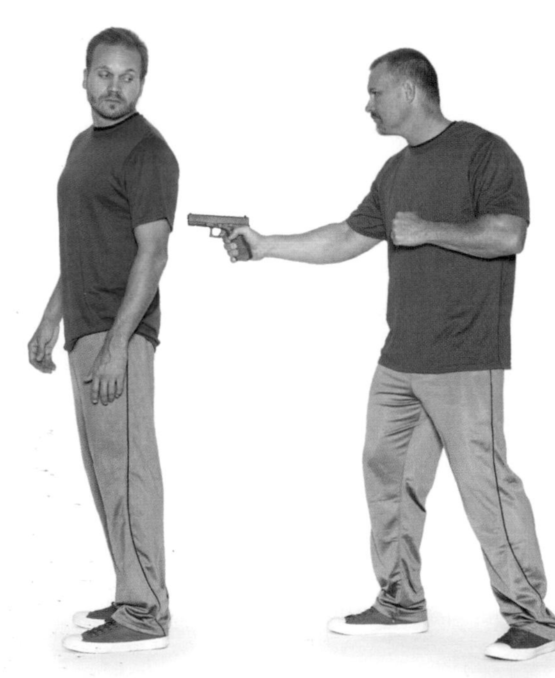

1 Look behind you to see with which hand your attacker is holding the gun. By looking over your shoulder, you gain a fuller picture of what's happening behind you and can then react more appropriately.

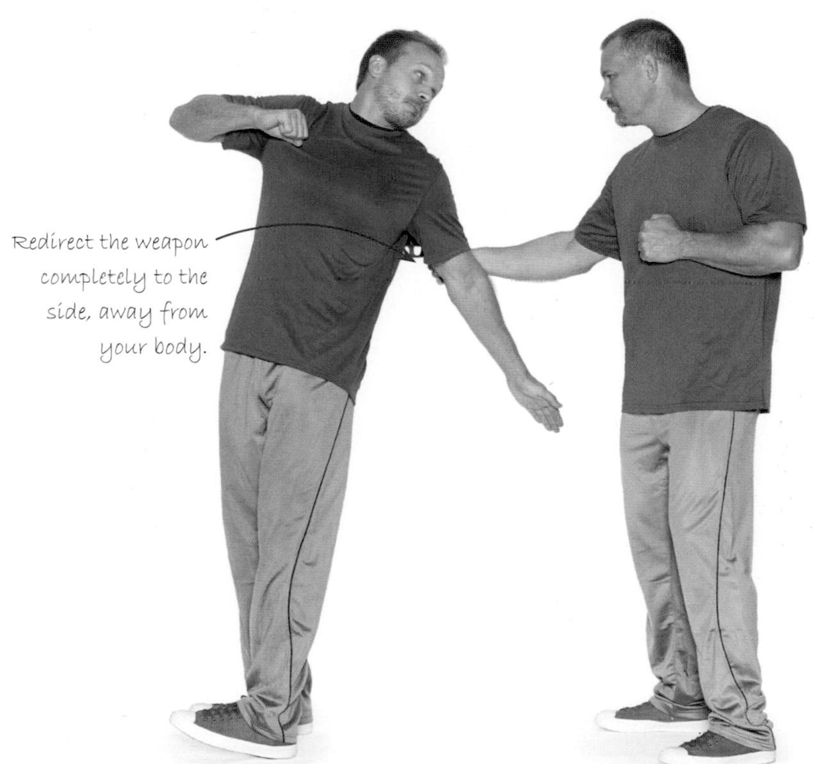

Redirect the weapon completely to the side, away from your body.

2 Keeping your arm straight and close to your body, turn in the direction you were looking. Use your arm to slightly push the weapon and redirect the line of fire.

DEFENSE TIP

Your instinct in this situation may be to turn completely around to face the attacker. If you react this way, just continue with the From the Front handgun defense technique.

3 Burst toward the attacker. With the hand of the arm that redirected the gun (deflecting arm), trace along the inside of your attacker's arm. Trap the arm holding the gun by wrapping your deflecting arm around your attacker's arm and bringing your hand to your shoulder. Simultaneously use your opposite arm to send an Elbow to your attacker's face and then quickly recoil your elbow.

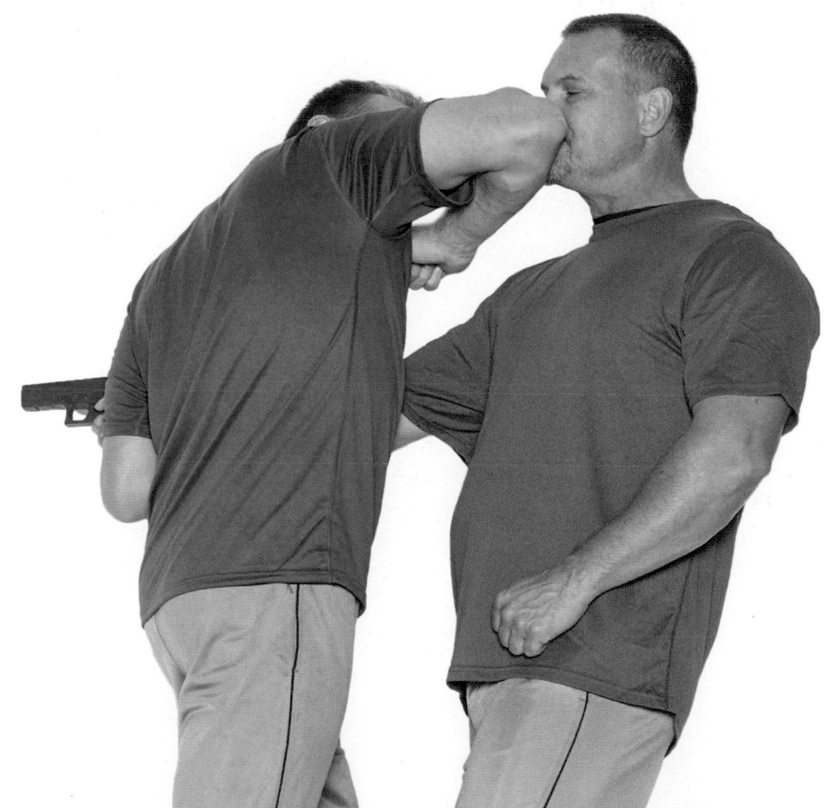

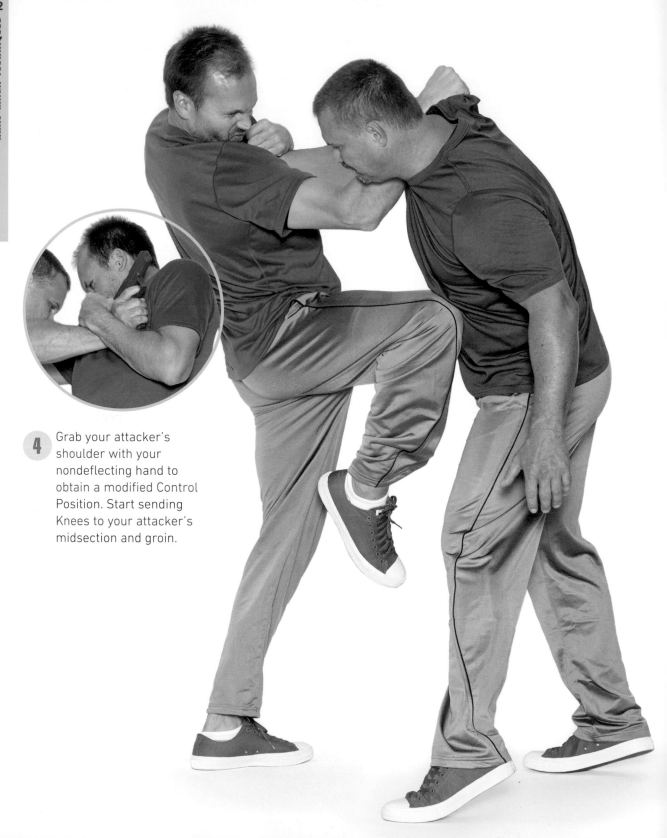

4 Grab your attacker's shoulder with your nondeflecting hand to obtain a modified Control Position. Start sending Knees to your attacker's midsection and groin.

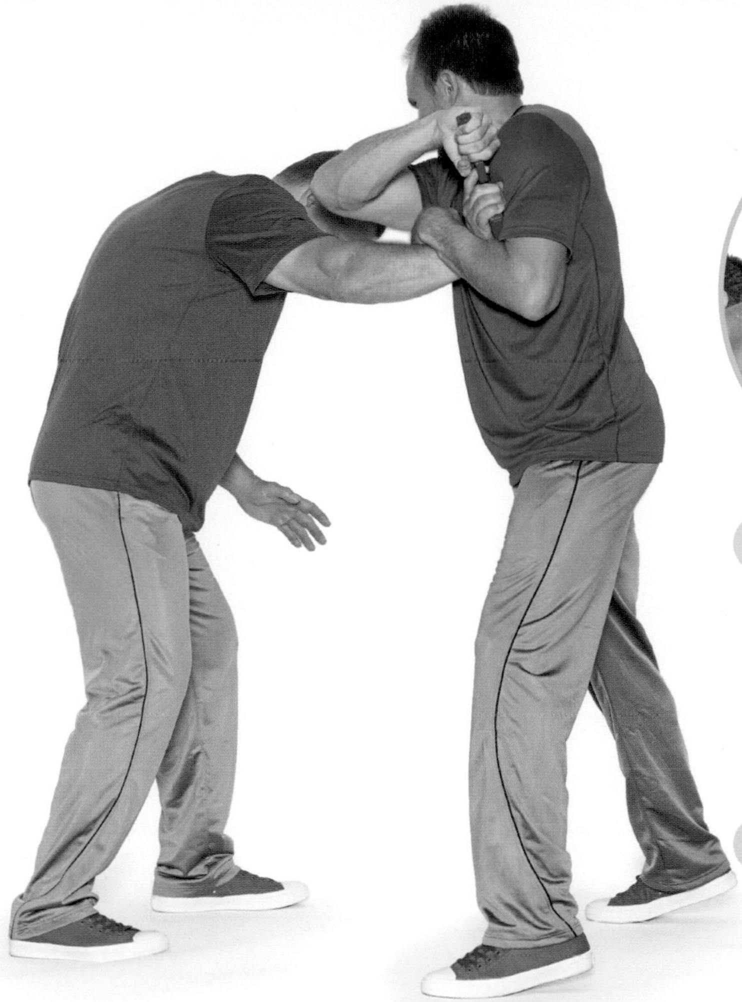

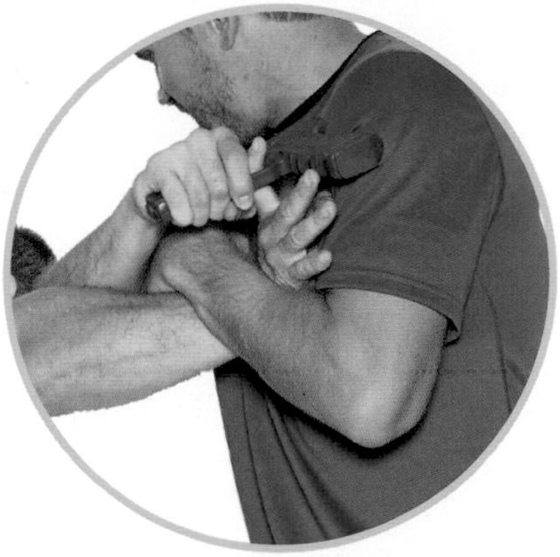

5 With your nondeflecting hand, reach over your deflecting shoulder. With your pinky finger on top, grasp the gun and break it down against your attacker's hand.

6 Pull the gun up and off your attacker's hand.

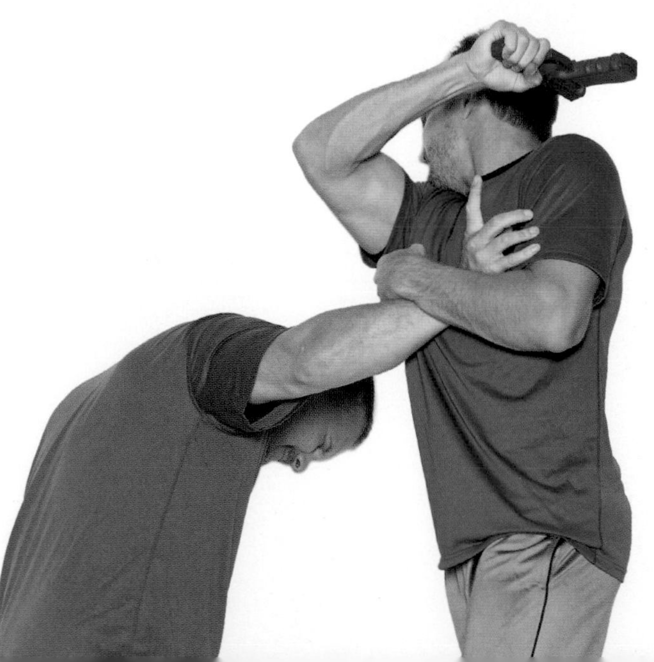

7 Deliver an Elbow to his or her head with the arm in which you're holding the gun. Immediately back up and move away.

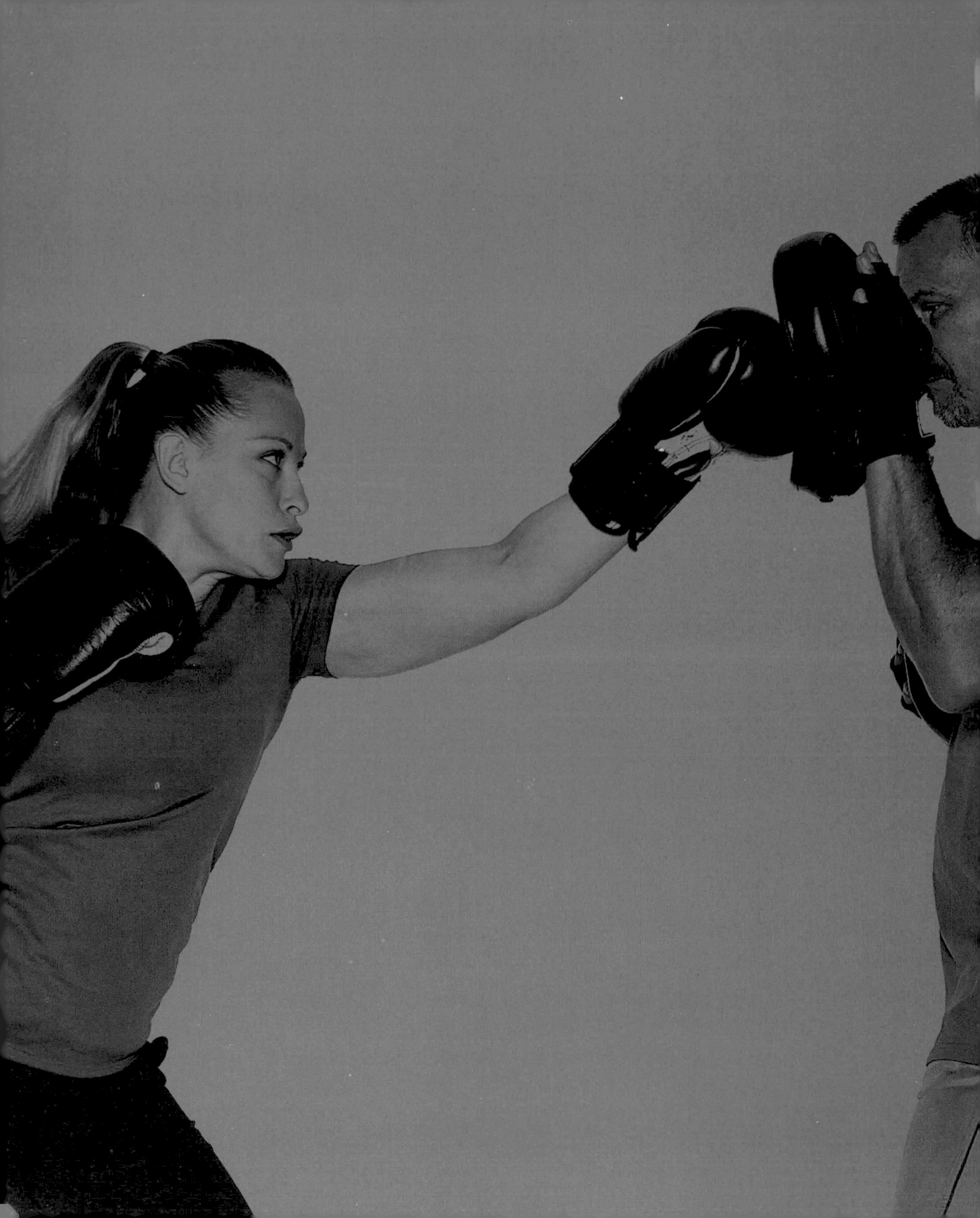

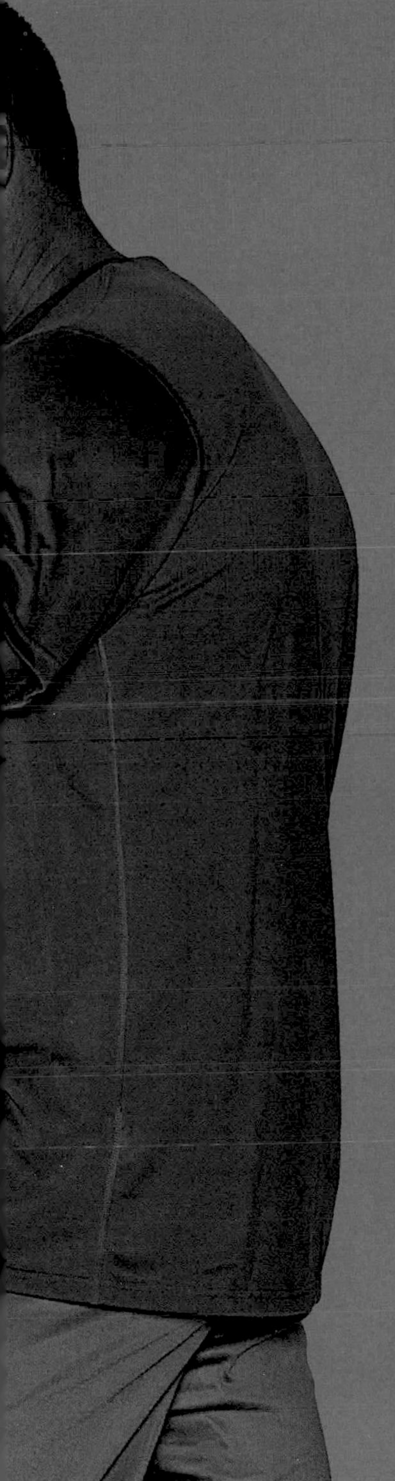

PART 4

KRAV MAGA TRAINING

PROTECTIVE GEAR AND EQUIPMENT

To build power, speed, focus, and repetition and to avoid injuring yourself or a partner, you have the option of purchasing some basic protective gear. The following are the different pieces of equipment we recommend.

A SOUND INVESTMENT

While you can spend as much or as little as you want, you'll probably want to invest a little more to ensure your equipment is durable over a long period of time (meaning you won't have to continually replace things).

Boxing Gloves

For matches and training, especially during repeated strikes to focus mitts or heavy bags, you can use boxing gloves to protect your hands. If you're less than 150 pounds (68kg), we recommend 14-ounce (400g) gloves; if you're more than 150 pounds (68kg), we recommend 16-ounce (450g) gloves.

Hand Wraps

As another option to protect your hands, you can train with hand wraps only. These keep the bones and tissues of your hands compressed to protect them from breaks and damage.

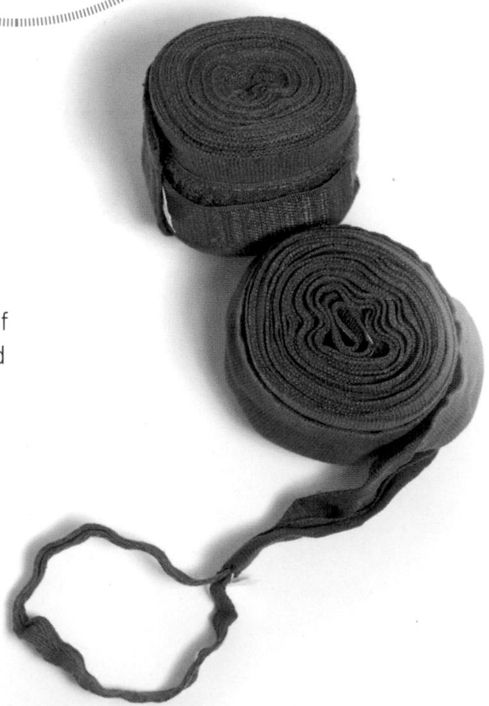

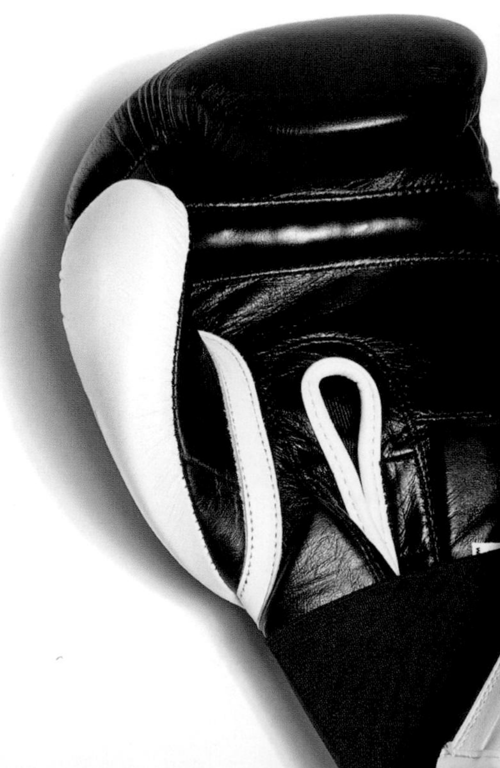

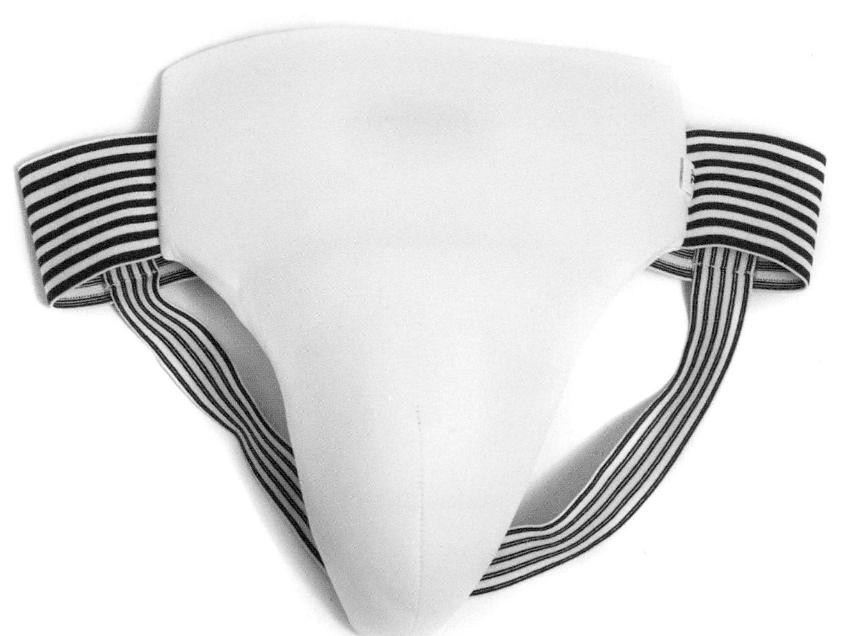

Groin Protector

Regardless of whether you're male or female, a groin protector will protect your groin during self-defense and sparring training. It distributes the shock of a strike, lessening the direct impact to the area.

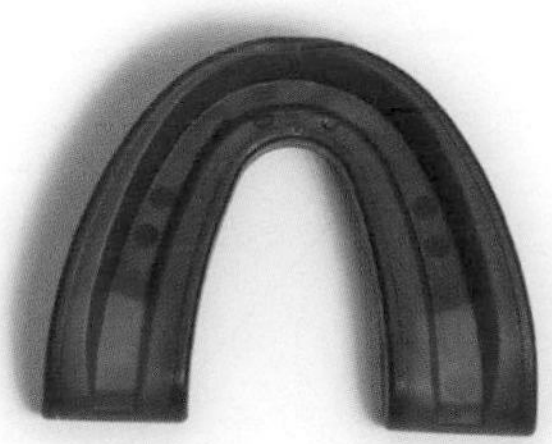

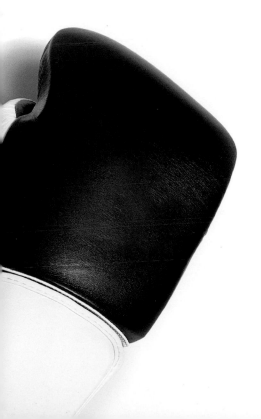

Mouth Guard

A mouth guard is a protective device that covers your teeth and gums to protect them against injury. We recommend wearing a mouth guard when training in Krav Maga in order to become more comfortable with the feeling before you begin more advanced training (such as full-speed partner work and sparring), where a mouth guard is a must.

Grappling Gloves

Grappling gloves are the light, open-fingered gloves used in Krav Maga training and MMA fights. They usually have 4 to 6 ounces (110 to 170g) of padding to protect the small bones in your hands while leaving your fingers free for making defenses.

Focus Mitts

Focus mitts are a versatile tool for developing speed and accuracy, as well as timing, distancing, and strategy. When using focus mitts with a trained partner, they help simulate a more realistic fight situation.

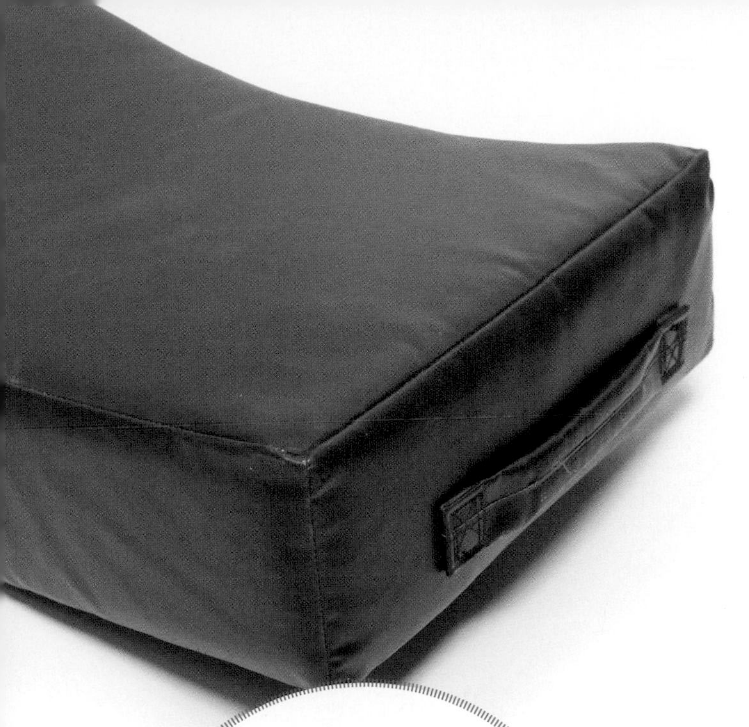

Kick Shield

The kick shield is a large pad used for stronger kicks, such as the Front Kick, Side Kick, or Back Kick. You can also use it to defend against stronger Knees or during ground and aggressiveness drills.

HEAVY BAG

You also have the option of a heavy bag for solo work—a large leather or vinyl stuffed bag ranging in weight from 50 to 200 pounds (23 to 90kg). Striking it develops your distancing, combinations, repetition, and power.

Tombstone Pad

Unique to Krav Maga training, the angles of a tombstone pad are developed so you can deliver combinations of Straight Punches, Palm Strikes, and Hammerfists without damaging your wrists. You can also use it when you're defending against Elbows, kicks, and light Knees.

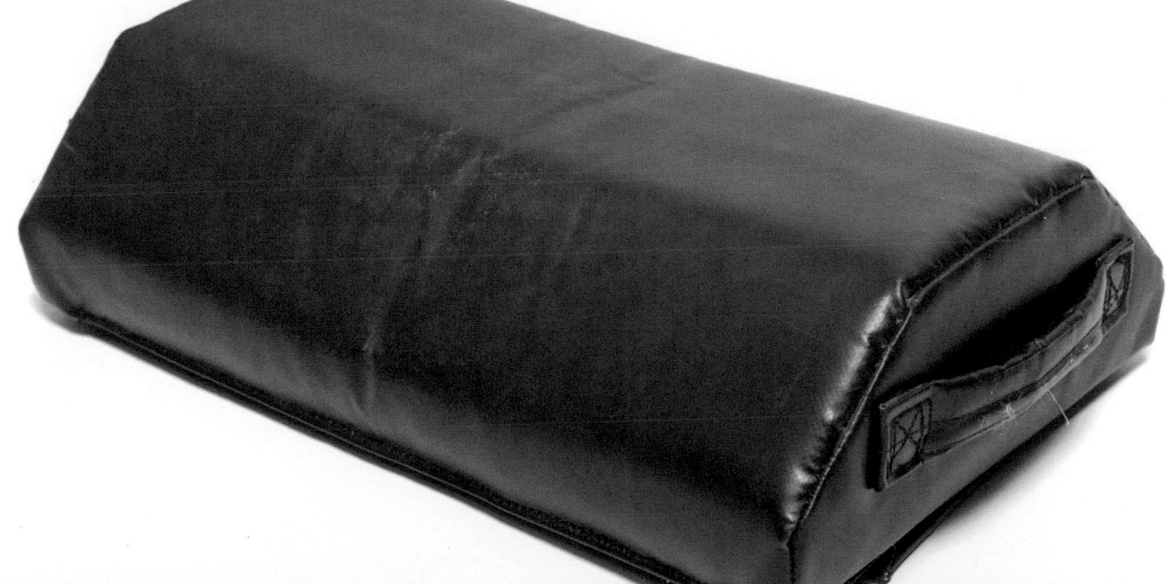

TRAINING WEAPONS

For training to defend yourself against weapons, you can use the following pieces. That way, you can simulate these dangerous situations in a safe, protected manner.

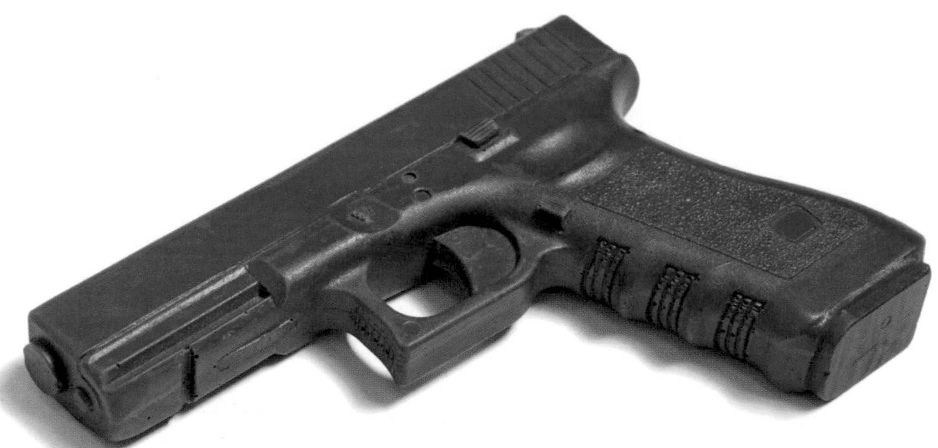

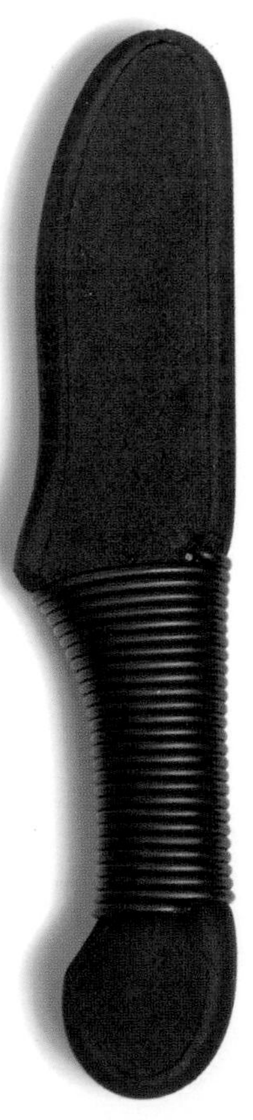

Training Gun

Training guns are a realistic and safe way to practice gun defenses. The risk of using a real weapon during training is always too high, but a quality training gun looks and feels similar to the real thing while avoiding any true danger in training.

Training Knives

Like training guns, training knives are a realistic and safe way to practice knife defenses. They're generally made from rubber or aluminum. We recommend starting with a softer rubber knife and progressing to a more realistic aluminum one for advanced training.

WARNING

Don't use real knives or guns to train, not even if alterations have been made to make the weapons "safer" (such as no bullets in a gun or a dull blade). You still have far more potential for injury when using the real thing versus prop weapons.

Rattan Stick

Use a rattan stick (the tough, pliable stem of a palm) or a padded stick as a substitute for a baseball bat. We recommend one that's 24 inches (61cm) long for a proper bat stand-in.

SOLO TRAINING

Your goal with solo training is to ingrain the Krav Maga techniques into your body and to develop coordination, conditioning, and control. Try setting aside at least three training sessions per week.

How to Train

To properly time your training, use a timer or stopwatch—even your smartphone's timer works well for this. In terms of your training area, set aside a space of at least 10×10 feet (3×3m), like a garage or patio. Be sure to clear the area of tripping hazards, and buy mats or put down some padding to cushion any potential spills you take. (After all, the number-one principle of Krav Maga is getting home safe!)

Warm-Up

To get your heart rate up, perform one to two 2-minute rounds of jump roping, calisthenics, or light jogging on a treadmill or in place.

Stretching

To warm up your muscles, perform two 2-minute rounds of basic stretching with emphasis on your joint mobility, hamstrings, Achilles tendons, hip flexors, and lower back.

Shadow Boxing Solo Drill

The repetition of shadow boxing is an effective way to practice your movement, striking, and defenses together in order to develop your coordination. It's also one of the best methods for developing your form similar to professional boxers, who spend hours shadow boxing to perfect the form of their punching and movements before a fight.

The following is a basic structure you can follow when training on your own. However, feel free to modify it to suit your individual needs.

FOCUS: **MOVEMENT AND STRIKE FORM**

ROUNDS: **6**

TIME PER ROUND: **2 MINUTES**

REST TIME BETWEEN ROUNDS: **1 MINUTE**

EQUIPMENT AND PROTECTIVE GEAR

Mouth guard and (optional) mirror to watch yourself

Rounds 1 and 2

Practice bursting forward in Fighting Stance and then changing direction as quickly as possible for 2 minutes for the first round. Maintain proper form by keeping your chin tucked and hands up as you move, and scan the area with your eyes. Rest for 1 minute, and repeat the routine for the second round.

MAINTAINING YOUR BALANCE

Never cross your feet as you shadow box. This can lead you to tangle them together and trip over them, putting you in a position of disadvantage in a real fight.

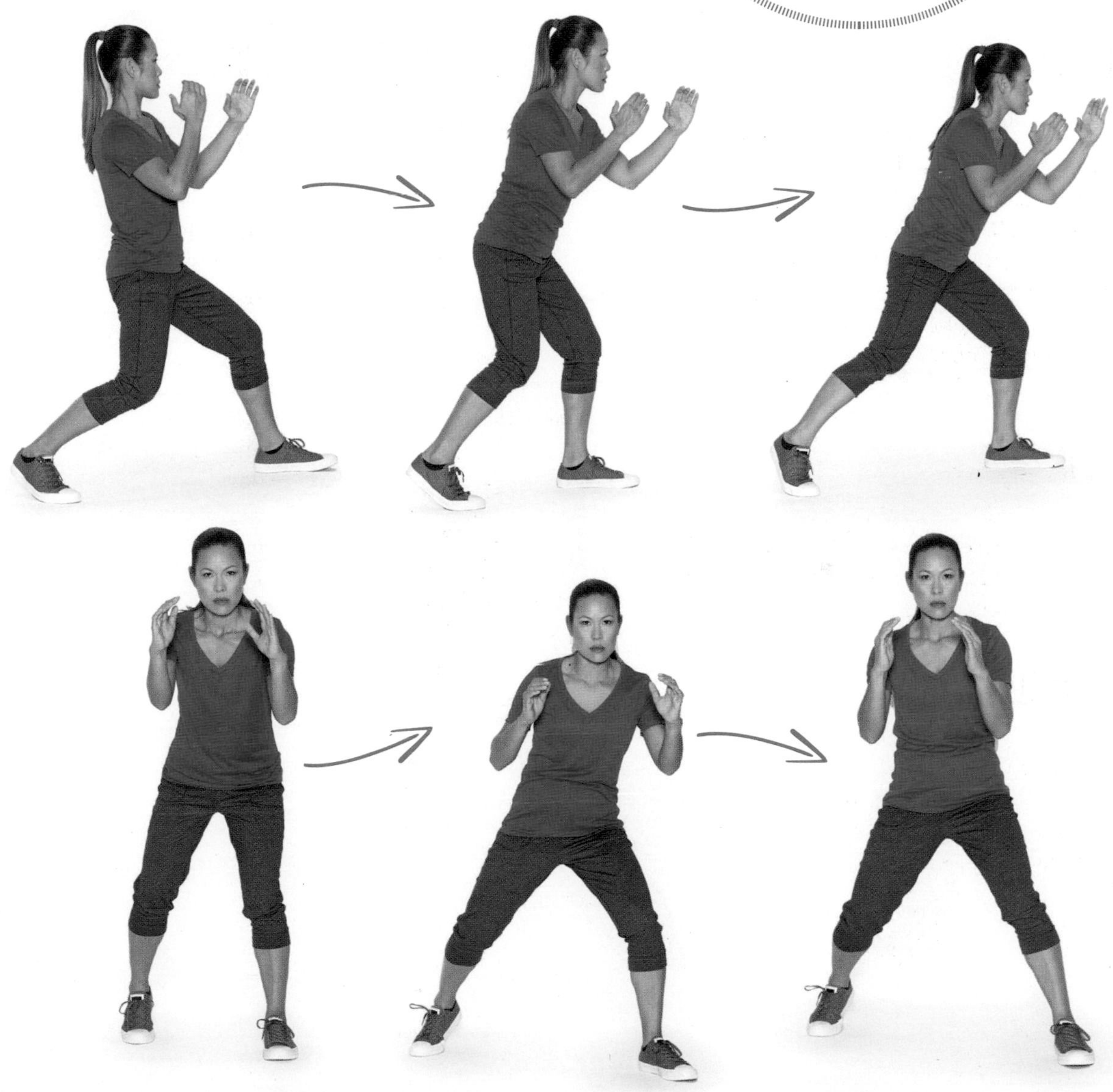

Rounds 3 and 4

Add Straight Punches, Hammerfists, Elbows, Knees, Front Kicks to the Groin, and Front Kicks to a Vertical Target (Defensive) to your movements from rounds 1 and 2. Do round 3 for 2 minutes, rest for 1 minute, and then do round 4 for 2 minutes. Don't forget to focus on continuous movement, balance, and form as you practice.

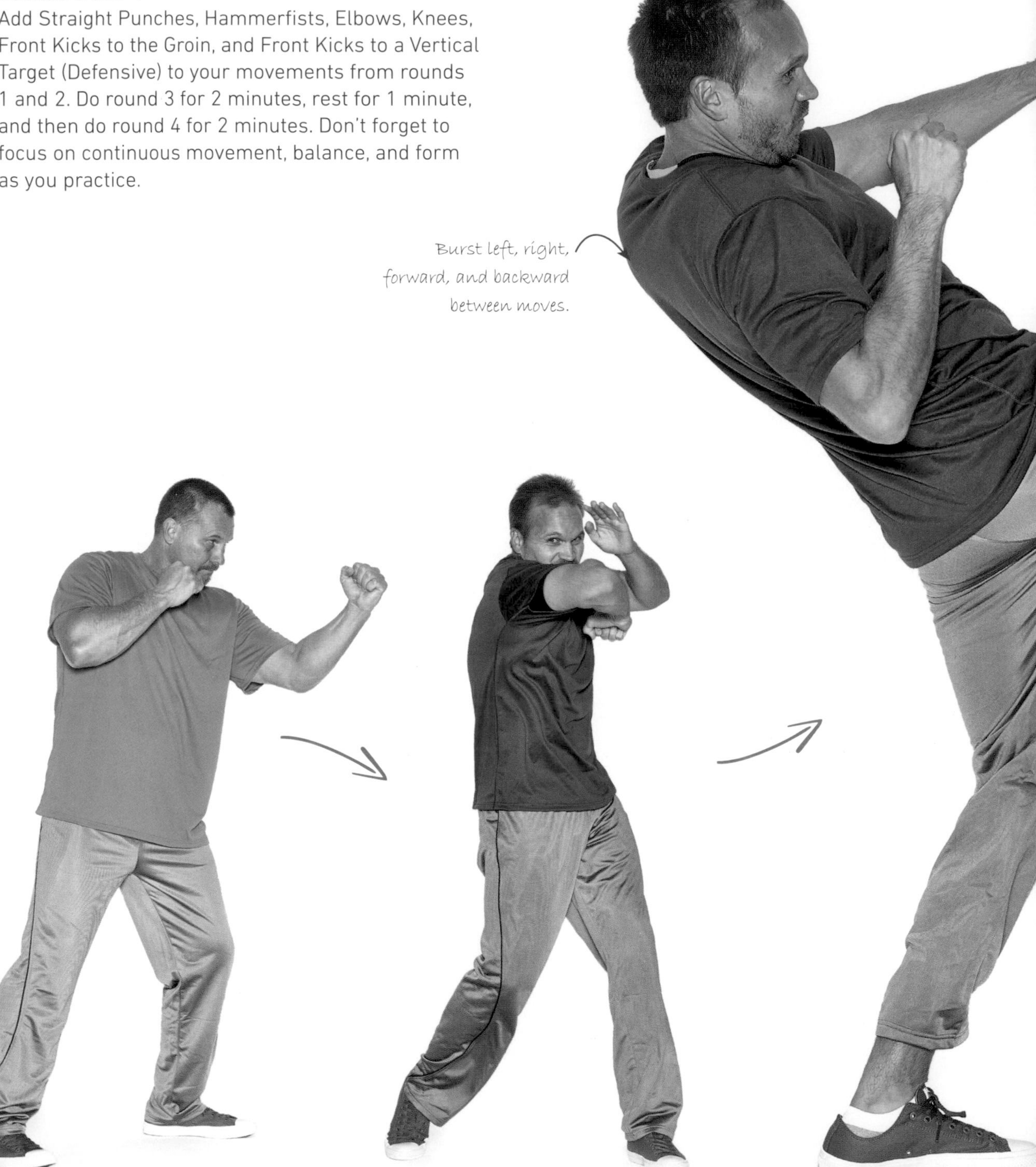

Burst left, right, forward, and backward between moves.

CUSTOMIZING THE DRILL

Feel free to individualize this drill based on your strengths and weaknesses. For example, if you're a strong striker, you may want to focus more on Knees or another weaker area. To avoid getting bored, alter your training every 4 to 6 weeks.

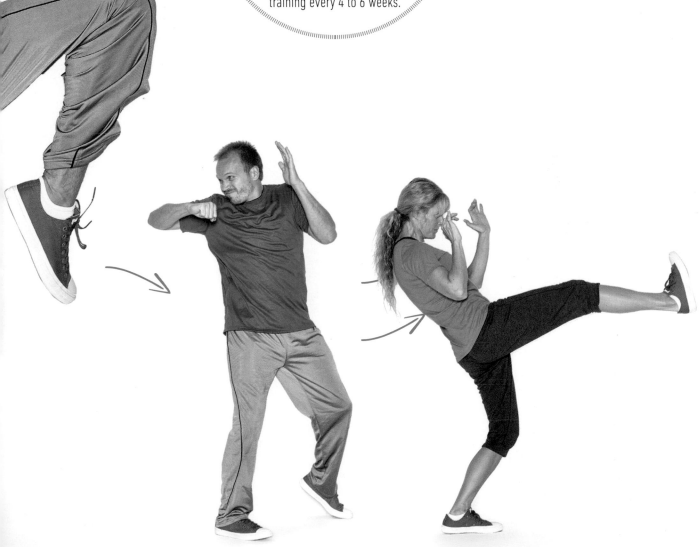

Rounds 5 and 6

Add Inside and Outside Defenses to your routine from the previous 4 rounds. Do the fifth round for 2 minutes, rest for 1 minute, and then do the sixth round for 2 minutes. Focus on smoothing out your movements and using them in different combinations. Your goal is to speed up implementing the techniques while maintaining proper form.

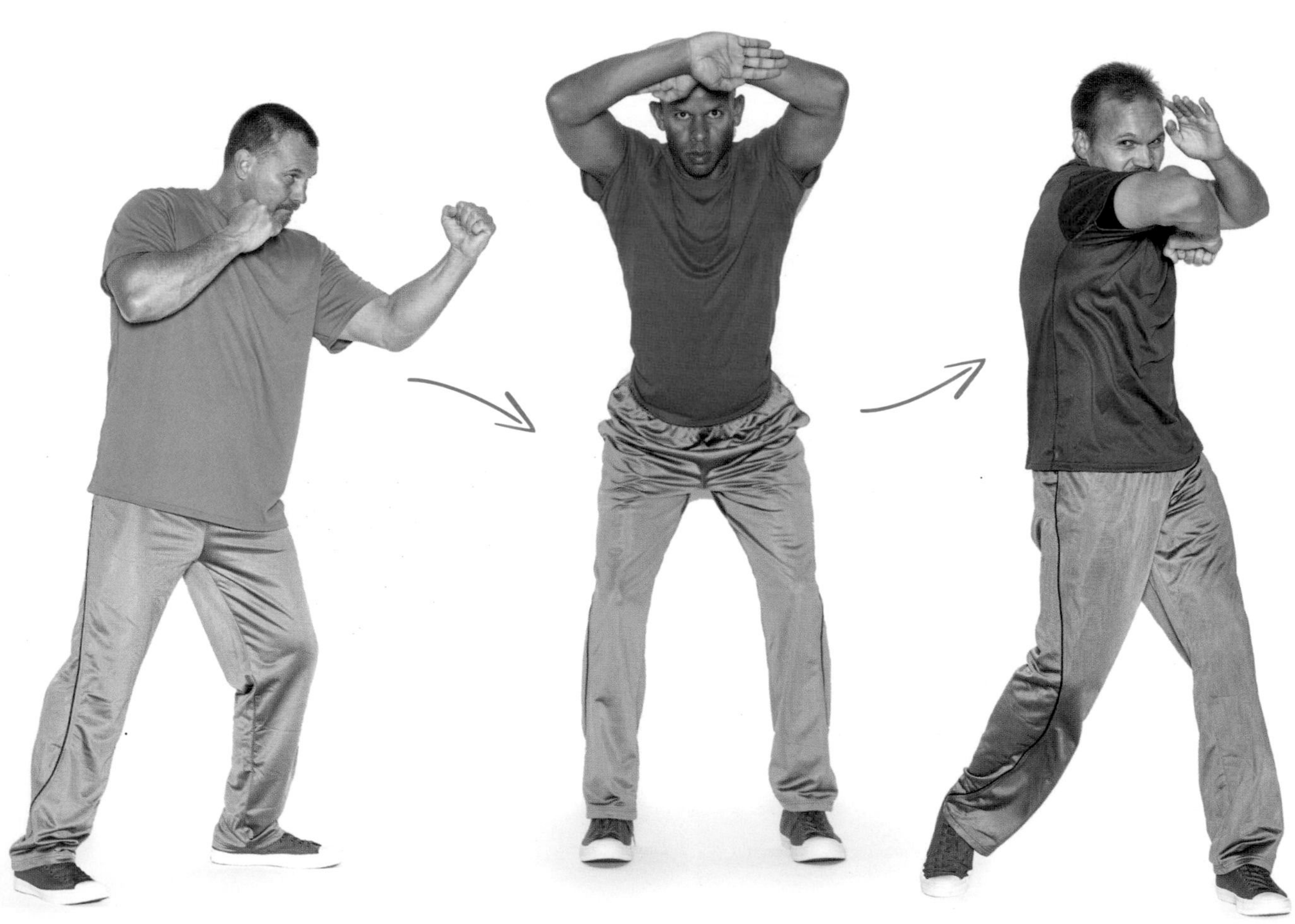

SLOWING THINGS DOWN

One variation for this drill is to slow it down. Break down your technique into each part—for instance, the initial Fighting Stance, your Inside Defense, and then your return to Fighting Stance. You can then do the entire thing slowly before finally moving back to a faster tempo.

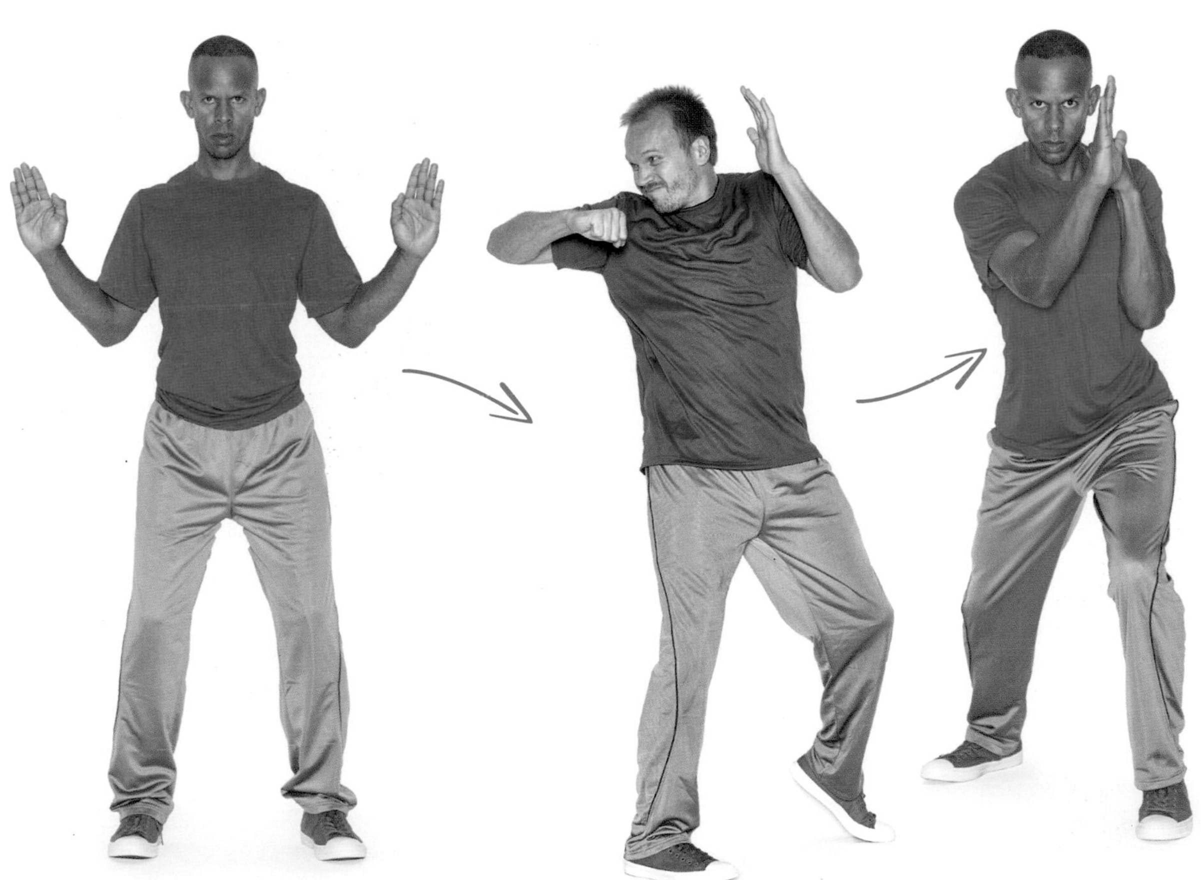

PARTNER TRAINING

To develop confidence in your self-defense techniques, it's essential to work with a partner. A good training partner should be giving you the proper amount of resistance so you can safely perform the technique and get in the repetitions you need to remember it.

Attack Drill

This version of the drill uses Choke from the Front, in which you use a plucking motion to remove a chokehold while your partner serves to demonstrate how you'd be held in such an attack. However, you can do this drill using any technique from earlier in the book.

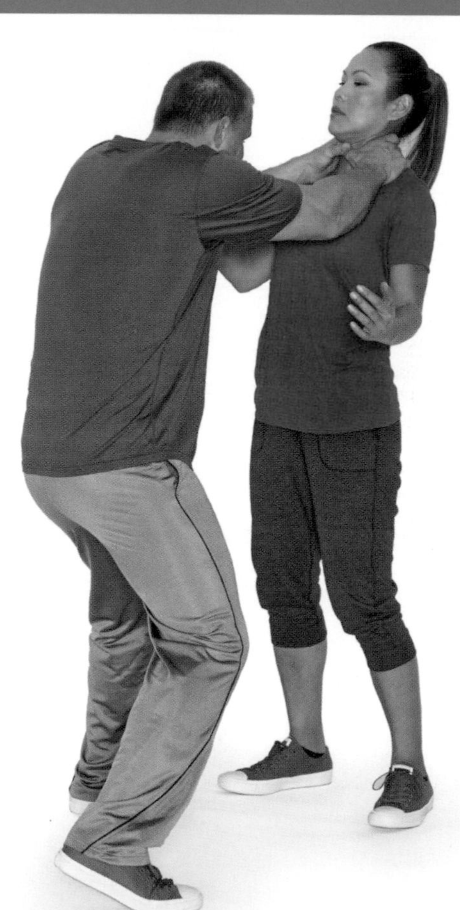

FOCUS: **MASTERING ESCAPES**

ROUNDS: **5**

TIME PER ROUND: **2 MINUTES**

REST TIME BETWEEN ROUNDS: **1 MINUTE**

EQUIPMENT AND PROTECTIVE GEAR

Mouth guard and grappling gloves, hand wraps, or boxing gloves

Attacker

1. Stand in front of the defender. Slowly reach up to the defender's neck with both hands and overlap your thumbs, if possible.
2. Begin to slightly tighten or wring your hands to increase the choke.

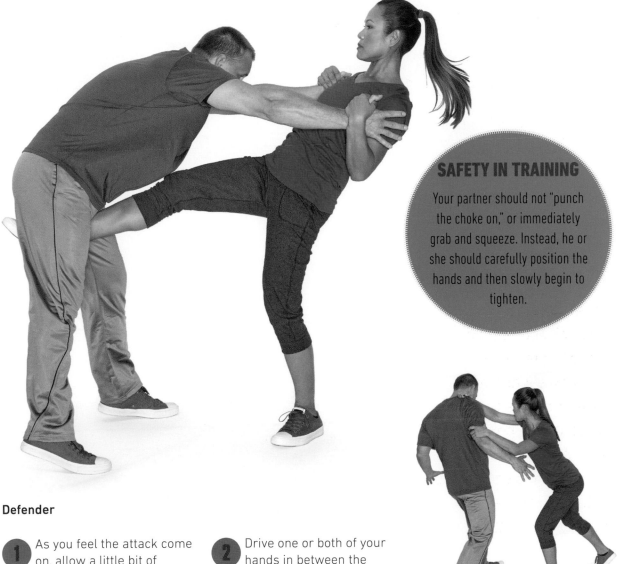

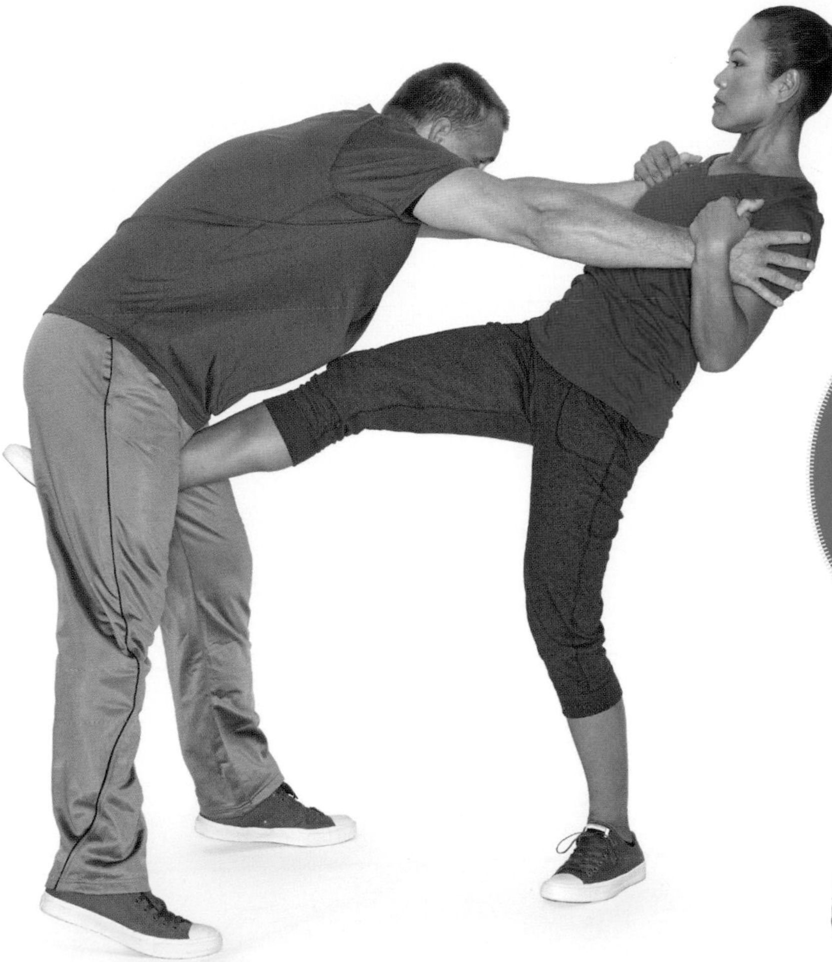

SAFETY IN TRAINING

Your partner should not "punch the choke on," or immediately grab and squeeze. Instead, he or she should carefully position the hands and then slowly begin to tighten.

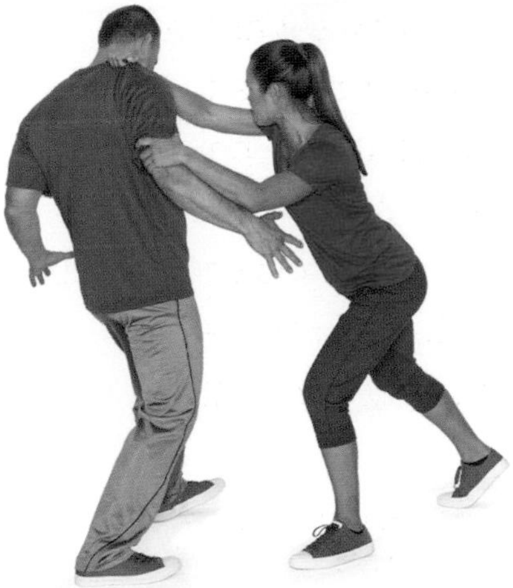

Defender

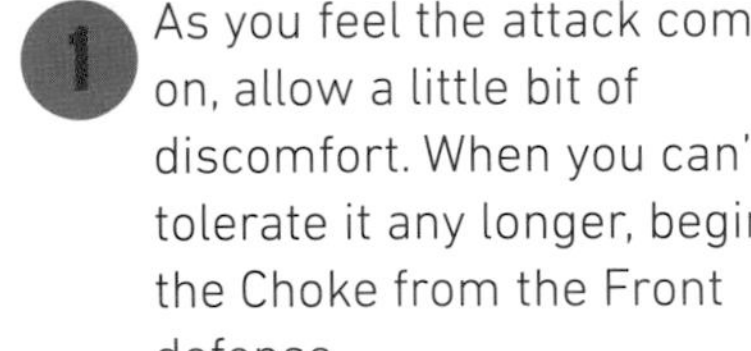

1. As you feel the attack come on, allow a little bit of discomfort. When you can't tolerate it any longer, begin the Choke from the Front defense.

2. Drive one or both of your hands in between the attacker's hands to his or her thumbs. Make the plucking motion by gripping at the thumbs and explosively trying to remove the hands around your neck. Simultaneously kick out at the attacker's groin while maintaining control of the hands.

3. Let go of the attacker's hands and use strikes and Knees to achieve the Control Position. Complete the exercise by disengaging from the attacker and resetting in Fighting Stance for the next round.

Focus Mitts Drill

Focus mitt training requires you and your partner to work together to develop and build in attacking combinations, movement to the dead side (otherwise known as the attacker's unarmed, impaired, or vulnerable side), and responses to specific common attacks.

FOCUS: **MOVEMENT, TIMING, AND ACCURACY**
ROUNDS: **5**
TIME PER ROUND: **2 MINUTES**
REST TIME BETWEEN ROUNDS: **1 MINUTE**

EQUIPMENT AND PROTECTIVE GEAR
Mouth guard, 14- to 16-ounce boxing gloves and hand wraps (for defender), and focus mitts (for trainer)

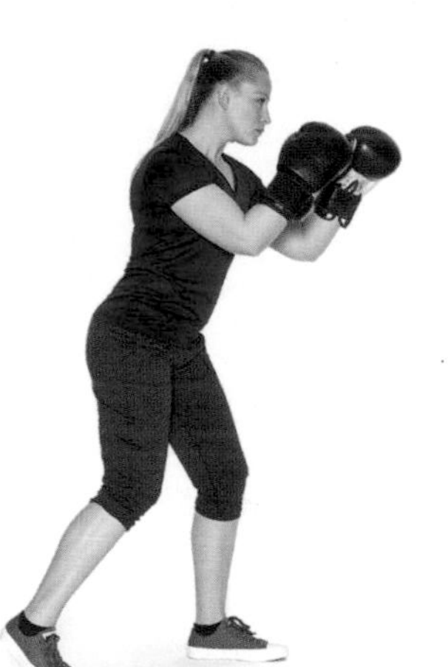
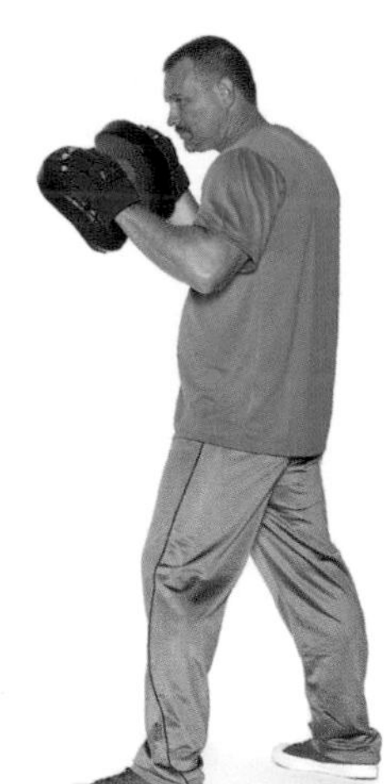

Trainer

1. Give a verbal indication for a Straight Punch combination by saying the number of punches you want. Use odd numbers for the left hand and even numbers for the right (for instance, "three" would be a straight left, straight right, and straight left).

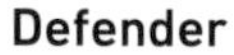

Defender

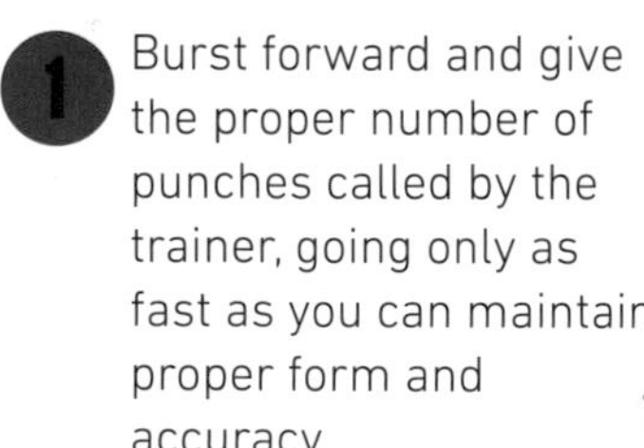

1. Burst forward and give the proper number of punches called by the trainer, going only as fast as you can maintain proper form and accuracy.

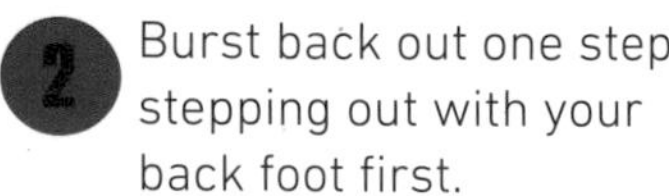

2. Burst back out one step, stepping out with your back foot first.

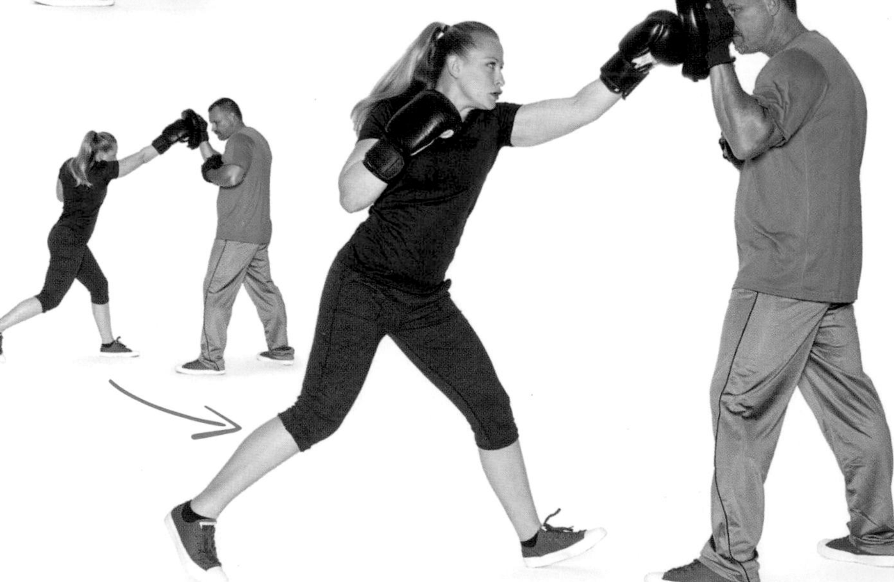

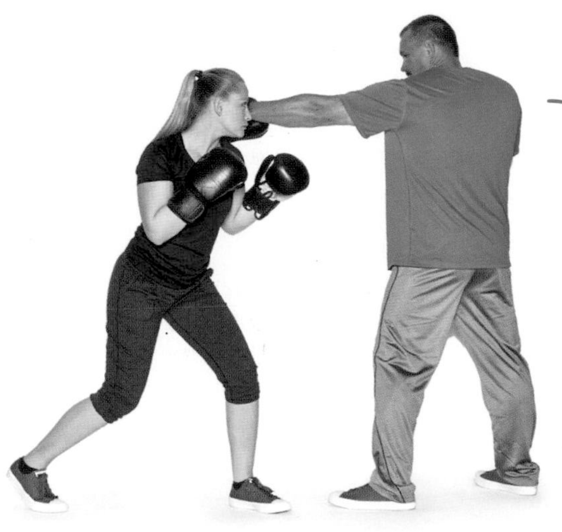

Trainer

1. Send your left hand out as if making a Straight Punch.

2. Leave it out and walk directly toward the defender.

Defender

1. As you see the trainer put his or her arm out, move off to the dead side. In this case, you move to your right and work to get behind the trainer.

Trainer

1. Turn and face the defender, who should now be behind you.

2. Give the next combination of punches you want him or her to perform. Don't call out single punches; instead, call out multiple punches.

Defender

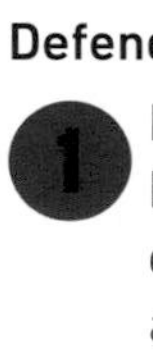

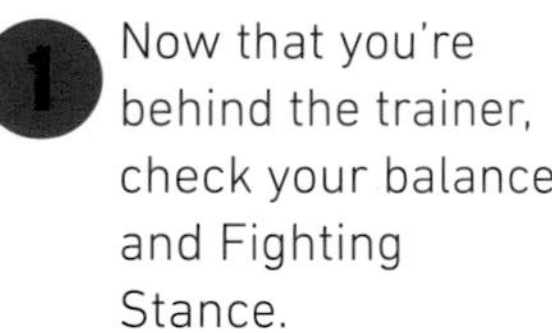

1. Now that you're behind the trainer, check your balance and Fighting Stance.

2. Work from the feet up to fix form or alignment. Prepare for the next punching combination and deliver it when it's called.

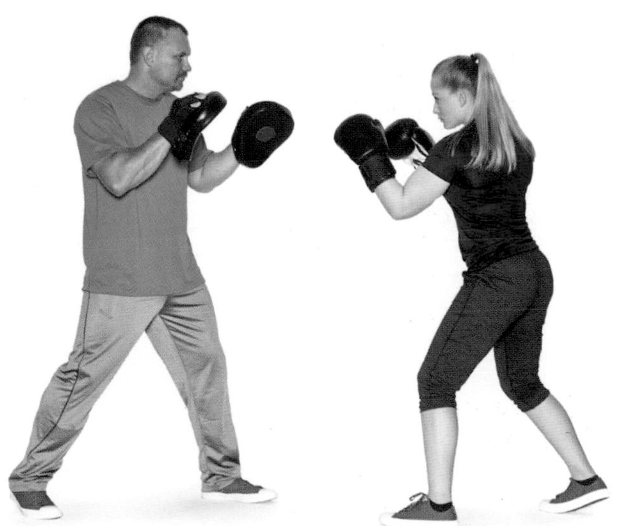

Inside and Outside Defense Drill

This defense blocks Straight Punches to the center and outside of your body. Partner work on this teaches you how to redirect an attack offline and defend your face and upper body.

FOCUS: **BASIC DEFENSE AND BLOCKING**

ROUNDS: **5**

TIME PER ROUND: **2 MINUTES**

REST TIME BETWEEN ROUNDS: **1 MINUTE**

EQUIPMENT AND PROTECTIVE GEAR

Mouth guard; grappling gloves, hand wraps, or boxing gloves (for defender); focus mitts (for trainer)

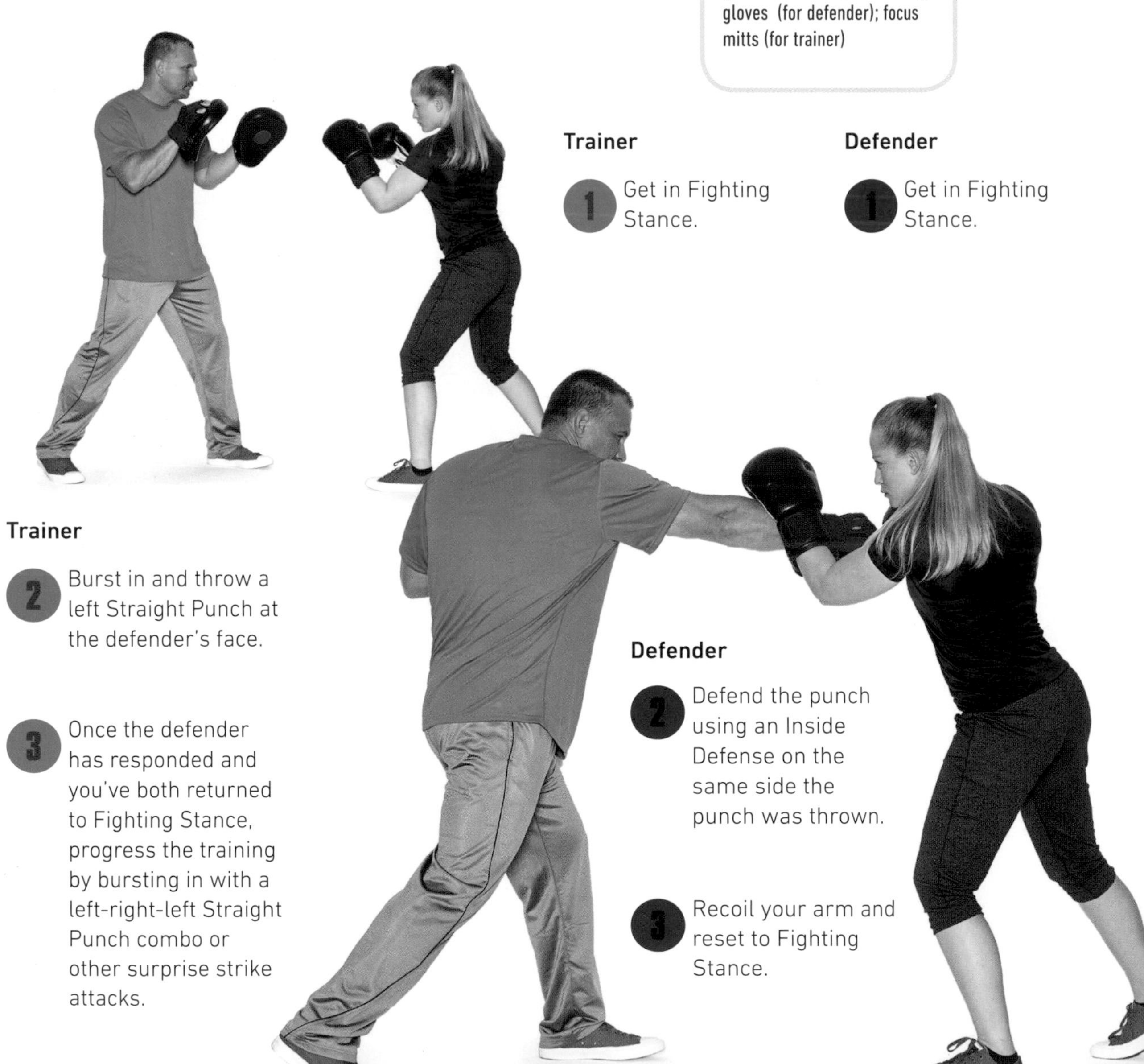

Trainer

1. Get in Fighting Stance.

Defender

1. Get in Fighting Stance.

Trainer

2. Burst in and throw a left Straight Punch at the defender's face.

3. Once the defender has responded and you've both returned to Fighting Stance, progress the training by bursting in with a left-right-left Straight Punch combo or other surprise strike attacks.

Defender

2. Defend the punch using an Inside Defense on the same side the punch was thrown.

3. Recoil your arm and reset to Fighting Stance.

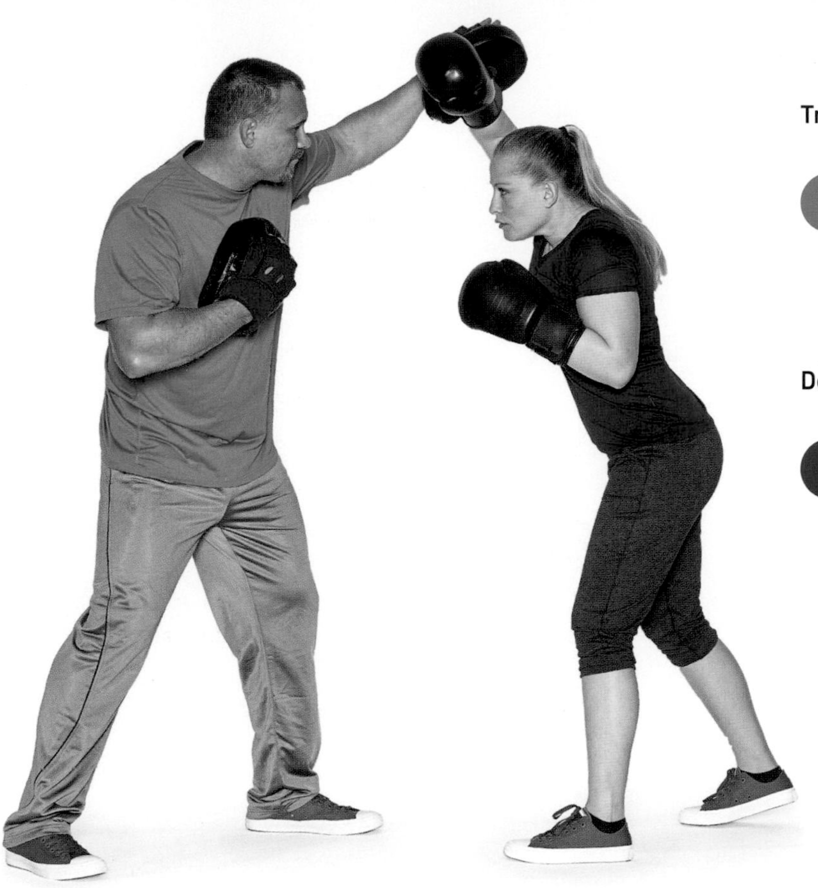

Trainer

4 Use a 360-degree attack to throw a looping strike coming from the outside.

Defender

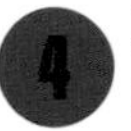

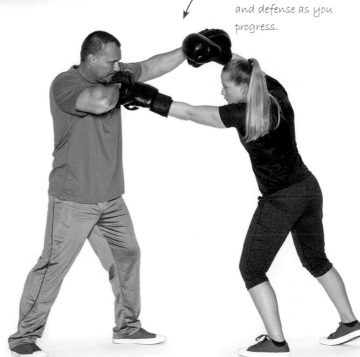

4 Use the appropriate Outside Defense to deflect the strike.

You can also integrate simultaneous attack and defense as you progress.

TRAINING TIP

Your partner can work on surprising you by throwing strikes to your head and then your body—for instance, a left punch to your head, a right punch to your body, and left punch to your head. The goal is to help prepare you for anything.

STRESS TRAINING

Being attacked is one of the most stressful situations that can happen to you. So it's absolutely essential to train your body and mind to be able to perform under that pressure. Combined, a solid mind with proper conditioning will increase your chances of getting home safe.

Ways to Increase Stress in Your Training

The goal of stress training is to progressively add stress to your mind and body so you can perform Krav Maga techniques in even the most harrowing situations. The following are a few general ways you can increase stress when training.

Incorporate speed into your attacks.
If you're practicing solo, you can work on going through your techniques while keeping proper form at an increasingly faster pace. When practicing with a partner, your partner can attack you not only at a faster pace, but with a stronger attack or even with multiple attacks one right after another. As soon as you disengage from one attack, he or she can immediately attack you again. By responding to faster or multiple attacks, which doesn't allow your mind to completely reset, you're adding stress.

Alter your environment.
When you train inside a secure location—such as your home, your garage, or your local self-defense school—you become accustomed to the sounds, lights, and comfort of the room. Disrupt this comfort by cranking the music up loud to make it harder for you to hear the attack coming or by flickering the lights on and off quickly to impair your vision. With this, you take one of your senses out of the equation, forcing you to use your other senses to think.

Train in uncomfortable or unstable conditions.
Try training in a smaller room or up against a wall, where you have fewer ways to escape after the attack. You could further disrupt the comfort of your environment by moving outside onto uneven terrain, to a sidewalk, or in a parking lot. By mimicking possible attack scenarios in a more controlled environment, you'll be able to react properly when attacked in that same or a similar scenario in real life.

Have your training partner disrupt your thought pattern with surprise maneuvers.
For instance, your partner could throw a straight punch or a kick and then immediately burst in with a choke. This doesn't allow your mind time to think—you must react! Once you learn to prepare for such manuevers, you're one step ahead of potential attackers.

Train from a position of disadvantage.
For instance, when training with a partner, put your hands in your pockets, talk on the phone, look through your purse, or bend down to tie your shoe before your partner engages you. This takes your mind off of the coming controlled attacks, so you can react as soon as you feel the pressure of an attack coming on.

Increase your heart rate through exercises.
You can mimic stress simply by getting your blood pumping. Try exercises such as running in place, performing burpees, jumping rope, and doing jumping jacks to get you in the right physical and mental state.

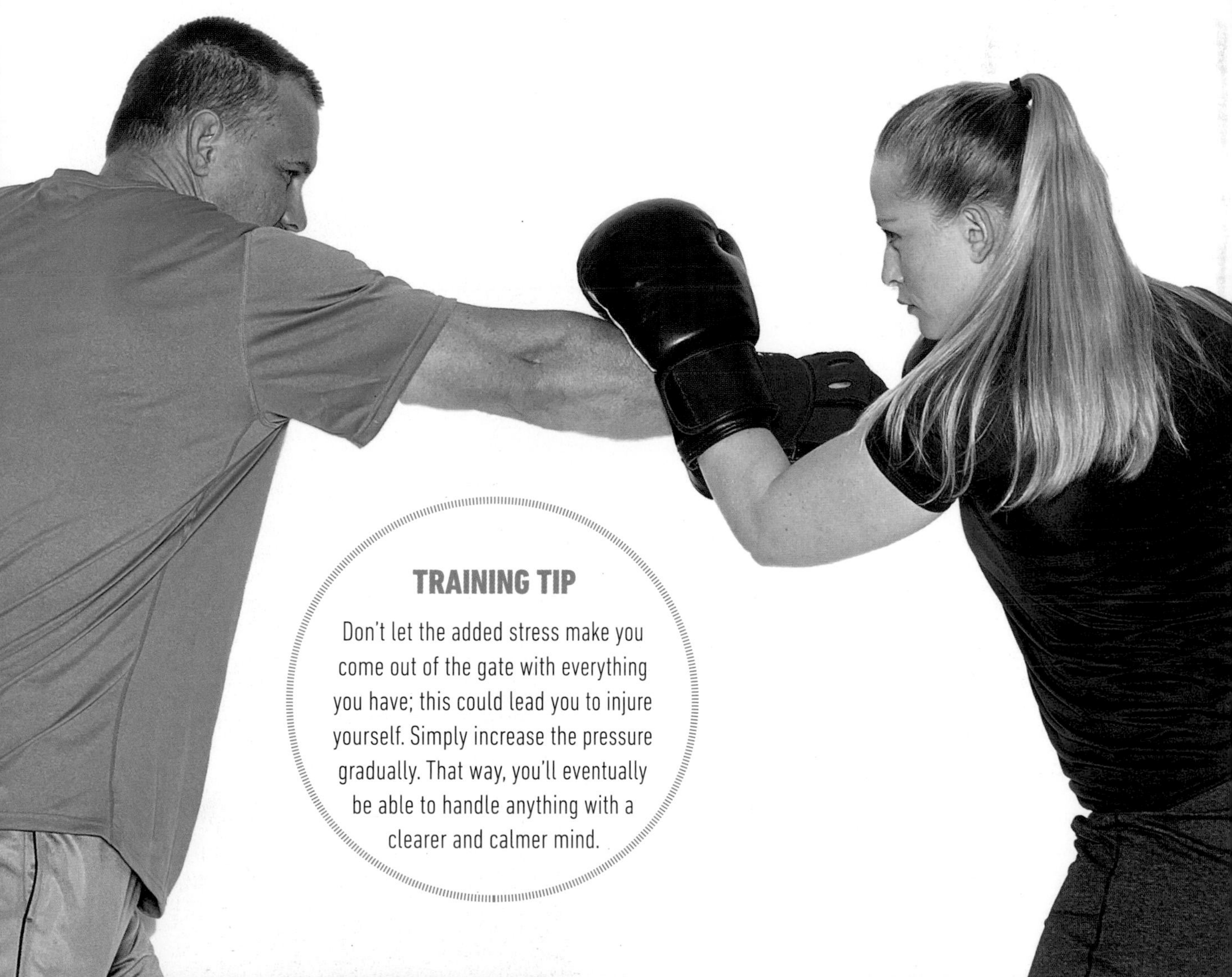

TRAINING TIP

Don't let the added stress make you come out of the gate with everything you have; this could lead you to injure yourself. Simply increase the pressure gradually. That way, you'll eventually be able to handle anything with a clearer and calmer mind.

Stress Drill

Up until now, your focus has been on getting the technique in your body by repitition and slowly adding resistance to the attacks. At this level, the goal is to to learn to recognize a threat already coming at you or to feel a threat and make the proper reaction.

FOCUS: **DEFENSE UNDER PRESSURE**

ROUNDS: **5**

TIME PER ROUND: **2 MINUTES**

REST TIME BETWEEN ROUNDS: **1 MINUTE**

EQUIPMENT AND PROTECTIVE GEAR

Mouth guard

Defender

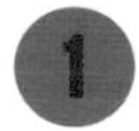

Stand in Passive Stance. Close your eyes and let your mind drift elsewhere, putting yourself in a maximum position of disadvantage.

Attacker

Position yourself to make your first attack at least a leg's length from the defender (in front of, beside, or behind).

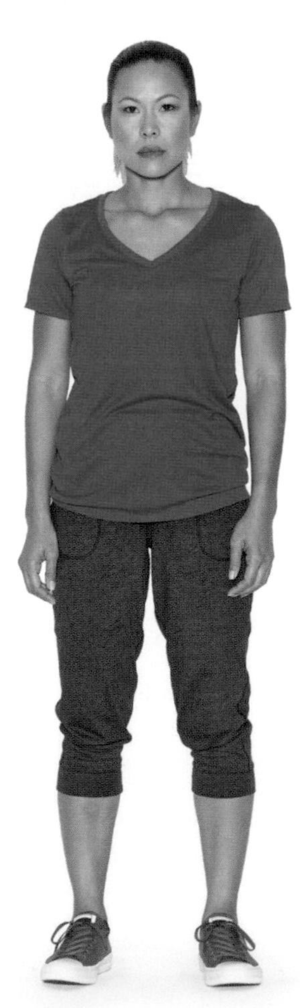

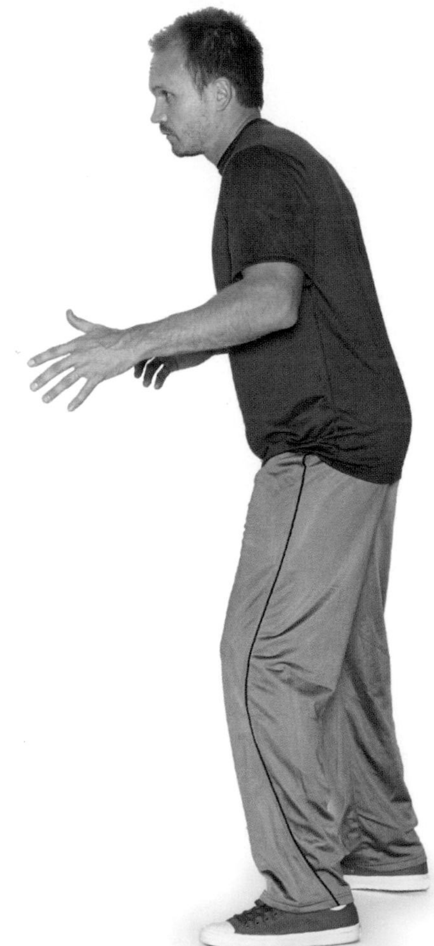

Attacker

2 Using any of the techniques the defender knows, yell "attack" and wait a beat for the defender to open his or her eyes before attacking.

Defender

2 When you receive a tactile cue or the attack alert, open your eyes, recognize the threat, and make the appropriate defense. Follow up with any counterattacks you need to disengage from the attacker.

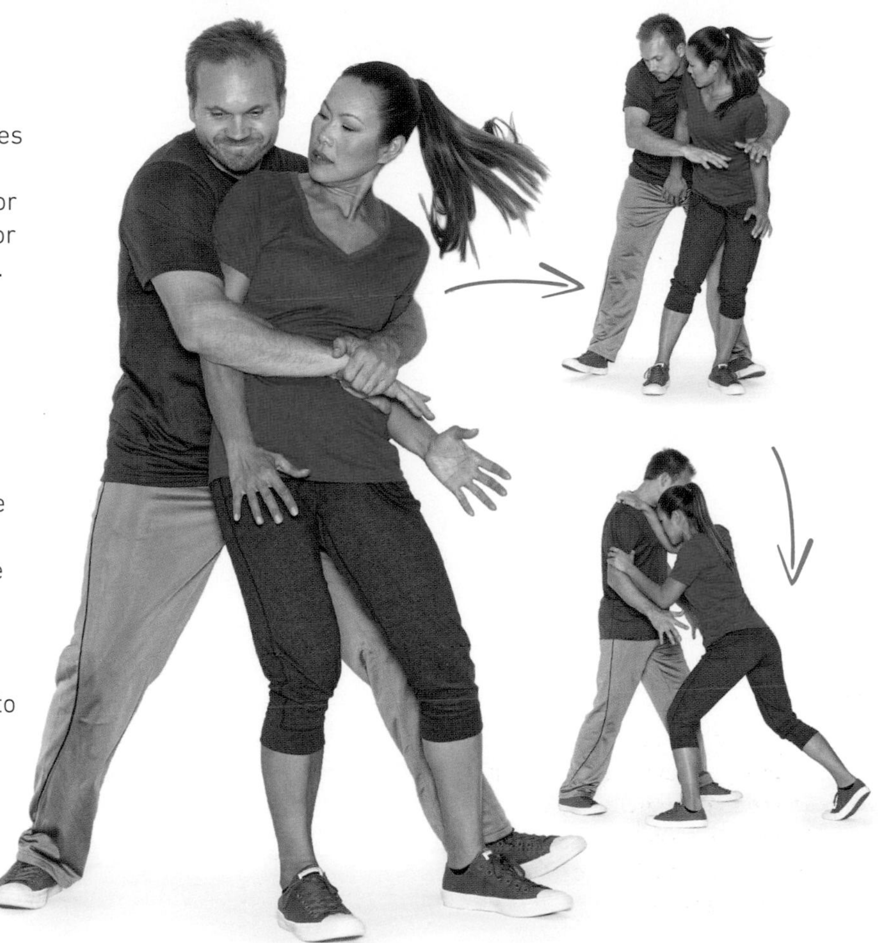

Attacker

3 Reset and do a different attack, rotating through all the self-defense and common attacks the defender has been trained in up to this point.

Defender

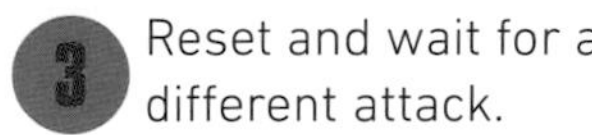

3 Reset and wait for a different attack.

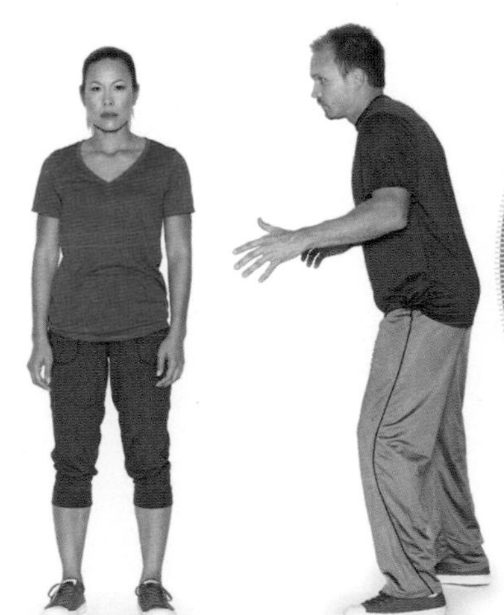

SAFETY IN TRAINING

The trainer should always make sure to yell "attack" before committing to a strike attack, as well as be at least a leg's length from you. This allows you to have time to open your eyes before you make the defense.

AGGRESSIVENESS TRAINING

Aggressiveness training with two partners is designed to teach you to let go of your social conditioning to hold back and learn how to bring out your aggressive side.

What You Accomplish with This Training

If you recall from earlier in the book, aggressiveness is the will to win the fight and stay in the fight no matter what happens. It's primal instinct to protect your life or the life of a loved one. While attackers expect you to freeze or try to run, you can instead learn how to stand your ground and fight back, no matter the odds. Aggressiveness involves pushing aside any thoughts of being outmatched physically and tapping into that instinctive, more-confident side of you that simply means to gain the upper hand.

Imagine a light switch. Turn it on, and the lights are on; turn it off, and the lights are off. That's how you should treat your aggression. When you're attacked, you need to throw the switch on and overwhelm your attacker with violence of action (counterattacks), explosiveness (bursting forward), and aggressiveness (combat mind-set). You want to hijack your attacker's OODA loop and leave him or her in a rumpled mess on the floor wondering "What just happened?" By the time that thought occurs though, you'll be long gone.

TRAINING TIP

It's easiest to perform upper-body strikes (such as punches, Elbows, and Hammerfists) for this drill, as the pull on you could make it difficult to land Knees and other lower-body defense techniques accurately.

Aggressiveness Drill

For this drill, you need three people: yourself and two trainers. Trainer A will hold a band or rope around your waist, while trainer B will hold a tombstone pad facing you. The goal of trainer A is to bring out your aggressive side by pulling you every which way as you try to defend yourself by hitting the tombstone pad held by trainer B.

FOCUS: **AGGRESSIVENESS**

ROUNDS: **5**

TIME PER ROUND: **2 MINUTES**

REST TIME BETWEEN ROUNDS: **1 MINUTE**

EQUIPMENT AND PROTECTIVE GEAR

Mouth guard, MMA gloves (for defender), tombstone pad (for trainer B), and rope or band (for trainer A)

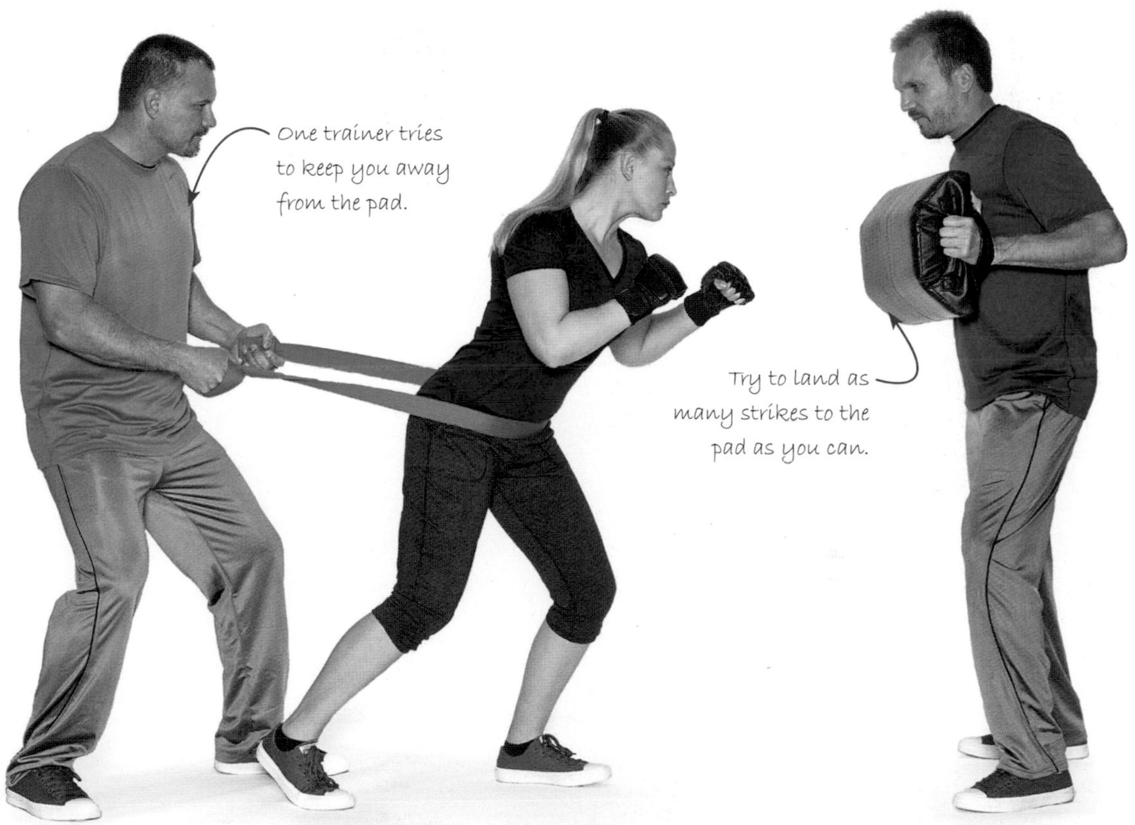

One trainer tries to keep you away from the pad.
Try to land as many strikes to the pad as you can.

1 Face trainer B, who's holding the tombstone pad, in Fighting Stance. Using the rope or band, trainer A pulls you back slightly from the tombstone pad—about one to two steps back works.

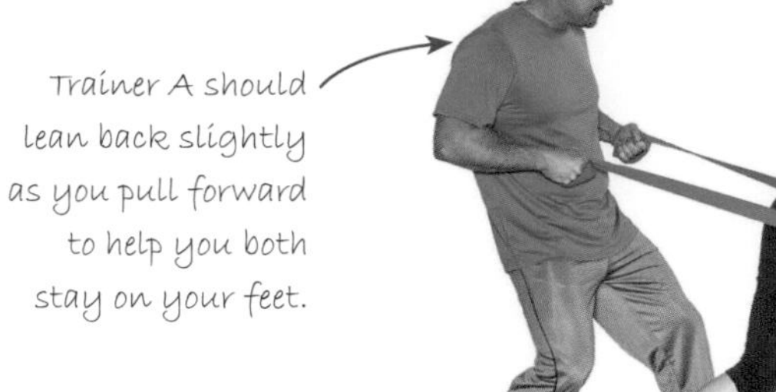

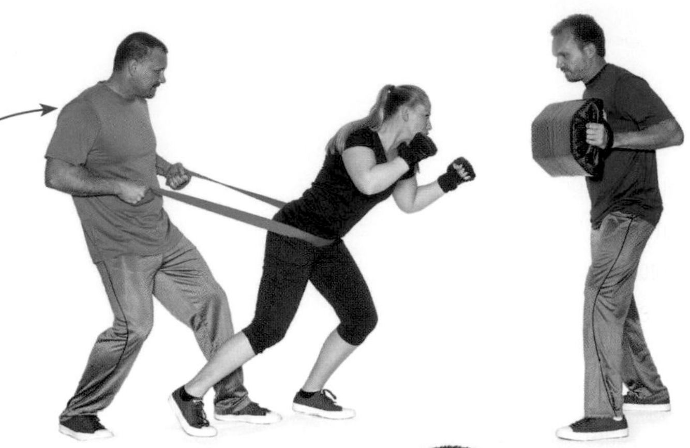

Trainer A should lean back slightly as you pull forward to help you both stay on your feet.

2 Trainer B says "Go!" On this cue, drive forward using your legs to try to put as many strikes on the pad as possible.

3 Trainer A starts pulling you left and right to further disrupt your balance. Continue to throw as many strikes as possible to the pad, such as Straight Punches, Hammerfists, Elbows, and Palm Strikes.

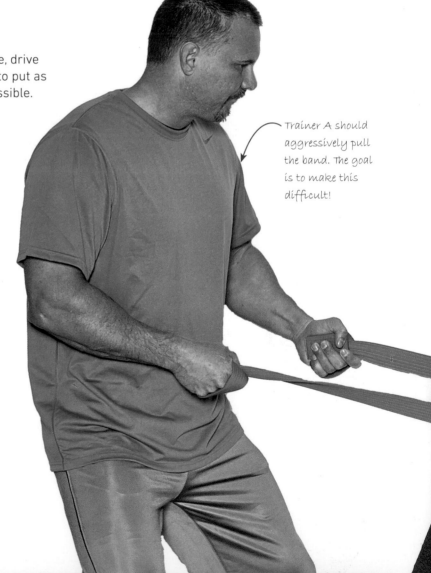

Trainer A should aggressively pull the band. The goal is to make this difficult!

TRAINING TIP

While your trainers shouldn't make the drill impossible to perform, they should gradually increase resistance to further test you. It shouldn't be too easy to connect your defenses, or you won't tap into your true aggressiveness.

Don't take your eyes off the pad.
Try to connect Hammerfists, Straight Punches, or Palm Strikes.

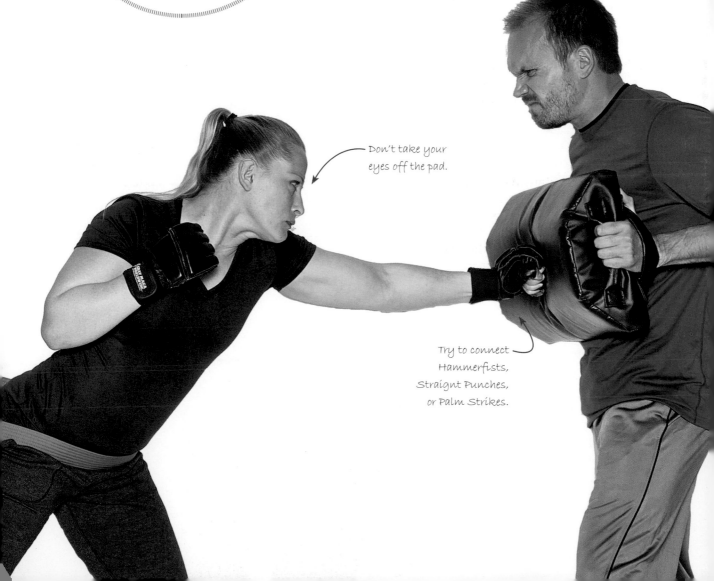

CONDITIONING

Because the average street encounter may only last a few seconds, you must condition yourself for a short-duration, high-intensity event like a fight. Accordingly, we have included training exercises that will condition your muscular and cardiovascular systems.

How It Works

We've broken down the following workouts into three levels: stability, strength, and power. While the examples start you from the stability level, if you have more experience, you can begin at a higher level. However, no matter what level you start with, the daily and weekly discipline of conditioning and training ensures you present a hard target for those who would do you harm.

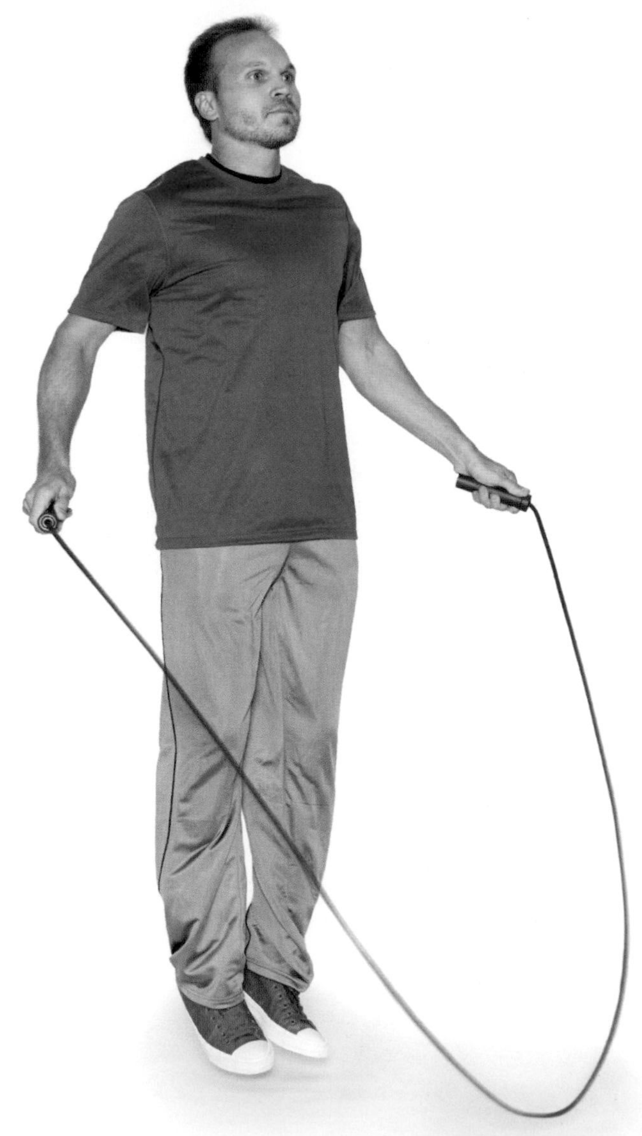

Jumping Rope

Jumping rope is a great way to train your anaerobic fitness, as well as gain better timing and agility. Professional fighters have been doing it for decades. The program is broken down into two sections, with basic conditioning for 2 weeks to build your jump rope technique and conditioning, followed by a 10-week program of jump rope sprints that develop your stability, strength, and power.

Basic Jump Rope Conditioning
For basic conditioning, you practice jumping rope forward and backward with both feet. As you jump, maintain proper alignment and focus on using only your wrists to spin the rope.

WEEK 1

This week simply works on reps and form.

DAY	FORWARD JUMPS	BACKWARD JUMPS
1	100	100
2	100	100
3	150	150
4	150	150
5	200	200
6	250	250
7	OFF	

WEEK 2

For this week, you do timed rounds with the goal of continuous motion. To add a challenge, each time you miss jumping over, switch directions.

DAY	ROUNDS	LENGTH OF ROUNDS
1	3	2 minutes
2	5	2 minutes
3	3	3 minutes
4	5	3 minutes
5	5	3 minutes
6	4	5 minutes
7	OFF	

Interval Training Jump Rope Sprints
Once you've worked on your basic conditioning with a jump rope, you can move on to doing jump rope sprints three times a week. For each level, focus on the following:
Stability: Two feet jumping
Strength: Alternating feet
Power: Double jumps

10-WEEK PROGRAM

The following is a program for jump rope sprints. Remember, you only complete the sprints three times a week.

WEEK	LEVEL	JUMP ROPE TIME	REST TIME	HOW LONG
1	Stability	30 seconds	30 seconds	10 rounds
2	Stability	40 seconds	20 seconds	10 rounds
3	Stability	1 minute	1 minute	10 rounds
4	Strength	30 seconds	30 seconds	10 rounds
5	Strength	15 seconds	15 seconds	20 minutes
6	Strength	30 seconds	30 seconds	10 rounds
7	Strength	40 seconds	20 seconds	10 rounds
8	Strength	1 minute	1 minute	10 rounds
9	Power	30 seconds	30 seconds	10 rounds
10	Power	15 seconds	15 seconds	20 minutes

Bodyweight Training

Some of the reasons we like to incorporate bodyweight training in a conditioning program are because it's effective, it burns fat, you can do it almost anywhere, and it doesn't cost you a thing. You should get great results by being consistent and continuing to push yourself every week.

Pushup
Assume a prone, face-down position on the floor. Place your hands approximately shoulder width apart, with your elbows pointed toward your toes. Raise yourself up and down using your arms while ensuring your elbows don't swing out to the sides.

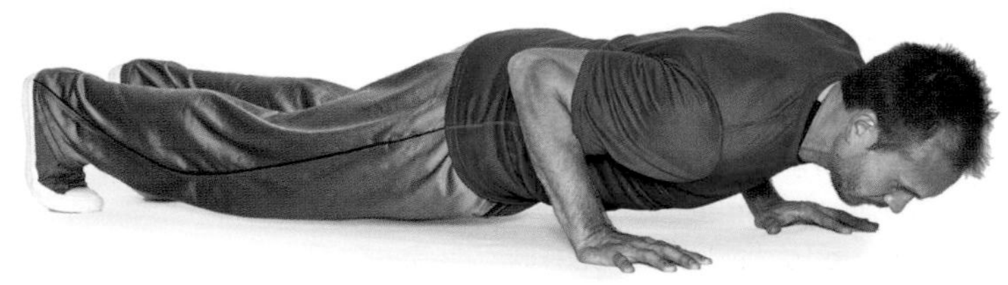

Full Squat
Stand with your feet a little wider than shoulder width apart, stacking your hips over your knees and your knees over your ankles. Roll your shoulders back and down, away from your ears. Extend your arms out so they're parallel to the ground. Bend your knees while bringing your hips backward and lower yourself as far as you can. Engage your core and, with your bodyweight in your heels, explode back up to standing.

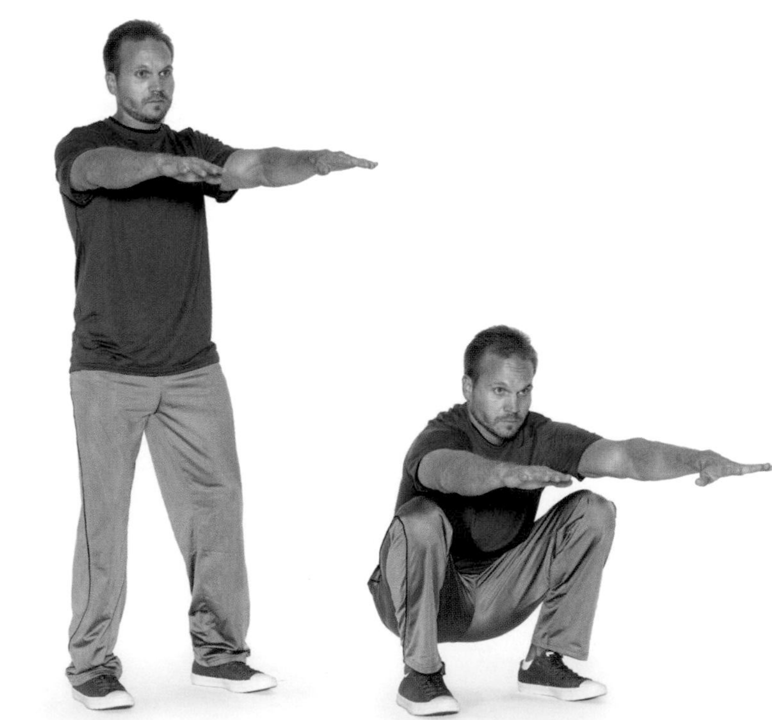

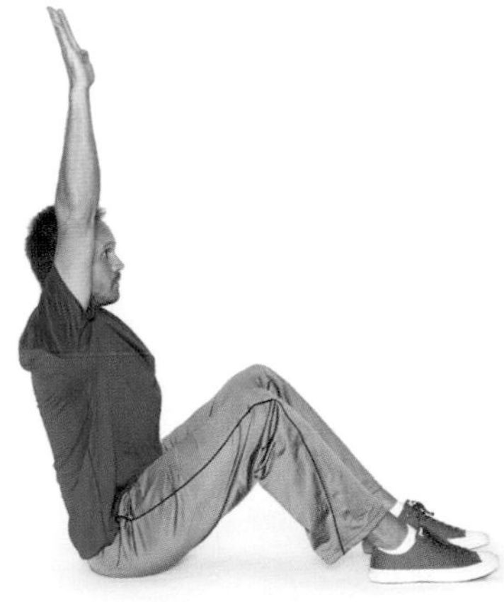

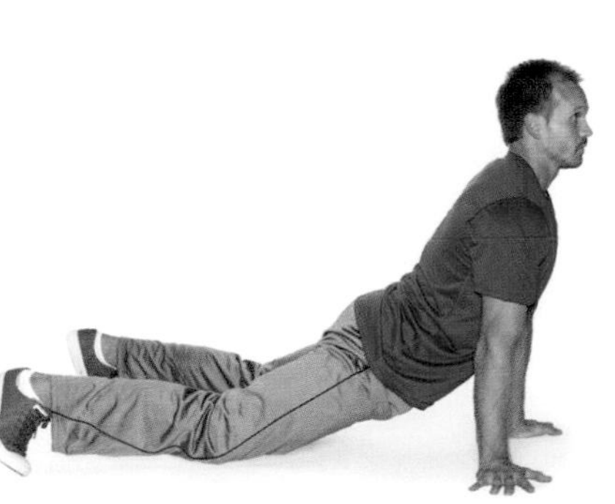

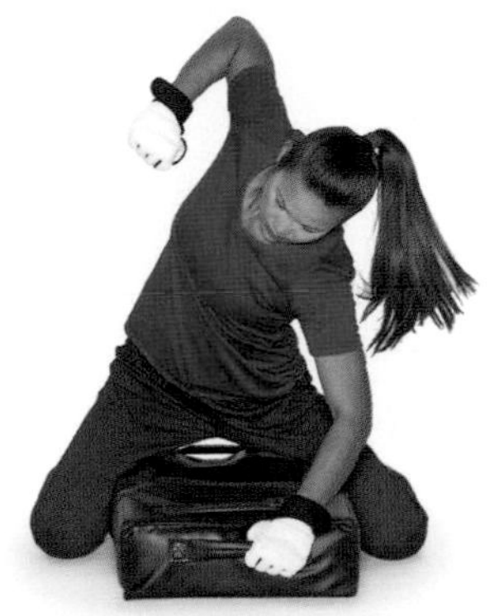

Sit Up and Reach
Begin on your back and place your hands behind your head. Plant your feet on the ground about shoulder width apart. Engage your core as you sit up and move your hands to reach forward and up toward the sky. Use your core to return your upper body to the ground.

Sprawl
Stand with your feet shoulder width apart and your hands relaxed at your sides. As quickly as you can, drop to the ground into a pushup position, kick your feet forward to move into a crouch position, and stand up.

Ground and Pound
Place a tombstone pad on the ground. Straddle the bag and deliver downward punches to the pad.

Bodyweight Training Drill
The following table shows you a typical bodyweight training drill. For each round, you do one of the exercises for the time provided, followed by a rest. Once you've reached five rounds, you move to the next level. For instance, the stability level calls for 40 seconds on and 20 seconds rest for 5 rounds; for that, you'll work as hard as you can for 40 seconds, take a 20-second rest, and immediately move on to the next exercise, rotating through all of them until the final round is complete. In the stability level, you'll focus on form. In the strength level, you'll focus on increasing your number of reps. In the power level, you'll focus on your intensity and really push yourself.

BODYWEIGHT TRAINING DRILL

Don't forget to do a warm-up before and cooldown after this drill; this will help you avoid injury by easing your body into and out of exercise.

LEVEL	EXERCISE TIME	REST TIME	NUMBER OF ROUNDS
Stability	40 seconds	20 seconds	5
Strength	50 seconds	10 seconds	5
Power	1 minute	none	5

GLOSSARY

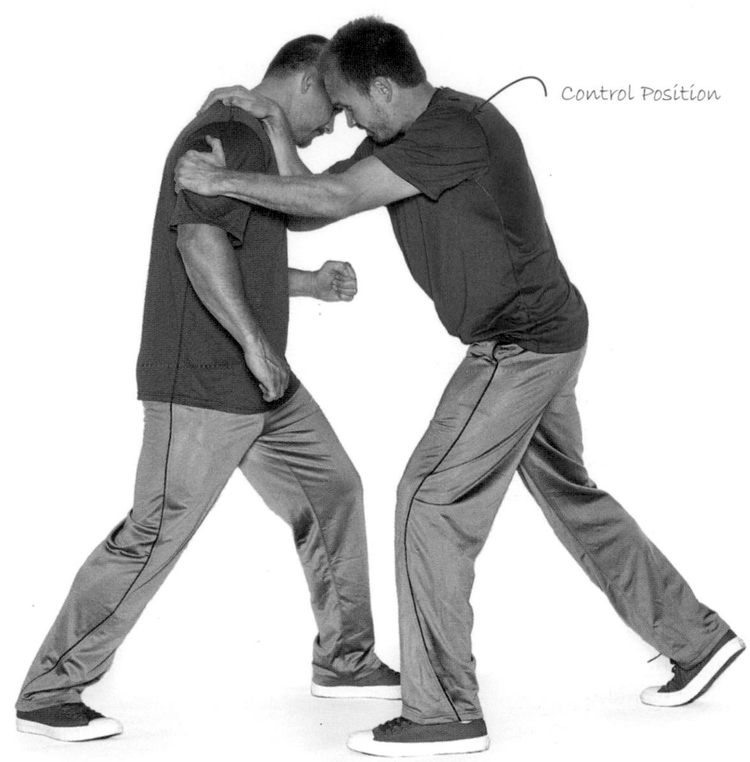

aggressiveness Making an all-out effort to win or succeed.

attacker An initiator who acts violently, aggressively, or forcibly toward someone.

base foot The leg providing support during the delivery of a kick or knee.

burst To launch yourself suddenly and forcibly toward an attacker to make a defense or counterattack.

chamber The action of loading a technique in order to create sufficient distance and to generate force.

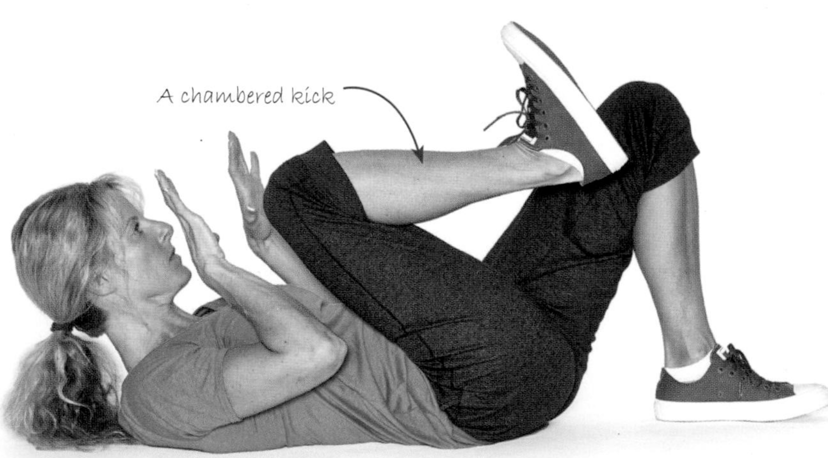

Control Position A physical position of advantage over your attacker. It's used for a brief period of time to assess the situation and your attacker's physical state prior to delivering more punishment or disengaging to a safe distance.

Cooper's color codes Introduced by Jeff Cooper as a way to determine your awareness as it relates to another person's preparedness to use deadly force. It allows you to move between increasing levels of awareness to properly handle a given situation.

counterattack The action of delivering an offensive technique after you've been attacked.

defender A person who defends himself or herself against an attacker.

defense A block, redirection, or body movement intended to protect you when attacked.

direct and decisive action Krav Maga principle that refers to focusing on using simple techniques with which you're confident to end a fight as soon as possible.

dead side The safer side of an attacker—usually your attacker's unarmed, impaired, or vulnerable side.

fatal funnel A hallway, doorway, or cone-shaped path that provides the defender no exits from an attacker. In close-quarters combat, it is a cone-shaped path leading from an entry (such as a doorway), where the assaulter is, to the defender in a room.

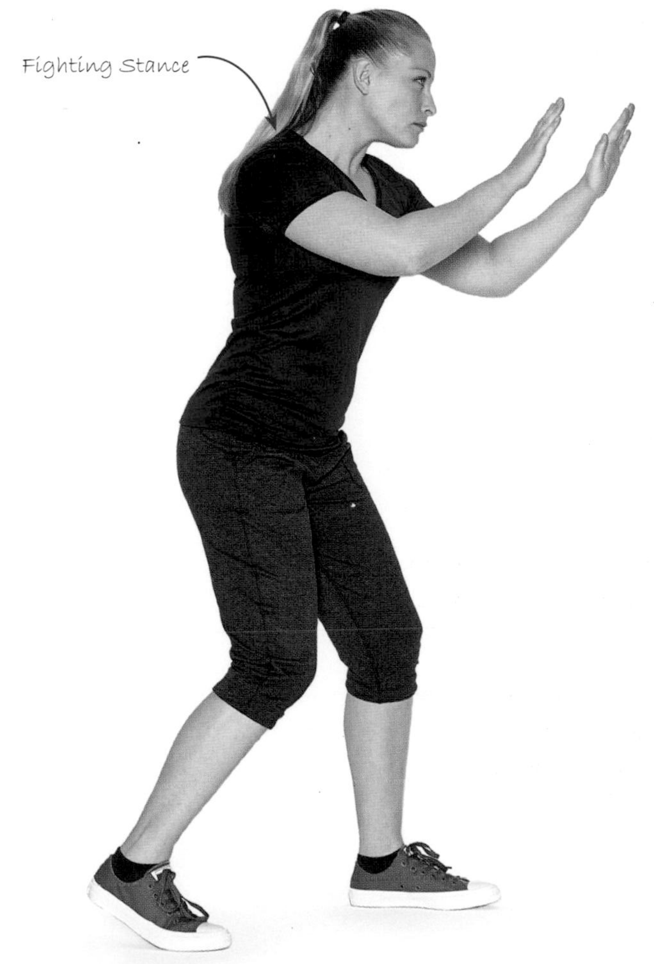

Fighting Stance A fight-ready position in which you are prepared to defend: one foot is in front of the other, the weight is on the balls of the feet, hands are up, the chin is tucked, and the shoulders are slightly raised.

guard Position in which one person has his or her back on the ground, holding another person between the legs in an attempt to obtain the Control Position.

hard target A location that has taken more than necessary precautions to prevent any breach in security of the location. People are considered hard targets when they have situational awareness, training to develop skill sets to protect, and confidence, making them an undesirable target for an attacker.

improvised weapon A device or object not designed to be a weapon but that's used that way.

Krav Maga A self-defense system created by Imi Lichtenfeld that emphasizes, simultaneous defenses and counterattacks, aggression, and ease of learning.

live side The more dangerous side of an attacker—usually your attacker's armed or mobile side—which is able to attack or strike.

martial arts Various arts of self-defense, such as judo and tae kwon do, usually practiced as a sport or path to enlightenment. Krav Maga is not a martial art.

mounted position A position in which one sits atop another person's torso with their legs on either side of the person mounted. It's typically a position of advantage in ground fighting.

OODA loop The decision cycle of observe, orient, decide, and act developed by U.S. Air Force Colonel John Boyd.

over speed A Krav Maga principle that emphasizes always exceeding the attacker's speed when defending yourself. Doing so causes confusion, as an attacker expects you to be caught off guard and resist, not to move into the attack and defend yourself.

Passive Stance A neutral standing position used in training as a realistic position of disadvantage.

pluck The action of explosively removing your attacker's grip with your hands by reaching deep inside where the wrists and thumbs meet and pulling up and out.

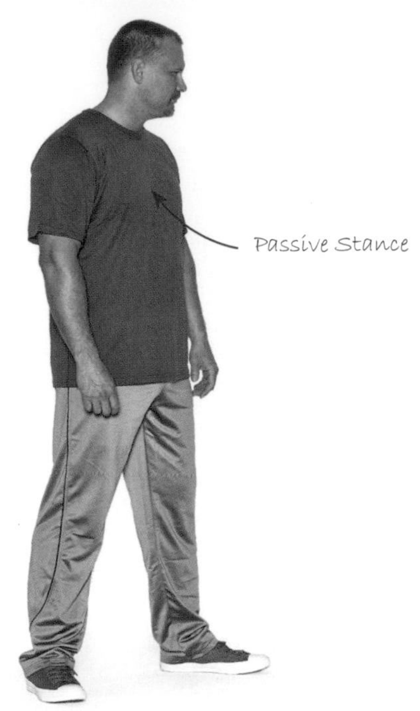

Passive Stance

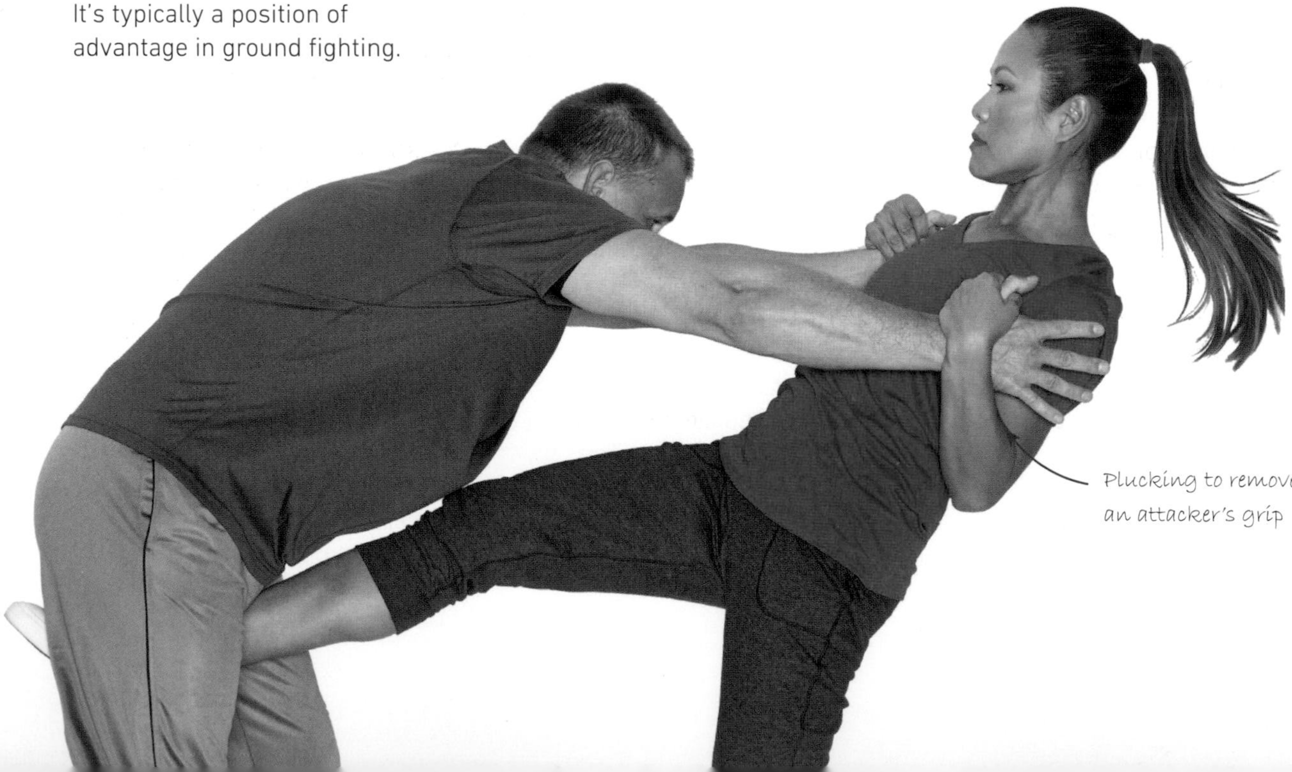

Plucking to remove an attacker's grip

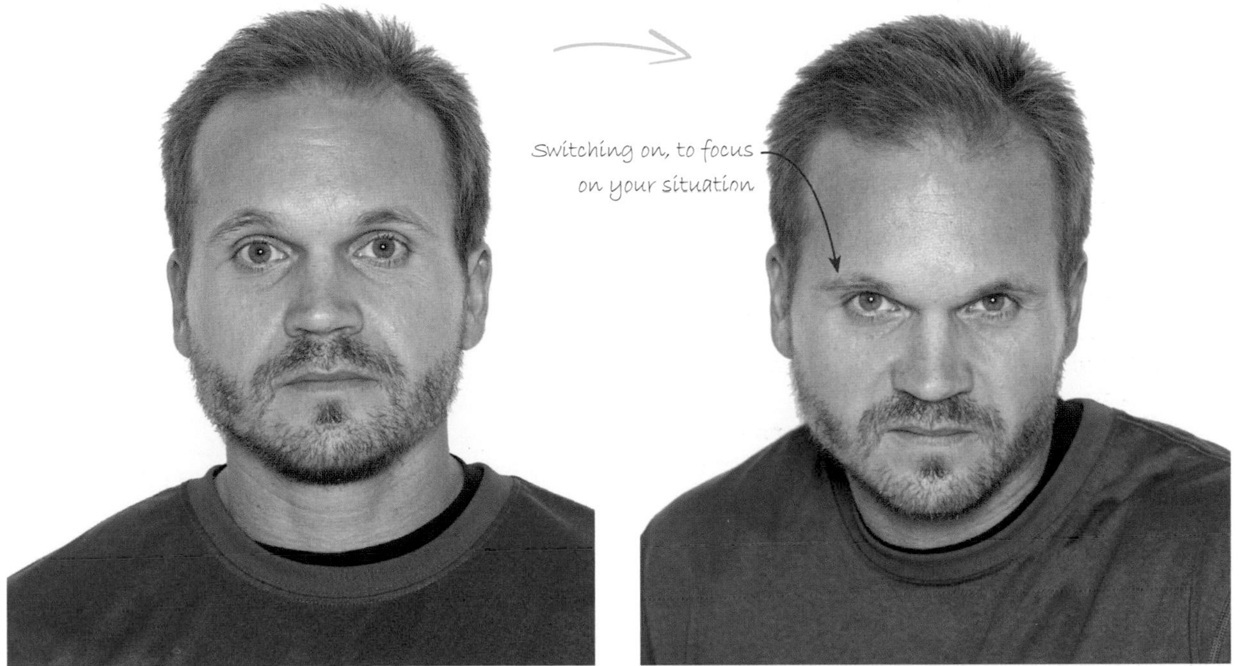

postfight All of the events that begin after the defender disengages and moves to a safe distance and the attacker has been neutralized.

prefight All of the events or actions that lead up to the first contact of an attack.

resistance The refusal as a training partner to accept or comply with a partner's movements. Gradually increase resistance to help a partner develop.

self-defense A countermeasure that involves defending yourself from attack.

situational awareness Your perception of the environment and how information, events, and your own actions will impact your safety.

smallest defender and biggest attacker (SDBA) The idea that a truly effective fighting technique succeeds even when the defender is smaller than the attacker.

soft target A location that doesn't have security measures in place or has easily defeated security measures. When used in reference to people, these are individuals who have little to no training or preparation for self-defense.

switch on Instantaneously heightening your situational awareness, narrowing your focus, and increasing your level of aggression in a fight.

tracing The movement of sliding your hand down a part of your body so your hand, arm, or body doesn't travel into the path of a weapon or projectile—for instance, tracing your right hand down your left arm, which controls your attacker's knife hand at the wrist.

wet check An initial first-aid check, specifically for bleeding or other bodily fluids.

INDEX

F

G

H

I

J-K

L

M

N-O

P-Q

R–S

T

U-V

W-X-Y-Z